Lance Vernon, DMD

Oral-Facial Emergencies

First Edition

First Edition 1994

International Standard Book Number 0-945892-05-5
Library of Congress Catalog Number 94-75601

Printed in the United States of America

JBK Publishing, Inc.
P.O. Box 69487
Portland, Oregon 97201
(503) 248-0717
FEIN: 93-0987705

Drug Notice

Every effort has been made by the authors, editors and publisher to ensure the accuracy of the indications of the drug dosages in the book. However, medical treatment is constantly evolving. The reader is advised to consult the product information insert included in the package of each drug they plan to administer for use and dosage approved by the Food and Drug Administration and for contraindications and side effects.

Oral-Facial Emergencies

Diagnosis and Management

EDITED BY

Michael T. Montgomery, D.D.S.
Chair, Department of Hospital Dentistry
Medical Center Hospital, San Antonio, Texas
Associate Professor, Department of General Practice
University of Texas Health Science Center, San Antonio

Spencer W. Redding, D.D.S., M.Ed.
Associate Professor, Department of General Practice
Associate Dean for Advanced Education and Hospital Affairs
University of Texas Health Science Center, San Antonio

JBK Publishing, Inc.
Portland, Oregon

PREFACE

The diagnosis and treatment of acute orofacial injuries are subjects that are rarely discussed comprehensively in a single text. Acute mucogingival problems are found in oral pathology texts, facial fractures and infections are covered in texts devoted to oral and maxillofacial surgery and otolaryngology, while a discussion of lacerations and basic suture techniques has been relegated to manuals. Similarly, acute and chronic facial pains, bleeding, dentoalveolar injuries, and acute odontogenic and periodontal disorders are reviewed in separate texts devoted to a variety of subject matter. Consequently, acute care clinicians, both dentists and physicians, must rely on portions of various texts to manage an assortment of orofacial injuries. Physicians and nurses are further handicapped by the scant amount of time devoted to acute orofacial injuries in their curriculum, although they are the first practitioners encountered in most acute care settings. Recognition of these shortcomings provided the impetus for and framed the goals of this text.

Acute care, both medical and dental, is a vital and substantive part of primary care, which often represents the initial and perhaps the only form of health care used by a large segment of the nation's population. The excessive dependence on acute health care management is, in part, a reflection of the design of our health care system. Health care systems designed to provide universal access should lessen the acute care needs of the population by promoting prevention, patient education and routine health screenings. In contrast, trauma-related injuries reflect the potential for accidents and violence in the society, and the solutions to these problems are more complex and less clear. The provision of acute care is universal and not confined to emergency rooms and acute care facilities, but is practiced by every dentist, physician and nurse. Orofacial complaints and problems comprise a significant portion of all acute care complaints.

This book attempts to thoroughly address a panorama of orofacial injuries that would likely be encountered in an acute care setting. The variation in the chapter formats employed reflects an attempt to present the differing topics in the most informative and accessible manner. Generally, each chapter defines the many types of problems that comprise the topic and then specifically discusses the management and treatment of each. The information presented is intended to be concise, with emphasis on tables and illustrations to promote the book's use as a quick clinical reference for acute care providers. Because the intended audience is exceptionally varied, including dentists, physicians, nurses, dental and medical ancillary personnel, the text devotes time to techniques that will be basic to certain disciplines, yet somewhat foreign to others. For example, information concerning oral anesthetic injections, dental anatomy, periodontal and odontogenic problems are more thoroughly understood by dental personnel, while medical personnel are much less familiar with these topics. The reverse statement can be made concerning many of the medical topics. For medical health care providers, especially those in acute care settings, the text is intended to be a much needed reference source for acute oral health problems. The text assumes that the medical practitioner will be a care giver rather than simply a source of patient triage. With regard to dental health care providers, especially residents receiving training in hospital dentistry and oral medicine, the text should uniquely bring together topics on acute orofacial emergencies.

The editors sincerely thank JBK Publishing for their unerring support and patience in the development of this book and to the many authors who contributed their time and expertise to their respective chapters. The text is, in essence, a compilation of their knowledge. Lastly, the editors wish to dedicate this text both to the University of Texas Health Science Center Dental School for providing a unique, rich environment for personal and professional growth, and to their parents and families for their innumerable sacrifices and unconditional love and devotion.

Michael T. Montgomery, D.D.S.

Spencer W. Redding, D.D.S., M.Ed.

CONTRIBUTORS

Brookie D. Armstrong, D.D.S.
(Lacerations)
Clinical Assistant Professor
University of Texas, Dental Branch, Houston, Texas
Private Practice, Houston, Texas

Robert M. Craig Jr., D.D.S.
(Mucogingival Inflammatory Conditions)
Chief, Dental Service
Audie L. Murphy Memorial Veterans Hospital
Clinical Professor, Department of Dental Diagnostic Science
University of Texas Health Science Center, San Antonio, Texas

Robert A. Dale, D.D.S.
(Dentoalveolar Trauma) (Lacerations)
Associate Professor, General Practice
University of Texas Health Science Center, San Antonio, Texas
Attending Staff, Department of Hospital Dentistry
Medical Center Hospital, San Antonio, Texas

Mary Kathryn Hagemeier, D.D.S.
(Extraoral Sources of Facial Pain)
Private Practice, Blanco, Texas

Jeffery L. Hicks, D.D.S.
(Odontogenic Pain)
Associate Professor, Department of General Practice
University of Texas Health Science Center, San Antonio, Texas
Attending Staff, Department of Hospital Dentistry
Medical Center Hospital, San Antonio, Texas

Ronald C. King, D.D.S., M.S.
(Orofacial Infections)
Assistant Professor, Department of Oral & Maxillofacial Surgery
University of Texas Health Science Center, San Antonio, Texas

Robert R. Lemke, D.D.S., M.D.
(Psychological and Behavioral Evaluations In The Acute Care Setting)
Oral & Maxillofacial Surgeon
Private Practice, San Antonio, Texas

Ernest B. Luce, D.D.S.
(Temporomandibular Disorders)
Assistant Professor, Department of General Practice
University of Texas Health Science Center, San Antonio, Texas

Michael T. Montgomery, D.D.S.
(Temporomandibular Disorders)
Associate Professor, Department of General Practice
University of Texas Health Science Center, San Antonio, Texas
Chair, Department of Hospital Dentistry
Medical Center Hospital, San Antonio, Texas

Gary J. Nishioka, D.M.D., M.D.
(Extraoral Sources of Facial Pain)
Resident Physician, Department of Surgery
Division of Otolaryngology
University of Missouri Hospital and Clinics, Columbia, Missouri

Spencer W. Redding, D.D.S., M.Ed.
(Oral Bleeding)
Associate Dean for Advanced Education and Hospital Affairs
University of Texas Health Science Center, San Antonio, Texas
Associate Professor, Department of General Practice
Medical Center Hospital, San Antonio, Texas

John D. Rugh, Ph.D.
(Psychological and Behavioral Evaluations In The Acute Care Setting)
Professor, Department of Orthodontics
Director of Research, Dental School
University of Texas Health Science Center, San Antonio, Texas

Scott D. Schumann, D.D.S.
(Lacerations)
Clinical Instructor, Ohio State University
Private Practice, Columbus, Ohio

Gerald W. Talcott, Ph.D.
(Psychological and Behavioral Evaluations In The Acute Care Setting)
Chief, Behavioral Health Psychology Service
Wilford Hall, U.S.A.F., Medical Center, San Antonio, Texas

B.D. Tiner, D.D.S., M.D.
(Facial Fractures)
Assistant Professor, Department of Oral & Maxillofacial Surgery
University of Texas Health Science Center, San Antonio, Texas

Gloria G. Vaughan, D.D.S.
(Dental Disease and Systemic Infections)
Assistant Professor, Department of General Practice
University of Texas Health Science Center, San Antonio, Texas
Attending Staff, Department of Hospital Dentistry
Medical Center Hospital, San Antonio, Texas

CONTENTS

Appedix A - INTRAORAL & EXTRAORAL INJECTION TECHNIQUES TO ACHIEVE LOCAL ANESTHESIA

Appedix B - A SUMMARY OF INTRAORAL AND EXTRAORAL DENTAL INJECTIONS

Appedix C - PHARMACOLOGICAL SEDATION FOR PEDIATRIC PATIENTS

Appedix D - TETANUS IMMUNIZATION SCHEDULE & PROPHYLAXIS RECOMMENDATIONS

1 Odontogenic and Periodontal Sources of Oral Pain

Jeffery L. Hicks, D.D.S.

Gloria G. Vaughan, D.D.S.

This chapter will present the essential information needed to diagnose and treat common acute odontogenic and periodontal problems. As this book is written for a wide audience with differing educational and clinical experiences, the examination of odontogenic and periodontal pain must first include a review of the pertinent anatomic structures and sensory elements.

I. GROSS ANATOMIC REVIEW

The sensory innervation of the oral cavity and surrounding structures is diagrammed in Figure 1-1.

The ***Trigeminal Nerve*** is the major sensory nerve to the oral cavity. As the fifth cranial nerve, its sensory component is a root that leaves the brain stem at the level of the pons. The nerve cells of the sensory root are located in the trigeminal ganglion within the middle cranial fossa. The trigeminal nerve yields three major divisions that are outlined in Table 1-1.

The ***Ophthalmic division*** consists of three branches: the lacrimal nerve, gives sensory fibers to the conjunctiva and skin of the upper eyelid; the nasociliary branch, supplies the skin and mucous membrane of the cartilaginous area of the nose; and the frontal branch, sends sensory elements to the skin of the upper eyelid, forehead, scalp and frontal sinus.

The ***Maxillary division*** leaves the cranium and enters the pterygo-palatine fossa, then crosses to the inferior orbital fissure where it becomes the ***Infraorbital nerve***. The ***Pterygopalatine ganglion*** receives fibers from the infraorbital nerve and is the site of origin for the ***Greater Palatine nerve***. This nerve supplies both the mucoperiosteum of the hard palate up to the palatal surfaces of the anterior teeth and the nasal mucous membrane of the inferior concha of nose and soft palate. The ***Lesser Palatine nerve*** branches from the infraorbital nerve supplying the mucous

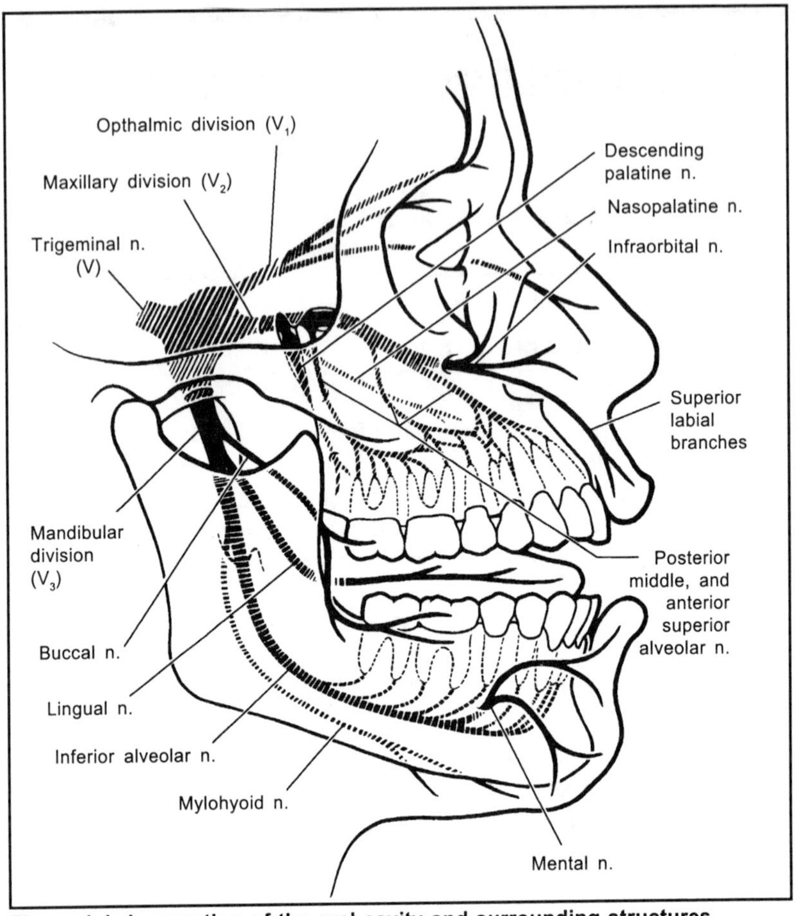

Figure 1-1: Innervation of the oral cavity and surrounding structures.

membrane of the soft palate and tonsils. The ***Nasopalatine*** (***or Sphenopalatine***) ***nerve*** supplies the mucous membrane of the nasal septum, the mucous membrane of the hard palate just behind the anterior teeth, and the mucous membrane of the superior and middle concha. Finally, the ***Zygomatic nerve*** supplies the skin superior and lateral to the zygoma.

There is overlap of the sensory fields of the next three maxillary division branches, namely, the Posterior, the Middle and the Anterior Superior Alveolar nerves. The ***Posterior Superior Alveolar nerve*** supplies the mucous membrane of the maxillary sinus, as well as the periodontium and pulps of the maxillary molar teeth. The ***Middle Superior Alveolar nerve*** supplies the periodontium and pulps of maxillary premolar teeth and the mesiobuccal root of the first molar. The ***Anterior Superior Alveolar nerve*** gives sensory fibers to the periodontium and pulps of the

Table 1-1: Trigeminal Nerve (CN V) Divisions

Opthalmic division
- Lacrimal Nerve
- Nasociliary Nerve
- Frontal Nerve

Maxillary division
- Pterygopalatine Ganglion
  - Intraorbital Nerve
  - Greater Palatine Nerve
  - Lesser Palatine Nerve
  - Nasopalatine Nerve
  - Zygomatic Nerve
    - Posterior Superior Alveolar Nerve
    - Middle Superior Alveolar Nerve
    - Anterior Superior Alveolar Nerve
  - Infraorbital Nerve

Mandibular division
- Nervous spinosus (meningeal branch)
- Nerve to the medial pterygoid muscle
- Anterior division
  - Massateric Nerve
  - Deep Temporal Nerve
  - Lateral Pterygoid Nerve
  - Buccal Nerve
- Posterior division
  - Auriculotemporal Nerve
  - Mylohyoid Nerve
  - Lingual Nerve
  - Inferior Alveolar Nerve
  - Mental Nerve

maxillary anterior teeth and the mucous membrane of the adjacent nasal cavity. The terminal branches of the ***Infraorbital nerve*** supply the conjunctiva and the skin of the cheek, upper lip, lower eyelid and sides of the nose.

The ***Mandibular division*** exits the cranium through the foramen ovale and gives off two branches that provide sensation to the dura mater and mastoid air cells before dividing into two divisions. The ***Anterior division*** contributes three motor nerves, the ***Masseteric nerve***, ***Deep Temporal nerve*** and ***Lateral Pterygoid nerve*** which innervate the corresponding muscles. The Anterior division then terminates in the ***Buccal nerve*** supplying sensory fibers to the skin and mucous membrane of the cheek. The ***Posterior division*** consists of five nerves. The ***Auriculotemporal nerve*** supplies sensation to the skin over the temple, the anterior part of the external auditory meatus, the tympanic membrane, the upper part of the pinna and to the temporomandibular joint. The ***Mylohyoid nerve*** gives motor fibers to its corresponding muscle and, some evidence suggests, sensory fibers to the mandibular teeth via communications that enter the mandible through accessory foramina on its inferior lingual border. The ***Lingual nerve*** innervates the lingual gingiva to the midline and provides taste and sensation to the mucous membrane of the anterior 2/3 of the tongue. The ***Inferior Alveolar nerve*** enters the mandible at the mandibular foramen and supplies the pulps and periodontal membranes of the mandibular teeth. A branch of the Inferior Alveolar nerve, the ***Mental nerve***, exits the mandible at the mental foramen and innervates the mucous membrane and gingiva of the anterior mandible along with the skin of the lower lip.

II. MICROSCOPIC ANATOMIC REVIEW

A. Pulpal histology and innervation

A histological examination of the tooth and its surrounding elements are summarized in Figure 1-2.

Enamel covers the coronal tooth surface and overlies the dentin, from which the majority of the remaining tooth is formed. Though enamel is relatively impervious, ***dentin*** is penetrable because of ***tubules*** that travel from its external surface to the pulp. The pulp tissue consists of ***odontoblasts***, nerves, circulatory elements (blood vessels, lymphatics), connective tissue (fibroblasts, collagen fibers), ground substance, and other cellular components (undifferentiated mesenchymal cells, histiocytes, and tissue lymphocytes). At the apex of each tooth, a ***common pulpal nerve*** is formed from branches of the alveolar nerve which then enter the root canal. Some fibers terminate in free nerve endings short of the pulp chamber, while other fibers branch repeatedly to form a plexus of nerves at the walls and roof of the pulp chamber. In the teeth of persons older than 40 years, a decrease in pulpal innervation has been reported. The mechanisms whereby electrical, thermal, chemical and tactile stimuli are transmitted through the dentin to the pulp are not completely understood. Odontoblasts, which line the pulpal chamber and form dentin, extend processes into the

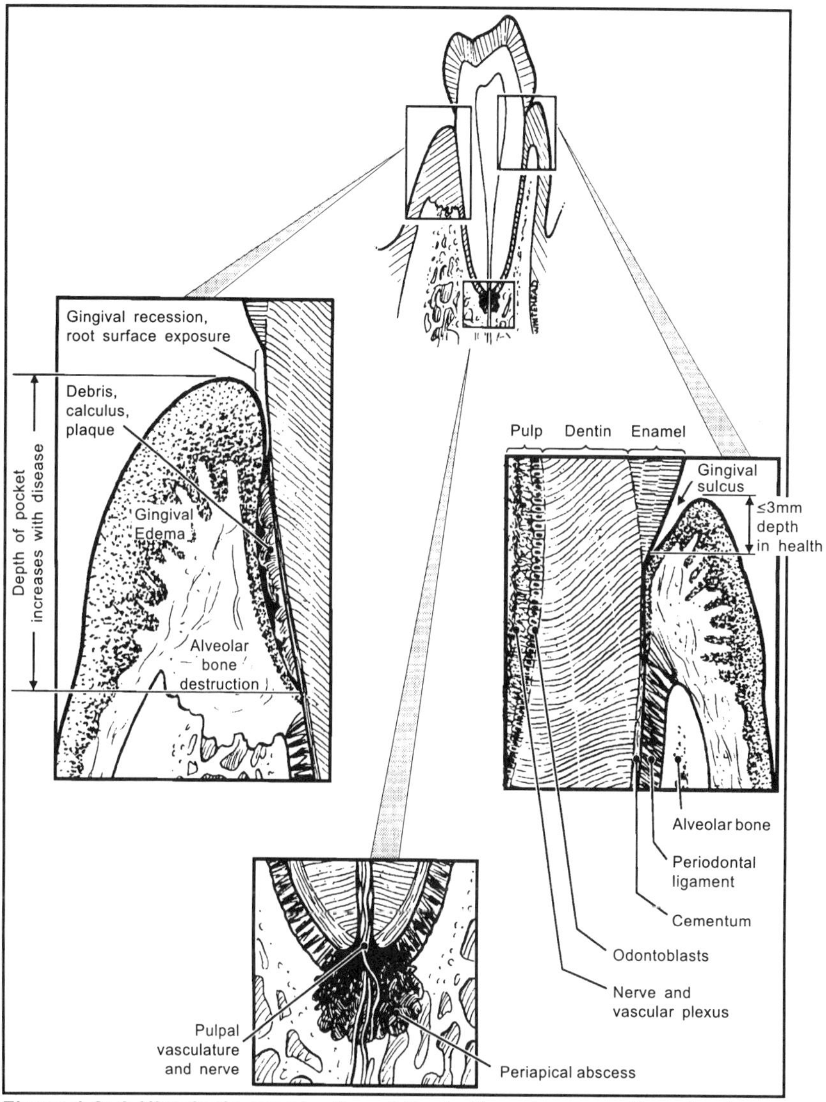

Figure 1-2: A Histologic examination of the tooth and surrounding structures.

dentinal tubules. Nerve fibers have been observed terminating between or onto odontoblasts in the pulp. Whether the dentin is directly innervated by fibers continuing through the dentinal tubules, or whether the tubules and odontoblasts are transducers for nerve impulses is controversial.

B. Periodontal histology and innervation

The supporting elements of the tooth are collectively termed the periodontium. The external root surface is covered by cementum, into which fibers from the supporting periodontal ligament are inserted. The opposite ends of the periodontal ligament fibers attach to the supporting bone of the tooth socket. Nerve fibers and circulatory elements are interwoven throughout the ligament (Figure 1-2). The periodontium is innervated by afferent fibers of the trigeminal nerve that enter the periodontal ligament (**PDL**) from mucosal and alveolar bone branches. These fibers terminate in two types of endings; free, uncovered nerve endings and encapsulated nerve endings. The free nerve endings are responsible for pain sensation and the encapsulated endings register pressure changes (***mechanoreceptors***). Many of these mechanoreceptors are concentrated in the apical portion of the PDL and some of these fibers appear to supply more than one tooth. The mechanoreceptors can precisely distinguish between forces of different magnitude, being especially sensitive to low forces. Receptors in the pulp serve little function in the tactile sensitivity of teeth.

III. RESPONSES OF THE PULP TO INJURY

Nerve fibers within the pulp are categorized as either sensory or motor. Motor nerves are responsible for vasomotor regulation by controlling the diameter of the vascular lumina. Stimulation of the vasomotor nerves results in changes in pulpal blood volume, blood flow and intrapulpal pressure. Sensory nerves in the pulp are either mechanoreceptors (touch, proprioception, pressure) or nociceptors (pain, temperature). The pulp is quite vulnerable to injury because it is a pressurized tissue enclosed in unyielding dentin. As such, simple ***edema*** can cause occlusion of its thin walled vessels and the resultant changes in pulpal circulation may modulate dental pain. Also, both heating of the tooth and inflammation of the tissue, pulpitis, can cause tissue pressure to increase significantly, while cold can cause intrapulpal pressure to drop. Although the exact mechanism is not fully understood, these findings suggest a relationship between changes in blood flow, pressure and dental pain.

A. Modified pulpal response

Studies indicate that the pathologic state of the pulp influences the degree of pain felt, to the point that non-noxious stimuli may produce pain. Chemical mediators are released in inflammation from injured cells which excite sensory nerve fibers and cause dilation of vessels. The increased vessel permeability that follows dilation allows plasma proteins and leukocytes to leak into the inflamed area in an attempt to remove or neutralize irritants. ***Pulp tissue pressure*** is thus elevated in acute and chronic inflammation, although pressures are lower in the chronic state. In severe inflammation, the lymphatic vessels are blocked, preventing a release of pressure and producing persistently increased fluid and pulp pressure. ***Pulp necrosis*** may result, although not by the process of self-strangulation that was once proposed. For example, pressures within the pulp do not rise high enough to completely occlude blood vessels at the tooth apex. Also, although the pulp can exhibit high pressures in the immediate area of inflammation, near normal pressures may exist elsewhere in the pulp. Finally, the presence of accessory foramina (and accessory circulation), common in molars, can provide ***collateral circulation*** allowing for continuation of blood exchange in the inflamed pulp which aids in the resolution of inflammation and the preservation of pulpal vitality.

Periodontal disease, trauma, dental operative procedures and caries can reduce pulpal circulation and, as a consequence, degenerative changes may take place. With periodontal disease, reparative processes are diminished and, as such, the pulp's reaction to dental operative injuries are more likely to result in necrosis. In older patients pulpal circulation is decreased because the concentration of blood vessels diminishes and secondary atherosclerotic changes occur in the remaining blood vessels. Increasing age may also reduce the number of nerve fibers in the coronal pulp. Circulation finally becomes sufficiently impaired to cause cell atrophy and death, accompanied by increasing fibrosis. With age the pulp becomes less cellular, more fibrous and its actual size diminishes because of further dentin deposition (i.e., secondary, reactive and sclerotic dentin). As the number of odontoblasts decreases, so does healing potential. In the mature tooth, although formation of the apical foramen is completed, ***secondary dentin formation*** continues at a slow rate. ***Reactive dentin*** is frequently, although incorrectly, called secondary dentin. Reactive dentin is formed quickly beneath dentinal tubules that are exposed to external insult to re-insulate the pulp. ***Sclerotic dentin*** is formed as odontoblasts die and their dentinal tubules become filled with mineral deposits. Sclerotic or transparent dentin may also be formed beneath carious dentin and commonly appears in the root.

Once ***caries*** has progressed through the enamel to the dentin, the pulp may be unaffected or the numbers of chronic inflammatory cells may increase. Reactive and sclerotic dentin form under the carious lesion causing a reduction in pulp volume and acceleration of the aging process. The pulp beneath deep caries, without pulpal exposure, is often chronically inflamed and painful, but contains no demonstrable bacteria. When reactive dentin is invaded, wide areas of dentinal tubules are demineralized, creating a pathway for microorganisms to enter the pulp. Once ***carious exposure*** of the pulp occurs, the pulp reacts at the site of exposure with an infiltration of inflammatory cells and the chronic pulpitis becomes acute. Clinically, a small ***abscess*** develops within the coronal portion of the pulp at the exposure. The remainder of the pulp may be uninflamed or may be converted to granulation tissue. If the pulp is open to the oral fluids and drainage occurs, the apical pulp tissue typically remains uninflamed or chronically inflamed. If the opening into the pulp is occluded as a result of food packing or the placement of a restoration, then the entire pulp may become rapidly necrotic.

Dental operative procedures can also cause pulpal irritation and acute pulpitis, whether anesthetic is used or not. Mediators of inflammation are released from odontoblasts damaged by heat and from dentinal tubule contents. These mediators increase vascular permeability, increase pulpal pressure and decrease pulp circulation. Edema results and pulpal blood flow is further impaired. After approximately one week the acute inflammation subsides and chronic inflammation ensues, characterized by the presence of ***granulation tissue***. Following irritation from dental operative procedures, the pulp may remain chronically inflamed for months or years. The persistence of chronic inflammation may explain why pulps that are symptomless after operative procedures may eventually exhibit painful symptoms. The effect of additional procedures is unknown, but it can be surmised that subsequent irritants will have a cumulative, damaging effect on the pulp. During ***pulp repair***, injured odontoblasts may recover from the trauma via the elaboration of reactive dentin, which seals off the dead odontoblasts and tubules. However, in pulps with poorer healing potential, a ***local necrosis*** may occur which can spread to the entire pulp. In addition to contamination by direct pulpal exposure, microorganisms may reach the pulp by anachoresis, a process whereby microorganisms from another site in the body are seeded to the pulp by the bloodstream. These microorganisms localize on inflamed pulpal tissue and the localization increases as the severity of pulp inflammation worsens. In most cases, the few microorganisms that reach the pulp are engulfed by the defense cells and phagocytized, however, pulp death has been attributed to anachoresis.

B. Referred pain

Pain from the teeth may be referred to other intraoral and extraoral structures, including other teeth, the eye, the temporomandibular joints and the ear, all of which hinder the diagnostic process. In contrast, ***sinusitis***, ***bruxism*** and ***trigeminal neuralgia*** cause pain that is commonly referred to the teeth. Besides being misleading with respect to the site of origin, the quality of referred pain is not characteristic of the tissue in which it appears to reside. For example, pulpal pain, a deep somatic type of pain, may be referred and appear to originate in deeper or more superficial structures. Despite the referral, the pain will continue to possess characteristics of pulpal pain. Referred dental pain rarely crosses the midline but may be referred to the ipsilateral, opposing arch of teeth. It is important to keep in mind that referred pain cannot be aggravated by stimulation of the site where the pain is felt, but rather is only heightened by manipulation of the true pain source. Likewise, anesthetizing the area where the referred pain is felt will not alleviate the pain. The reasons for referred pain are poorly understood, but it seems likely that dental referred pain results from the inability of the nervous system to accurately localize afferent nociception from teeth. This poor localization and subsequent referred pain may in part be secondary to convergence of afferent nerves from orofacial structures onto ***trigeminal neurons*** which relay pulpal sensations to higher centers. Studies have demonstrated that the localization of pulpal pain is poorer in posterior teeth than in anterior teeth, and that the stimulation of a single tooth is less well discriminated by patients than is the simultaneous stimulation of several teeth.

IV. DIAGNOSTIC METHODS

Pain arising in the teeth is often poorly localized, referred to other orofacial sites and difficult for patients to describe. In contrast, pain arising from oral soft tissues is more localizable than pulpal pain and is characterized as dull or burning. These ***pain descriptors*** are common and are indicative of ***deep or visceral pain***. Pulpal pain is often described as sharp or stinging, which is characteristic of ***superficial or cutaneous pain***.

In many studies clinical signs and symptoms correlate poorly with the ***histologic diagnosis***. Several problems account for the difficulty in categorizing pulpal disease by either histologic or clinical examination. First, histologic categorizations are arbitrary and definitions of specific stages of disease vary from one proposed scheme to another. Second, an apparently healthy pulp may demonstrate atrophic changes or other signs of disease on histologic examination. Third, a diseased pulp will often demonstrate histologic evidence of more than one disease category, thus, it is not possible to define the histologic condition of the pulp based on a limited microscopic examination. Fourth, diseased pulpal tissue will demonstrate transition stages from one histologic classification to another. Fifth, clinical symptoms correlate poorly with the histologic findings and the severity of disease present, confusing the clinical diagnosis. Sixth, symptoms are often the result of an acute exacerbation of an underlying, frequently unsuspected chronic condition. As such, it is clinically impossible to accurately classify the pulpal condition of all painful teeth based on histological findings or even to reliably differentiate clinically salvageable and non-salvageable teeth. With the advent of conservative procedures that attempt to preserve the vitality of the pulp or to resolve pulpal inflammation, the need for accurate assessment of pulpal disease is more critical. The diagnostic examinations of oral structures can be grouped into categories as described in Table 1-2. A discussion of these categories follows.

Table 1-2: Categories of Diagnostic Information

A. History
B. Clinical Examination
    1. Percussion
    2. Pressure and Occlusion
    3. Palpation
    4. Pulp Testing
    5. Radiographic Examination
    6. Illumination
    7. Dyes

A. History

The history is probably the most important item in the diagnostic process, yet it is often the most overlooked tool by the novice clinician. In one study of incompletely fractured teeth, 25% of the patients diagnosed the fracture themselves and 37% gave a history of a previously cracked tooth. The experienced clinician will take the time to elicit a thorough history in addition to interpreting patients' signs. Table 1-3 lists the essential questions for an adequate history. Based on the patient's responses, further questions may provide valuable information. For example, if the patient is able to localize the pain to a specific tooth, the patient's recollection of prior restorative or endodontic therapy involving that tooth would be beneficial.

Table 1-3: Typical Questions Regarding Odontogenic Pain

1. Where do you feel the pain?
2. What does the pain feel like? Sharp? Dull? Throbbing? Burning?
3. How long has the pain been present?
4. Is the pain constant or intermittent?
5. Does anything make the pain worse?
6. Does anything decrease the pain?
7. Does the pain wake you from sleeping or prevent you from going to sleep?

The patient's description of the pain is also useful in the diagnosis and generally the severity of pain is directly related to the severity of the problem. However, the absence of pain does not imply the absence of disease. Pain characteristics that indicate a greater chance of irreversible pulpal damage are listed in Table 1-4. Each of these items describes a pulp that has sustained greater damage and has less chance of recovery.

Table 1-4: Aspects of Pain Associated with Irreversible Pulpal Damage

- A previous occurrence of pain
- A long duration of pain
- The presence of lingering pain after a stimulus is removed
- The presence of spontaneous pain (pain occurring without a stimulus)

B. Clinical Examination

After gathering historical information, a clinical examination and indicated adjunctive tests should be performed. The first step in the clinical examination is inspection. An extraoral and intraoral visual scan of the soft tissue and teeth should be performed. Intraoral soft tissues to be inspected include the cheek mucosa, gingiva, hard and soft palate, tonsillar folds, pharynx, uvula, tongue, inner lips and floor of the mouth. The presence of lesions, fistulas, lacerations, swellings and inflammation should be noted. Extraoral soft tissue inspection should include the skin of the head and neck, lips, nose, eyes and ears. Intraoral and extraoral palpation should follow to determine the presence of tumors, infections and lymphadenopathy. Extraoral palpation should include those areas of head and neck lymphatic drainage, (i.e., preauricular, submandibular, submental, and superficial and deep cervical chains). Bimanual palpation of the cheeks, floor of the mouth, tongue, and perioral tissue should also be performed. Finally, the teeth should be grossly inspected for carious lesions, fractures and large or defective restorations.

Percussion

Percussion may uncover pathologic changes in the tooth or supporting periapical structures. Percussion is accomplished using the end of an intraoral mirror handle and the desired effect is a sharp rap delivered to the tooth crown. Buccal and lingual tooth surfaces and the cusp tips can be percussed to help identify an occult fracture. In percussing the tooth begin gently at first, then increase the magnitude of force used if the previous attempt did not elicit a painful response. The sound produced with percussion can also be important. A fractured tooth or one with a periapical lesion may yield a dull, thudding sound rather than the normal solid and higher pitched response. When percussing several teeth, vary the sequence in subsequent repetitions so that the patient's response is blinded to which tooth is being tested. Thus, if the patient erroneously believes that a certain tooth is the culprit, they will be less likely to anticipate the percussion of that tooth and a truer response will be obtained. A positive percussion sensitivity reaction usually indicates the presence of apical inflammation, however, a negative response does not rule out periapical inflammation.

Pressure and Occlusion

Biting forces (***mastication***) or occlusal pressures transmit axially directed forces to the tooth. Sensitivity to mastication may indicate an occlusal prematurity, recent trauma, tooth fracture or the presence of a periapical lesion. Mild or absent pain with pressure accompanied by increased pain on release of the pressure is suggestive of an incomplete coronal fracture (cracked tooth). Movement of a tooth segment on mastication or percussion can reveal a displaced or fractured tooth, while noticeable changes in the occlusion may indicate an alveolar or jaw fracture (See Chapters 8 & 9). Occlusal pressure may also elicit muscle pain in patients with TMD (See Chapter 9).

Palpation

Tenderness to palpation of the mucosa over the tooth apices will be present with periapical abscess formation that has perforated the buccal and/or lingual plates. Soreness of the mucosa or periosteum over the roots of a tooth may also indicate inflammation and/or infection of the periodontal ligament. The presence of mucosal swelling may indicate cellulitis, abscess formation or alveolar plate expansion associated with periapical or periodontal disease. The presence of a sinus tract usually indicates significant infection secondary to a necrotic pulp, although other infections (periodontal and alveolar) may also produce a sinus tract. Muscle tenderness because of splinting may also be present and can also be elicited by palpation of those muscles or the mucosa overlying them.

Palpation of a tooth (an attempt to move a tooth buccolingually or mesiodistally) can uncover a periapical infection, an abscess, trauma, the loss of tooth support or edema in the tooths supporting structures. Palpational tenderness can also signal fractures of the tooth, alveolus or jaw. The distraction of tooth parts is associated with a complete fracture of the tooth, and the independent movement of maxillary or mandibular alveolar segments indicates an alveolar or jaw fracture. Finally, the presence of foreign objects in the soft tissues may also be determined by palpation.

Pulp Testing

Pulp testing with currently available means does not quantify disease and does not measure pulp vitality. This type of testing measures the ability of the pulp's nervous tissue to respond to a stimulus. However, vital pulps can exist without vital nervous components. Apparently, nervous tissue is more susceptible to injury and may necrose while the remainder of the pulp remains vital. Despite this lack of correlation between test responses and the pathologic state of the pulp, there is a statistically significant relationship between the absence of a response to the pulp test (i.e., a very high reading to electric pulp test) and the presence of a completely necrotic pulp. Therefore, pulp vitality should be based on the gross response parameters of presence or absence. A response to testing signifies vital pulpal tissue, while the lack of a response implies a non-vital or severely inflamed pulp. The use of control teeth either adjacent to the suspected tooth or on the contralateral side may be helpful in establishing a range of responses that are 'normal' for a particular patient. However, this practice can be criticized as there is no way of knowing the pulpal status of the control teeth and because apparently normal teeth can exhibit pulpal pathosis. To further complicate pulp testing, traumatized pulps may not respond to electrical pulp testing for up to two months following injury and yet recover fully. The development of testing devices that use ***flow popplerometry*** to measure intrapulpal blood flow should improve diagnostic accuracy in determining pulpal status.

One method of pulp testing involves subjecting the tooth to a hot or cold stimulus. However, the responses obtained with ***thermal*** pulp testing are not quantifiable since variable temperatures are delivered to the tooth for differing lengths of time. The only reliable correlation between thermal tests and the pulpal response is the lack of response in non-vital teeth. Cold has been shown to be a more reliable indicator of pulp vitality than hot and some investigators have shown that cold is a more accurate indication of a prolonged pain response than is electrical pulp testing. However, there are inherent problems associated with the use of cold since ice is difficult to handle and is not cold enough for testing some teeth. Also, the use of some of the pressurized chemicals that deliver an extremely cold agent (CO_2 at -78° C) can cause crazing of the enamel and may induce pulpal damage. A hot stimulus is normally delivered by heating up an instrument tip and placing it on the crown of the tooth. The use of ***pressurized air/water*** is a simple thermal test that can detect existing cavities, exposed dentin from a tooth fracture or exposed dentin, or cementum secondary to gingival recession. In this test, a stream of air, air and water or water alone from either the air-water syringe or the dental handpiece is directed onto the tooth. As the tooth is cooled, exposed dentin or cementum is stimulated and pain is produced.

In ***electrical*** pulp testing (EPT) a direct current is passed through the tooth and supporting structures. A sliding analog or digital scale records a number which is directly related to the delivered current strength. The EPT is inaccurate because there is no standardization among different machines and current strength is not reproducible within a single machine. Also, variations between teeth, such as the presence of secondary dentin or reactive dentin, reduce response reliability. With higher machine settings the current transmission may occur through the periodontium instead of solely through the dentin, resulting in a false negative response. Another problem is that the sensation from the EPT may be unpleasant and patients fearing a painful stimulus may over react to anticipated stimulation. As previously stated, the EPT does not correlate directly with pulpal pathosis. Although judicious interpretation of EPT results may qualitatively identify pulpal status (no response = possibly necrotic), the quantification of pulpal status is not possible.

A ***test cavity*** involves penetrating the enamel of a non-anesthetized tooth with a dental drill to elicit a pulpal response from dentinal stimulation. A sensation of pain when dentin is reached is indicative of some degree of pulp vitality. While useful, reponses may be unreliable or unattainable in anxious patients. The test's utility is also limited by the fact that it creates a breach in the enamel or restoration that requires restoration. However, the test may be useful when a prosthetic crown is present.

The ***anesthetic test*** is useful when pain is present at the time of examination. A small amount of local anesthetic is deposited directly over the tooth root or roots immediately against or under the periosteum. The relief of pain identifies the symptomatic tooth. The technique may also make use of an intraligamentary injection as a method of local anesthesia.

Radiographic Examination

A radiographic examination can greatly facilitate clinical diagnosis. However, the absence of radiographic evidence consistent with periapical pathosis does not exclude a positive diagnosis because pulpal and/or periapical disease may occur in the absence of radiographic changes. Radiographic evidence of inflammation, infection or trauma may include: widening of the periodontal ligament space, a decrease in density or obliteration of the lamina dura, obliteration of the pulp, prolonged enlargement of the pulp canal due to failure of the pulpal system to mature, internal resorption of the pulp, external resorption of the dentin at the periodontal ligament space, or an apical radiolucency.

Illumination

Illumination of the tooth may be helpful in detecting coronal fractures as well as caries, which are occult to conventional viewing methods. The fiberoptics in operative handpieces can act as the light source by using the handpiece lighting without a bur in place or by using the terminus of the handpiece tubing without the handpiece attached. The latter allows for easier placement of the light against or proximate to the tooth. When viewing an operative or root canal access cavity with the fiberoptic placed against the external enamel or dentin, the identification of fractures and canal locations is facilitated. Also, illumination of the intact tooth from the facial or lingual surfaces may demonstrate changes in tooth color or areas of reduced light transmission consistent with pulpal injury or death.

Dyes

Placing methylene blue or iodine containing dyes into a cavity preparation is another method of detecting a previously undisclosed fracture. Regarding fractures, however, it is important to remember that teeth can exhibit small fractures without symptoms and may exhibit symptoms without signs of fracture. As such, the visualization of a fracture line is not incontrovertible evidence of pulpal disease.

V. DIAGNOSIS AND TREATMENT

The remainder of this chapter will address the most common causes of odontogenic and periodontal pain and their treatment. Also discussed will be other maladies that are not strictly dental in origin, but which may be considered either a sequelae of dental treatment or may affect the dentoalveolar tissues. Recognizing that even under the best circumstances diagnosis is uncertain and much is still to be learned about the treatment and subsequent repair of injured pulpal tissue, undertreatment or overtreatment of pulpal disease is inevitable. However, from an analysis of the symptoms, the objective findings, and the immediate dental history, a useful categorization of clinical entities is possible. The most common clinical categories responsible for odontogenic and periodontal pains are summarized in Table 1-5.

Table 1-5: Common Causes of Odontogenic and Periodontal Pain

A. Pulpal Disease
B. Periodontal Disease
C. Occlusal Trauma
D. Dentinal Sensitivity
E. Tooth Fractures
F. Pericorinitis
G. Alveolar Osteitis

A. Pulpal Disease

Pulpal disease is described as reversible or irreversible depending on the severity of the insult to the tooth. Both reversible and irreversible pulpal damage can occur from caries, trauma (mechanical or thermal), operative procedures or for unknown reasons. The accompanying discomfort will vary depending on the severity of the pathology. Reversible pulpitis is characterized by intermittent pain which usually requires a stimulus for initiation. The tooth may be hyperreactive to thermal stimuli, but the pain is not lingering. Clinical and/or radiographic evidence of caries, large restoration or trauma may be apparent. Because the insult to the tooth is usually mild and indirect, the pulpitis will resolve with time or with correction of the insult (i.e., restoring caries, eliminating occlusal trauma)(Figure 1-3).

Signs and symptoms of irreversible pulpitis include spontaneous pain, percussion and thermal sensitivity, a non-vital pulp test, radiographic evidence of a carious lesion that encroaches on the pulp, a periapical radiolucency or thickening of the apical periodontal ligament and fistulous tracts, if present. Evidence of tooth trauma such as fractured crowns (deep dentinal and pulpal fractures) and root fractures, as well as tooth subluxational injuries are additional signs of irreversible pulpitis. Teeth which have suffered injuries resulting in irreversible pulpal damage will require either endodontic therapy and restoration or extraction. Emergency treatment can consist of medications alone or in combination with partial or complete

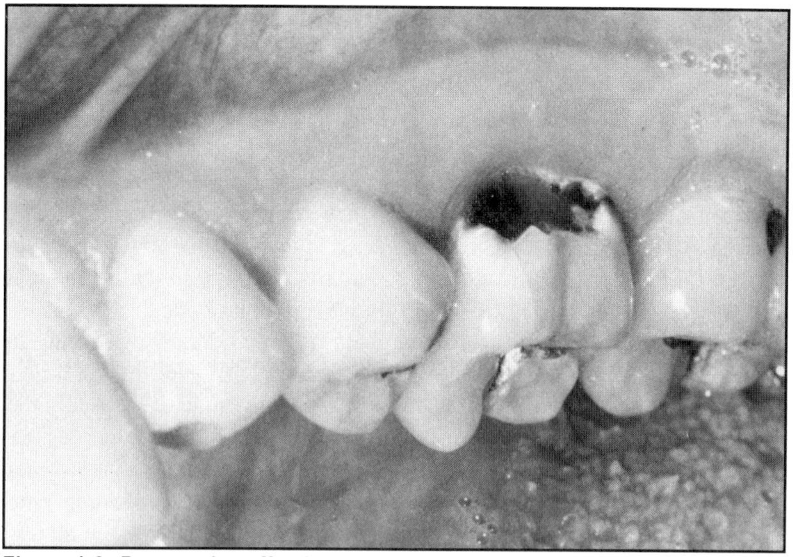

Figure 1-3: Deep caries affecting pulpal health.

pulpal extirpation or extraction. This decision will be determined by the patient's ability and desire to save their teeth. Patients who demonstrate past attention to their oral health and have the desire and financial ability to retain the tooth are good candidates for medication and pulpal therapy. Recommended medications can include analgesics such as non steroidal anti-inflammatory drugs (NSAID) or a narcotic/NSAID combination and antibiotics when signs and symptoms of infection are present. The pulp therapy can consist of a pulpectomy or a partial pulpectomy. Pulpal therapy or endodontic therapy consists of partial or complete removal of the pulp chamber contents and filling the emptied pulp chamber. Filling the chamber and root canal system prevents the reseeding of infectious organisms via anachoresis and subsequent abscess recurrence. Commonly used filling materials are gutta percha and pastes of various compositions. Following the root canal therapy, the tooth will require restoration with a filling (usually amalgam or composite resin) or a crown. The decision to perform pulp therapy will depend on the severity of the signs and symptoms (i.e., in cases with severe pain or infection). Patients who have poor oral health and are not predisposed to improve their oral hygiene or are financially unable to afford pulpal therapy and the needed restorative dentistry are candidates for extraction. It is recommended that a dentist be consulted to make these decisions and to render the appropriate care.

Untreated, irreversible pulpitis can proceed to pulpal necrosis. In the early stages of pulp necrosis, a moderate amount of pain or no pain may be present. However, as a periapical abscess forms, significant pain develops until the resulting infection achieves an avenue of escape (Figure 1-4). When a tooth has a pulpal exposure through the crown, secondary to a fracture or carious exposure, the infection can escape through the coronal opening. In the absence of a coronal exposure, the infection will seek release through the root apex and then through the hard and soft tissues supporting the tooth. After exiting the apex, the infection can traverse to the external surface of the jaw resulting in a fistula, or the infection can drain into deeper tissues resulting in a fascial space infection (Figure 1-5). External drainage may occur through the periodontal ligament to the sulcus (sinus tract) or laterally through alveolar bone to the mucosa (fistula). The fistula may persist for years. Internal drainage resulting in fascial space infections are discussed in Chapter 2. Which of the aforementioned outcomes occurs is dependent on tissue resistance. Usually the infection will follow the route of least tissue resistance. Once the pressure of the infection has obtained release to the external surface, a great relief of pain is noticed, usually accompanied by a foul taste. If no treatment is sought (i.e., extraction or root canal therapy), the tooth will be slowly exfoliated. During this time, the tooth will decay and only a very small piece of root may remain to be exfoliated. Throughout this process, the infection and fistula may remain. Should the fistula become obturated at any time prior to exfoliation, the pressure again would build and the pain resume. This seemingly benign course should not generate a false confidence, as the infection that does not find an external surface commonly spreads to deeper structures with more rapid and morbid consequences.

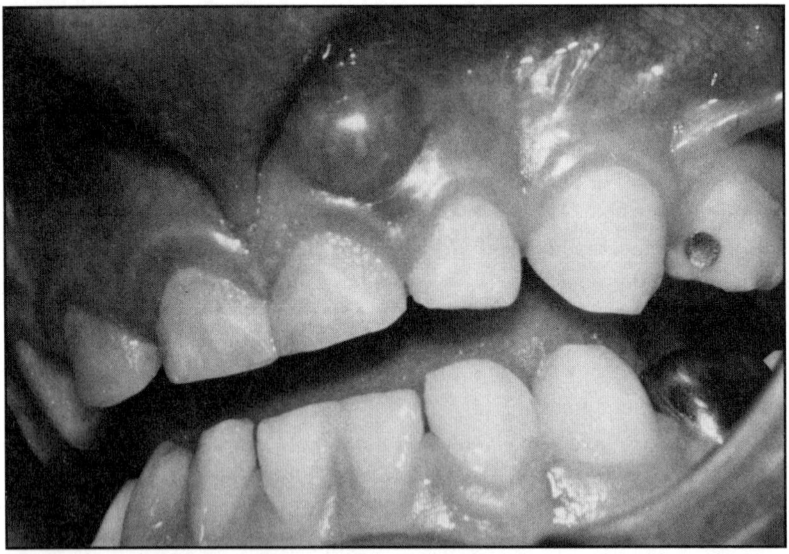

Figure 1-4: Periapical abscess associated with pulpal disease of deciduous incisor.

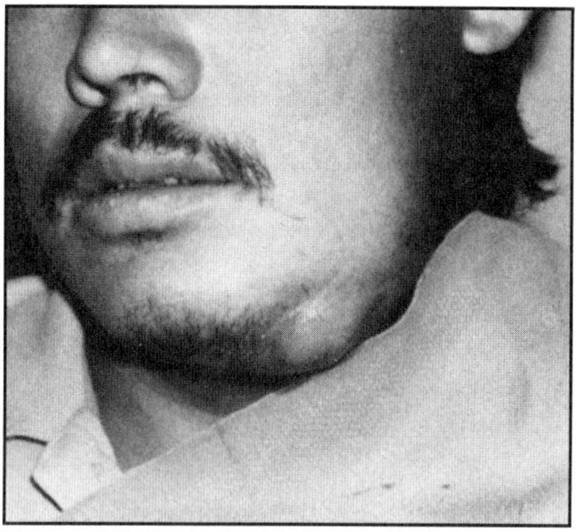

Figure 1-5: Periapical infection/dental abscess seeking release below lower jaw.

B. Periodontal Disease

Periodontal disease is one of the most common oral cavity diseases, affecting nearly all adults to some degree. To understand the pathophysiology of periodontal disease, the anatomy of the normal adult periodontium must be understood (Figure 1-2). In a healthy state, gingival and periodontal health, the gingiva is firm, reddish-pink in color, fitting snugly against the tooth surface with mild stippling of the keratinized zone. The gingiva forms a cuff or collar around the teeth and the most coronal aspect is called the free gingival margin. At the depth of the sulcus is the attachment apparatus of the gingiva termed the epithelial attachment. In health, the distance from the free gingival margin to the base of the sulcus is minimal, usually less than 3 mm. Gingivitis is an inflammation of the gingiva caused by bacterial plaque. With chronic exposure to bacterial plaque the gingivae become red and inflamed, tend to bleed easily and may be tender to the touch. Increased inflammation and edema causes a loss of the normal gingival contours, resulting in bulbous interdental papillae and rolled free gingival margins. As gingival size increases, there is an increased collection of debris and bacteria resulting in a self-perpetuating cycle of inflammation (Figure 1-6). Gingivitis affects only the gingival tissues, leaving the underlying bone intact. Although systemic factors can play a role in gingivitis, most cases are the result of local irritating factors. Removal of the local factors usually results in the rapid resolution of gingival inflammation.

If gingivitis is left untreated it may progress to periodontitis. In contrast to gingivitis, periodontitis involves the gingivae, the alveolar bone and the

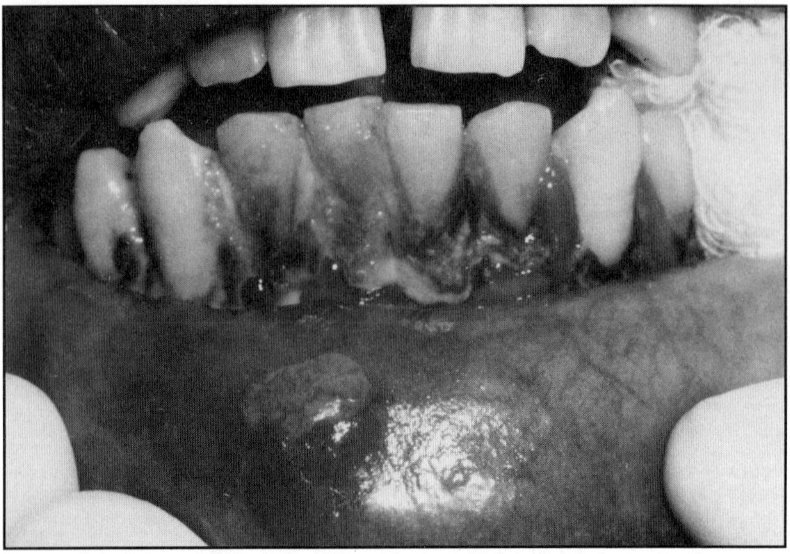

Figure 1-6: Advanced periodontitis with accumulated debris on teeth.

periodontal ligament. As gingival inflammation increases, ulceration of the crevicular epithelium increases, and apical "migration" of the epithelial attachment occurs. The ulcerated crevicular epithelium is easily detached from the tooth surface. This combined with the edematous enlargement of the marginal gingiva results in deepening of the sulcus and the formation of a periodontal "pocket." Accompanying the soft tissue changes is destruction of the underlying bone. The earliest radiographic sign is blunting of the alveolar crest, however, with disease progression, horizontal and/ or vertical bone loss occurs. Clinical signs of periodontal disease may include gingival inflammation, gingival recession, increased periodontal pocket depths, bleeding, halitosis, tooth mobility and suppuration through the sulcus. Subjective symptoms can include a bad taste in the mouth, bleeding gums, and tooth hypersensitivity. Hypersensitivity results from exposed cementum at the necks of the teeth secondary to gingival recession. If left untreated, destruction of the soft tissue and bony support may be so severe that tooth loss results.

A condition frequently associated with chronic periodontal disease is the periodontal abscess (Figure 1-7). A true periodontal abscess arises when diseased tissue and debris become trapped in the periodontal pocket. Microorganisms in the debris produce pus which normally escapes through the sulcus. Inflammation can cause the gingiva to close about the tooth, thereby obturating the pocket opening and preventing the normal escape of infectious material. As a result, the infection traverses the pocket

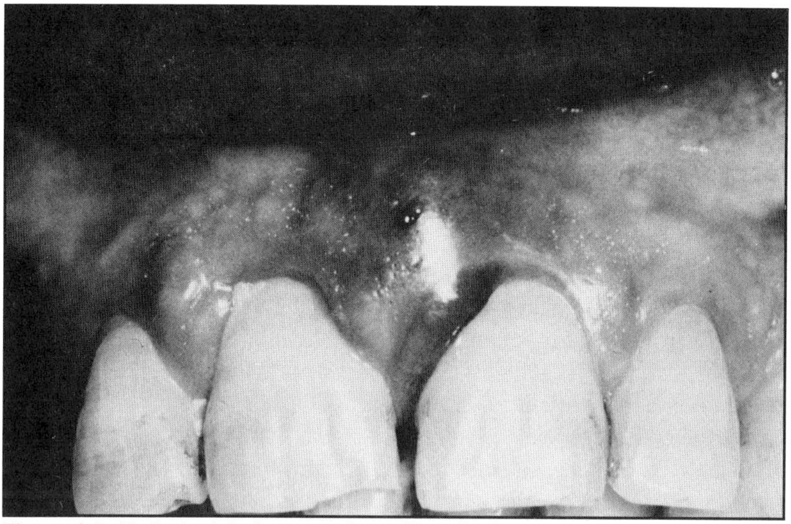

Figure 1-7: Periodontal abscess of maxillary incisor.

epithelium and invades the supporting tissues. The lesion may spread to involve the periapical tissues and form a combination lesion termed a periodontal/periapical abscess. A periodontal abscess appears as a red and painful swelling in the unattached gingiva immediately over the abscess and the swelling may be fluctuant. The gingival surface over the abscess will be shiny because the normal gingival texture is obliterated. Other signs and symptoms can include throbbing pain and sensitivity to palpation. If the abscess is severe, enlargement of lymph nodes draining the affected area and fever may be present.

If the lesion has not yet consolidated to form a central area of pus (pointing), hot rinses every two hours will help to accomplish this. If the lesion has pointed but has not yet drained through the sulcus or gingival surface, drainage will need to be created by incision. Under local anesthesia, a small incision over the center of the lesion can provide drainage and access for curettage of the lesion without affecting gingival anatomy. Aggressive debridement and curettage of the periodontal pocket is essential, however, to remove the source of the problem. Afterwards, the pocket should be irrigated with saline solution, chlorhexidine or water. Warm saline rinses several times a day may aid in the resolution of the lesion. When the degree of the infection or the patient's condition warrants, antibiotics are recommended for 10 - 14 days (Table 1-9). If left untreated, the periodontal abscess will invariably recur. Following successful resolution, definitive treatment (i.e., elimination of the periodontal pocket) is recommended to prevent a recurrence.

Mastication, oral hygiene maneuvers or trauma (including dental treatment) may lead to the imbedding of food or debris within an otherwise healthy sulcus. The tissue irritation and infection that results, termed a gingival abscess, will usually swell the attached tissue, although the unattached mucosa may also be affected. The surface of the tissue will be red and shiny from the swelling and infiltration of blood. Enlargement of the lesion may also involve the sulcus and mimic a periodontal abscess. Patients may report localized pain or no pain, depending on the severity of the inflammation. The gingiva will be tender to palpation and the tissues may be fluctuant. In severe cases, the associated teeth will be sensitive to palpation, percussion and mastication. Radiographs are of minimal value, but may assist in ruling out a periodontal abscess. Recommended treatment includes elimination of the source of infection by debridement of the sulcus using local anesthesia. Aggressive curettage of the abscessed area is essential to insure complete removal of the offending debris. Antibiotics may be prescribed if the infection has physically progressed beyond a simple localized infection or if systemic signs and symptoms are present (i.e., fever and malaise).

C. Occlusal Trauma

The pain associated with occlusal trauma may range from a limited discomfort to severe pain. The pain usually has a dull quality except for the sharp pain experienced when the affected tooth is stimulated. Degrees of trauma exist and the magnitude of pulpal and periodontal irritation appears proportional to the severity of the trauma. As a consequence of the trauma, the supporting structures of the tooth, and sometimes the pulp, become irritated and hypersensitive. Symptoms typically mimic mild periodontal or pulpal irritation, but can be severe enough to mimic a periodontal abscess. The affected teeth may be sensitive to chewing, thermal stimulation, speaking or to other normally non-noxious stimuli during acute episodes.

The patient's history will often reveal a precipitating event such as recent dental restoration, orthodontics or bruxism (clenching or grinding of the teeth). Patients can usually localize the pain to a specific tooth or teeth due to the involvement of the periodontal ligament and its proprioceptive fibers. Thin occlusal indicating tape or ribbon is of great help in identifying the problematic teeth. Also, the practitioner may perceive excessive movement of teeth in occlusal trauma (fremitus) by placing a fingernail perpendicularly on the buccal surface of a tooth at the gingiva and having the patient lightly tap the teeth together. At times the occlusal trauma may be so significant that movement of the teeth is visible when the patient lightly taps the teeth together (Figure 1-8). Some hyperocclusive

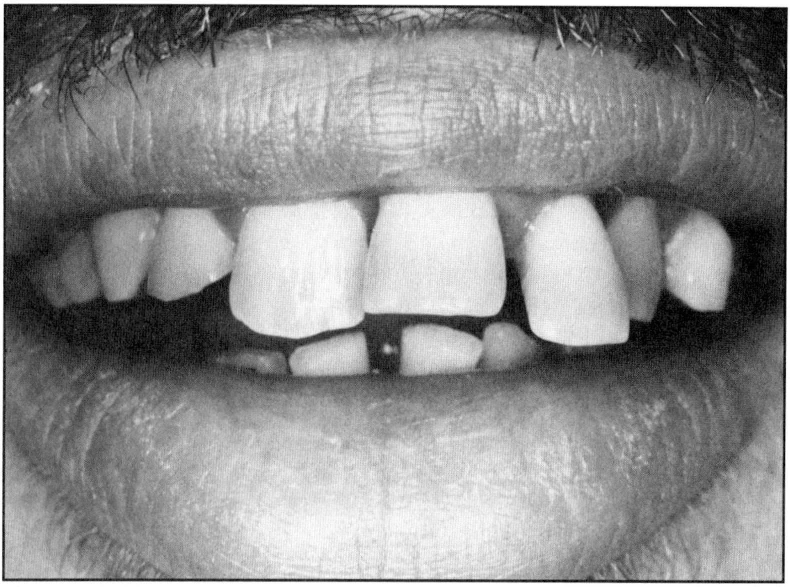

Figure 1-8: Displaced incisor and resulting hyperocclusion.

contacts do not occur in centric occlusion and the patient must be observed when moving the mandible side to side and forward with the teeth in contact. When the contact causing the discomfort is identified it must be noted if the contact occurs in centric, lateral or protrusive contact positions or a combination of these. Minimal occlusal adjustment of the symptomatic tooth or teeth is most often all that is necessary to permanently alleviate the pain. Sometimes the offending tooth is so sensitive that local anesthesia is required prior to occlusal adjustment. If the nature of the contact allows, the opposing tooth or teeth may be adjusted instead of the symptomatic tooth. The pulpal or periodontal irritation associated with occlusal trauma is usually reversible and, therefore, relieved by occlusal adjustment. Uncommonly, occlusal trauma results in irreversible pulpitis, whose signs, symptoms, diagnosis and management were discussed in the previous section.

D. Dentinal Sensitivity

The stimulation of exposed dentin or cementum by cold, heat, chemical or mechanical means may also result in pain. The communication of odontoblastic processes through the dentinal tubules is thought to be the means whereby the pulp can perceive changes in the external environment. Deformation or damage to the processes stimulates the nervous elements around the odontoblasts. A second theory is that the fluid within the tubule is able to conduct ionic changes to the odontoblastic process, effecting cellular changes and causing the perception of pain. Pain from sensitive dentin or cementum is typically sharp and may be described as an electric shock. Upon questioning, the patient can usually identify the specific stimulus that causes the discomfort. Patients may relate that a specific food (often high acid foods), thermal or mechanical stimulation (toothpick, brushing teeth, inhaling air between the teeth) gives rise to the pain. The causes of dentinal sensitivity include poor marginal adaptation of restorations, fractures of the enamel, gingival recession and gingival erosion or abrasion (Figure 1-9).

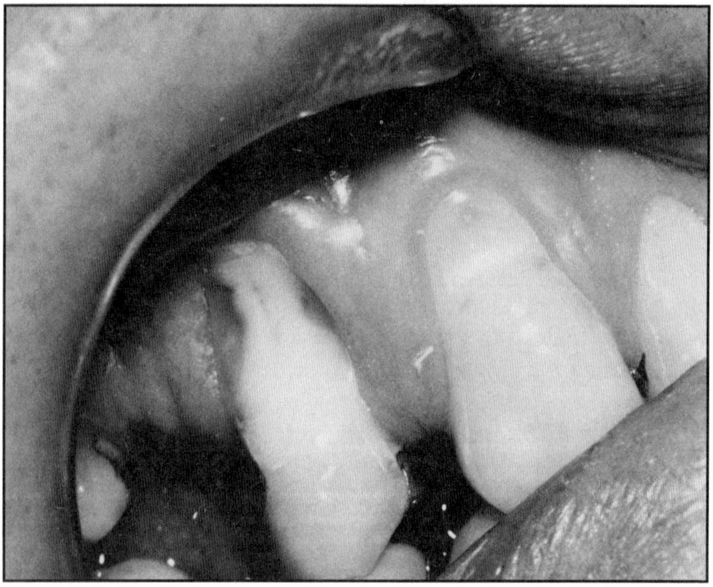

Figure 1-9: Gingival recession from toothbrush abrasion and exposure of root (dentin) surface.

Treatment is directed at protecting the tubules and their contents from the external environment. Such treatments include: covering the dentin surface with dental varnish, a resin or other restorative materials; deposition of oxalate salt crystals in the external tubule openings; and fluoride applications to the dentin via a gel or iontophoresis. Immediate, but temporary, relief may be obtained by covering the exposed dentin surface with copal varnish or a resin bonding agent. Permanent therapies include restoration of the dentin with composite resin, amalgam or glass ionomer filling materials with or without surgical preparation of the dentin (Table 1-6). Surgical preparation is irreversible and may aggravate the condition if surgically prepared dentin is left unrestored. Promoting the deposition of crystals in the lumen of the dentinal tubules to act as a physical barrier has proven effective, but the chemicals used must be reapplied on a regular basis. Commercially available oxalate salt solutions, fluoride gels and desensitizing toothpastes are used for this purpose. The oxalate salt solutions provide relief of discomfort more quickly than the fluoride or toothpastes but the results with oxalates may be more short lived.

Table 1-6: Treatment Modalities for Dentin/Cementum Sensitivity

Agent	Material	Method of Application
Copal varnish	Copal	Direct application
Resin bonding agent	Various	Direct application
Oxalate salts	Na, K or Fe oxalate	Direct application
Flouride	Sodium fluoride, Stannous fluoride	Rinse, direct application, toothbrushing, iontophoresis
Desensitizing toothpaste	Strontium chloride, Potassium nitrate	Toothbrushing
Restoration of tooth	Amalgam, Composite, Resin, Glass ionomer	As per requirements of the restorative material

E. Tooth Fractures

Fractures of the tooth crown and/or root are a common occurrence and may arise from trauma, bruxism, loss of supporting tooth structure, previous dental restorations, thermal cycling, root canal treatments or combinations of these factors. Several classification schemes have been devised to segregate fractures according to their location (e.g., involving only coronal tooth structure, involving the root, or involving both the coronal structure and the root). Fractures may also be classified based on the direction of the fracture (e.g., vertical, horizontal and oblique), and the loss of tooth structure; (e.g., incomplete and complete). The incomplete fracture is one in which the tooth has been divided to some degree, but the parts are held in place by either the remaining tooth structure, periodontal tissues or pulpal tissues (Figure 1-10). A complete fracture is one in which a portion of the tooth has been completely separated from the tooth and a discussion of this subject can be found in Chapter 7.

The diagnosis of ***incompletely fractured teeth*** (cracked teeth) is difficult because the diagnosis cannot usually be made until other more likely causes have been excluded. Also, the diagnosis is commonly made

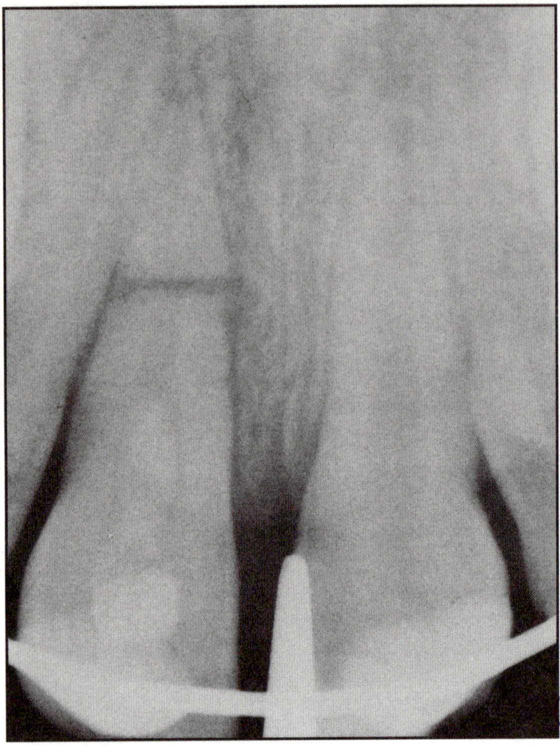

Figure 1-10: Complete fracture of incisor root. Tooth splinted with wire to adjacent teeth.

without actually visualizing the fracture itself. However, the diagnosis is often facilitated by findings in the dental history. One researcher reported that 25% of patients make their own diagnosis and 35% give a history of a previously cracked tooth. The history is also important for revealing recent etiologic events and symptoms characteristic of a fractured tooth.

The resulting symptoms are dependent on these circumstances: the thickness of the remaining dentin over the pulp, whether the pulp or periodontal tissues are involved and the degree of movement allowed of the fractured portion. The pain may be intermittent or constant and may be sharp or dull in quality depending on the tissues affected. The pain may not be present except when the tooth is stimulated by biting pressure, thermal or ionic changes (e.g., eating sweets). The most reliable symptom is the generation of pain upon the sudden release of a slow and steady biting pressure. Presumably, the biting pressure forces the fractured portions of the tooth outward and the sudden release of this pressure generates intrapulpal pressure and pain. The amount and quality of the pain produced is dependent on the extent of the fracture, the tissues involved and the presence of a vital or diseased pulp. In early fractures, teeth are usually not percussion sensitive because percussion does not force the fractured parts of the crown or root sufficiently apart to cause pain. The pulp may survive for months and there generally is no spontaneous pain unless the fracture has allowed ingress of microorganisms into the pulpal tissues. Other pain complaints may include a constant, vague discomfort which indicates a greater degree of pulpal irritation.

Upon clinical examination, the diagnosis of completely fractured teeth is facilitated by the missing coronal tooth structure. Completely fractured teeth may also have the fractured portions still somewhat attached to the bulk of the tooth by soft tissue. Firmly held, but completely fractured portions may require pressure delivered from an instrument such as a mirror handle to demonstrate free movement. In contrast, incomplete fractures cannot be discerned by this method. The use of fiberoptics to illuminate the tooth may be helpful in demonstrating fractures. However, finding fracture lines in enamel does not lead incontrovertibly to a diagnosis of a fractured tooth. Many teeth normally demonstrate craze lines or small fractures in the enamel and yet do not exhibit symptoms. Therefore, this test is very non-specific.

A more reliable use of fiberoptics is in the diagnosis of a significant fracture that extends into dentin. After removing an intracoronal restoration (amalgam, casting) or opening into the coronal pulp chamber, fiberoptics can be placed against the side of the tooth to transmit light through the enamel and dentin. This technique may reveal a fracture line in the floor of the pulp chamber or in a line angle of the cavity preparation. Another visualization technique is the placement of methylene blue or iodine into a tooth preparation. Both of these dyes will creep into the slightest fracture allowing easy detection. Radiographs are of limited help in demonstrating fractures as only 15 to 36% of incomplete fractures are visible radiographically. It is important to make radiographic exposures from two or more angulations as fractures are often occluded by superimposed tooth structure and/or restorations. Fractures may be demonstrated if the path of the x-ray beam is within 15 to 20 degrees of the parallel of the fracture. If the fracture extends to the supporting tissues, radiographs may reveal pathologic changes in the periodontium or apical tissues (75% of such cases), such as widening of the periodontal ligament space or loss of interseptal bone (Figure 1-11).

Clinically, most incomplete fractures occur in a mesiodistal direction following a path of least resistance. Sufficient occlusal force to fracture a tooth is often created by the removal of an adjacent tooth which increases occlusal forces. Additionally, caries and dental restorations may substantially weaken a tooth so that a fracture occurs with normal occlusive forces. Another common cause of incompletely fractured teeth is traumatic injury.

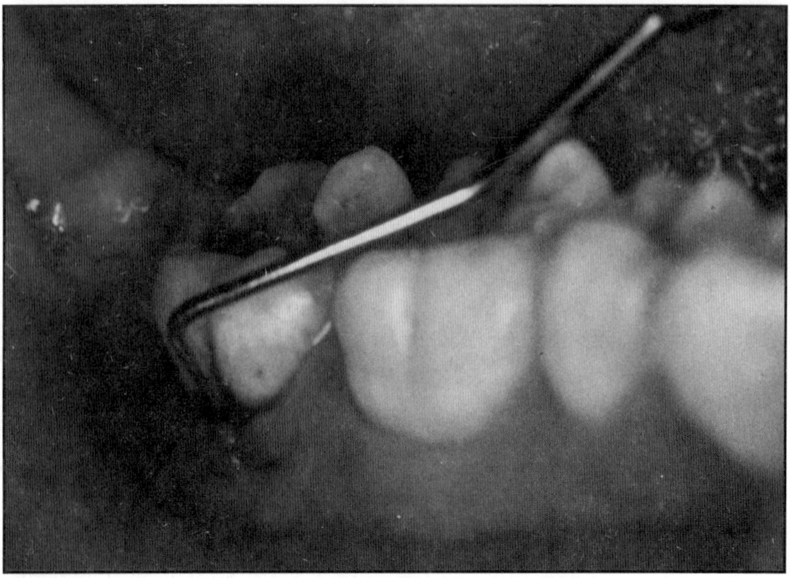

Figure 1-11: Mandibular molar with suspected vertical fracture. Periodontal probe is inserted into sulcus to a depth of 10 millimeters.

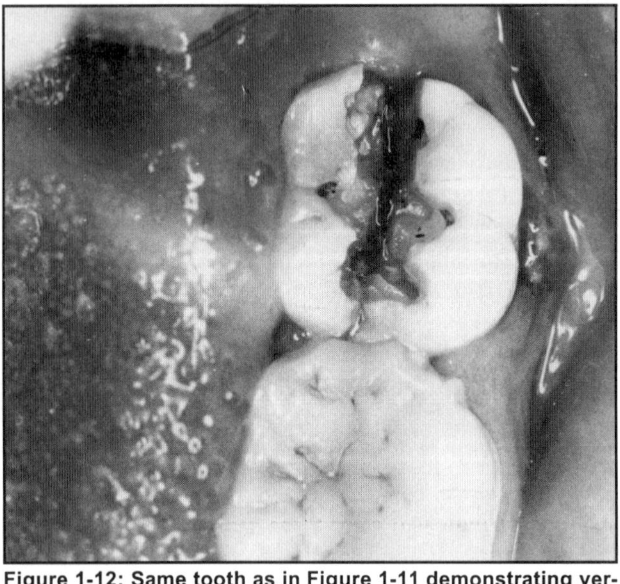

Figure 1-12: Same tooth as in Figure 1-11 demonstrating vertical fracture. Molar was determined to be non-saveable.

The treatment of odontogenic fractures is dependent on type (i.e., traumatic versus secondary to caries), their extent (complete versus incomplete), and the tissues involved (Figure 1-12).

Traumatized teeth should be tested for responsiveness to stimuli, which is a relative measure of pulpal injury. It is believed that damage to the tooth is more severe when the crown or root has not fractured and the majority of the force has been absorbed by the pulp and periodontium. Injured pulps may respond in either an exaggerated manner or less quickly and severely. Recently traumatized teeth may not have had time to suffer significant inflammatory changes and, therefore, may respond normally. A normal response should also be expected from minimally traumatized teeth reflecting a healthy pulp. These patients, however, should be informed that pulpal irritation has occurred despite the lack of clinical signs and that the tooth should be protected from further insult (thermal, mechanical) for several weeks after the trauma. The patient should also be advised of the potential for endodontic therapy in the future. Following traumatic odontogenic injuries, radiographs should be made at regular intervals to evaluate the development of subsequent pathosis. Every three months is suggested for the first year following the injury and annually thereafter. If signs of pulpal necrosis or resorption are noted, endodontic therapy should be initiated. Traumatic injuries to younger teeth have a better prognosis for healing, compared to older teeth, because of their greater relative pulpal vascularity, wider apical foramina and less pulpal fibrosis.

The treatment of non-traumatic odontogenic fractures varies depending on the extent of the fracture. If chewing produces symptoms consistent with an incomplete fracture, the placement of an orthodontic band or temporary crown is indicated. The band or crown will prevent movement of the coronal portions of an incompletely fractured tooth and should alleviate symptoms elicited during mastication. This treatment modality is especially useful when an incomplete fracture is suspected, but the fracture cannot be located. If symptoms abate, restoration of the tooth with a crown is indicated after sufficient time has elapsed to allow for pulpal healing (i.e., three months following resolution of symptoms).

When the fracture extends into the pulp allowing bacterial ingress, binding the tooth will not completely alleviate the discomfort. In such cases, the next step would be to extirpate the pulp and observe for improvement in symptoms. If symptoms cease, completion of the root canal treatment and crown construction are indicated after three months. If symptoms persist following pulp removal, then periodontal inflammation from a fracture extending into the periodontal ligament (PDL) should be suspected. The only recourse at this juncture is extraction of the tooth, if the fracture cannot be identified, or if located, the fracture position renders the tooth unrestorable (Figure 1-13).

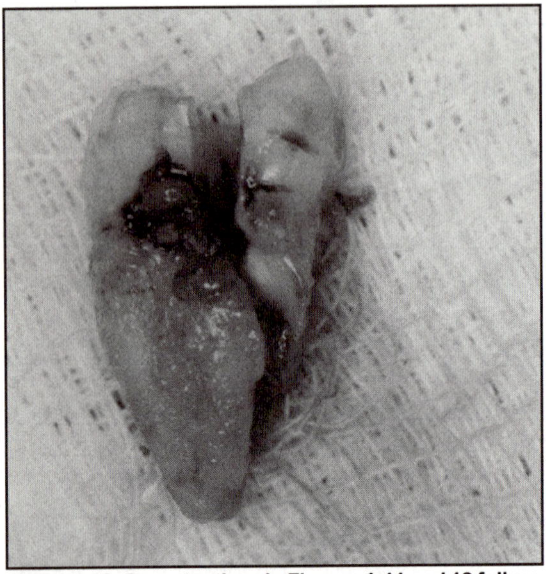

Figure 1-13: Same tooth as in Figures 1-11 and 12 following extraction. The fracture extends from the crown a significant distance down the root into the periodontium.

F. Pericoronitis

Because true periodontal attachment will not occur between the enamel of a tooth crown and the surrounding gingiva, partially erupted teeth are variably covered by an operculum (gingival flap). Such teeth have potential spaces about the crown of the tooth not caused by disease (pseudopocketing). The operculum is frequently traumatized during mastication and the pseudopocketing is prone to food impaction and plaque accumulation which irritates and infects the gingiva. The irritation and infection of the coronal periodontal tissues is termed pericoronitis (literally, inflammation around the crown). If the tooth is partially within non-keratinized gingiva (loose mucosa), it is more prone to pericoronitis because non-keratinized tissue is less resistant to trauma and infection. Third molars are particularly prone to pericoronitis, however, any tooth can be affected during eruption than is keratinized tissue. Patients presenting with pericoronitis commonly report previous episodes, and the severity of the pericoronitis appears to worsen with each occurrence. Typically, weeks or months separate episodes of pericoronitis.

Signs of infection are often seen, especially if foreign material has become impacted in the pericoronal gingiva. Swelling, erythema, edema, pus and foul breath may all be present (Figure 1-14). Patients generally report moderate to severe pain which may be referred to the ear. As tissue swelling increases, the operculum will become more prone to trauma from the opposing dentition. Regional lymphadenopathy is often detected in the nodes that drain the affected area and the patient may have an elevated temperature. Tenderness to palpation on the affected site is also common and patients may have limited opening of the jaw (trismus) if the infection involves the masticator spaces. Infections in the third molar regions pose the additional threat of spreading through the fascial planes of the face and neck. Radiographically, a pericoronal radiolucency or thickening of the pericoronal space may be visible.

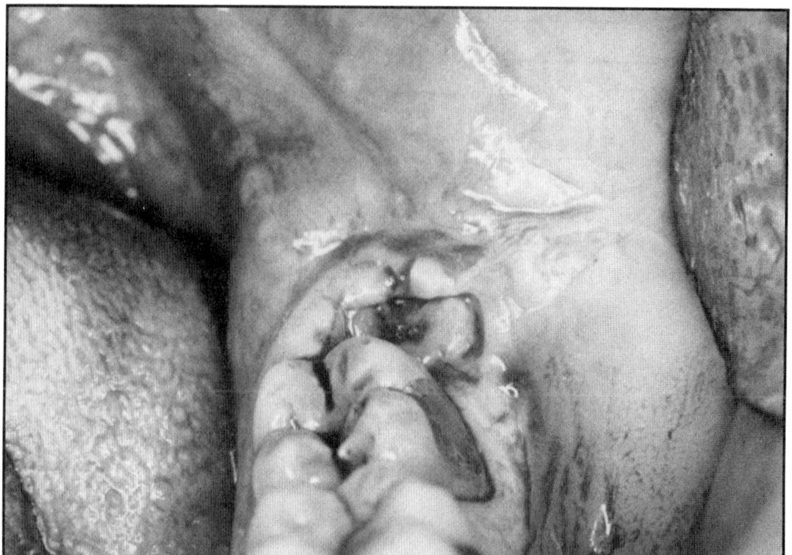

Figure 1-14: Partially erupted mandibular third molar with trauma from opposing molar on overlying, edematous mucosa.

If the tooth involved is not a candidate for retention (e.g., most third molars), extraction of the tooth is recommended when possible. However, the presence of infection in the soft tissues is a relative contraindication to immediate extraction, especially in the presence of severe trismus when access is limited. As an alternative treatment, the area under the operculum can be mechanically debrided and irrigated with saline, chlorhexidine or water under local anesthesia. As a temporary measure or as a definitive treatment for a tooth to be retained, the operculum may be removed to permit hygiene and prevent masticatory trauma. In these cases, electrosurgery is recommended to facilitate hemorrhage control and minimize the chance of spreading the infection. Operculectomies are temporary measures because the excised tissue will recur unless the tooth erupts or the tooth is extracted. Another approach is to extract the opposing maxillary third molar, lessening the likelihood of further trauma to the operculum. Hot compresses or hot rinses applied several times a day will aid in the resolution of the initial lesion and decrease the trismus. The patient should be given an irrigating syringe for home use to maintain hygiene until removal of the tooth is possible. If significant infection is present, antibiotic therapy is suggested for approximately one week before extracting the tooth (Table 1-9).

G. Alveolar Osteitis

A common occurrence following the extraction of teeth is delayed healing and the premature loss of the blood clot within the socket. A variety of terms exist for this condition, the most common being alveolar osteitis or dry socket. Dry socket is characterized by the presence of intense pain at the extraction site which often radiates to other areas such as the ear. The pain typically develops two to four days post-operatively and lasts from five to seven days. Clinically, the extraction site has lost the protective blood clot leaving a hypersensitive exposed bony surface which may be covered with a grayish yellow exudate. A fetid odor is usually present and the patient may also complain of a foul taste. Dry socket most often occurs following the extraction of mandibular third molars, especially impactions, but may occur following the extraction of any tooth. Treatment is palliative, and involves irrigation of the extraction site with saline to remove necrotic tissue and debris. A medicated guaze strip (typically impregnated with eugenol and/or a topical anesthetic) is gently and loosely placed into the socket to cover the exposed bone surface and provide relief from the discomfort. Medicated guaze should be removed and replaced at least every two days as needed to control the patient's discomfort. When it is not feasible to have the patient return frequently, a drop of eugenol applied to an absorbable gelatin sponge may be placed in the extraction socket. Pain medication may also be prescribed if needed (Table 1-11). Antibiotics are of little benefit in treating alveolar osteitis and are not recommended unless signs or symptoms of infection are present.

VI. ANTIBIOTICS

In the presence of infection, the first goal of treatment is to remove the source of infection. Antibiotics can be used as an adjunct in the control of infection either before or following the extraction. Overuse or misuse of antibiotics can unnecessarily add to the cost of medical treatment, increase the chances of allergic reaction and increase the growth of antibiotic resistant microorganisms. As such, the decision to use antibiotics should be based on well defined objectives and should be limited to cases in which antibiotics will help resolve or prevent the spread of infection. Antibiotics are indicated in many cases of acute and chronic infection, especially when the infection is poorly localized. An exception to this use includes acute alveolar osteitis (dry socket) in which antibiotics are of no benefit. Other dental indications for antibiotics are for the prophylaxis of patients at risk for endocarditis and for invasive procedures in patients who are immunocompromised as a result of medications or medical conditions (e.g., IDDM, AIDS, post-organ transplantation). In these cases, antibiotics may prevent opportunistic organisms from infecting a susceptible host.

A. Selection of an antibiotic

A gram stain can be performed in the dental office to identify the morphologic characteristics of organisms and thereby aid in the selection of an appropriate antibiotic. Also, culture and sensitivity testing can be used to identify the offending organisms and assist in antibiotic selection. Determining the need for microbiological identification and the sensitivity of an appropriate antibiotic are dependent on the size and location of the infection, its clinical history and the patient's medical status. Because of time and financial limitations, culture and sensitivity testing is rarely beneficial. For example, 4 - 7 days are required for anaerobic culture results and the offending organisms are predominantly anaerobic in cases of cellulitis. Because of this, the selection of an antibiotic is made empirically, in most cases, based on the organisms known to cause most dental infections. Culture and sensitivity testing is reserved for infections that fail to respond to initial antibiotic therapy

When collecting a sample for culture and sensitivity testing, it is best to use aspiration to prevent exposing the sample to oxygen and thereby inhibiting the growth of anaerobic organisms. Ideally, the sample should be collected before antibiotics are prescribed, since antibiotic therapy may skew the culture results. As illustrated in Table 1-7, odontogenic infections are most often caused by a mixture of organisms. In early infections aerobes predominate, while in later infections anaerobes increase are dominant. Most often, antibiotics chosen for odontogenic infections will need to be effective against aerobic and anaerobic organisms.

Table 1-7: Odontogenic infections

In general:

- 70% - are mixed aerobic and anaerobic organisms
- 25% - are pure anaerobic
  - most common are Streptococci, Peptostreptococci, Bacteroides, Fusobacterium
- 5% - are pure aerobic
  - most common are streptococci

Cellulitis	-	early infection	-	aerobes predominate
Abscess	-	later infection	-	anaerobes predominate

Penicillin is the antibiotic of choice because of its wide spectrum of activity, the sensitivity of oral microorganisms and the cost. However, additional factors in drug selection must be considered including patient allergies, current patient medications and the potential for penicillin-resistant bacteria such as ß-lactamase producing bacteria. Table 1-8 lists the most common organisms present in oral infections, their morphological characteristics and antibiotic sensitivities.

Table 1-8: Commonly Occurring Bacteria in Oral Infections

Gram stain	Oxygen Demands	Incidence(%)	Antibiotic of choice: First choice	Antibiotic of choice: Second choice
gram positive cocci				
Streptococcus	facultative anaerobic	60	Penicillin	Cephalosporin, Erythromycin
Staphylococcus		5	Cloxacillin,	Cephalosporin, Clindamycin Dicloxacillin
Peptostreptococcus	anaerobic	18	Penicillin	Clindamycin
gram positive rods				
Actinomyces	mostly anaerobic	5	Penicillin	Tetracycline, Erythromycin
Lactobacillus	anaerobic	7	Penicillin	Cephalosporin, Clindamycin
gram negative cocci				
Neisseria	aerobic	10	Penicillin	Amoxicillin, Tetracycline
Veillonella	anaerobic	20	Penicillin	Cephalosporin
gram negative rods				
Klebsiella	aerobic	15	Gentamicin	Cephalosporin
Eikenella	facultative anaerobic	9	Penicillin	Ampicillin, Tetracycline
Bacteroides	anaerobic	50	Penicillin	Cephalosporin, Metronidazole
Escherichia		15	Gentamicin	Cephalosporin
Fusobacterium		5	Penicillin	Cephalosporin

Table 1-9: Antibiotic Administration Regimens for Oral Infections

Antibiotic	Route	Mechanism of Action	Dosage and Frequency	Indication
Aminoglycosides		Bactericidal		
Gentamicin	IM or IV		3 mg/kg/day in equal doses q 8 hours	Component of bacterial endocarditis prophylaxis** for patients at high risk
Cephalosporins		Bactericidal		
cefaclor	PO		250 - 500 mg q 8 hours	Useful when broader spectrum is needed
cephadroxil	PO		500 mg to 1 gram q 12 to 24 hours	
cephalexin			250 - 500 mg q 6 hours	
Penicillins		Bactericidal		
amoxicillin	PO		1 gram initially, then 250 - 500 mg q 6 hours	Bacterial endocarditis prophylaxis**
cloxacillin	PO		250 - 500 mg q 6 hours	
dicloxacillin	PO		125 - 250 mg q 6 hours	Staphylococcus infection
*penicillin G	IM or IV		600,000 - 1,200,000 units q 12 - 24 hours	Drug of choice for serious infections
penicillin V	PO		1 gram initially, then 250 - 500 mg q 6 hours	Drug of choice for most infections
Macrolides		Bacteriostatic		
erythromycin	PO			Useful for mild infection and bacterial endocarditis prophylaxis** if patient is penicillin allergic
sterate			250 - 500 mg q 6 hours	
ethylsuccinate			400 - 800 mg q 6 hours	
Tetracycline		Bacteriostatic		
doxycycline	PO		Initially 100 mg q 24 hours or 50 mg q 12 hrs	Mild infections when need broad spectrum, periodontal disease
oxytetracycline	IM		250 mg q 24 hours	
tetracycline	PO		500 mg q 6 hours	
Clindamycin	IV or PO	Bactericidal and Bacteriostatic	150 mg q 6 hours	Instead of metronidazole for penicillin allergic patients with serious infections, or endocarditis prophylaxis** if cannot use penicillin or erythromycin
Metronidazole	IV or PO	Bactericidal	500 mg q 6 hours	Second line of therapy for odontogenic infections, ANUG, HIV periodontitis
Vancomycin	IV	Bactericidal	1 gm infused over 1 hour starting 1 hour before procedure	Component of bacterial endocarditis prophylaxis for patients at high risk**

*400,000 units = 250 mg **See Chapter 3 for bacterial endocarcitis prophylaxis regimen

For most oral infections, penicillin V will be effective when administered orally every 6 hours in 500 milligram doses for 7 to 10 days. When the patient's condition, the size or location of the infection warrants, parenteral administration (IM or IV) of crystalline penicillin G 300,000 to 4,000,000 units every 4 hours is recommended. In-patients and patients in observation could be candidates for repeated parenteral administration because of its rapid absorption intramuscularly and its rapid excretion, crystalline penicillin G may be administered initially, followed by the more slowly absorbed procaine penicillin G (600,000 to 1,000,000 units every 12 to 24 hours). This intramuscular approach coupled with subsequent oral dosing may be indicated for out-patient management of severe infections. Table 1-9 specifies dosages for commonly prescribed antibiotics.

General antibiotic prescribing rules for infections in which culture and sensitivity tests have not been performed are: 1) If there is no improvement after two days of initial antibiotic therapy, a second antibiotic should be added that is more effective against anaerobic organisms (approximately 48 hours is required to observe a therapeutic response from antibiotic administration). This action attempts to control the infection and prevent the rise of antibiotic resistant organisms. 2) If it becomes necessary to prescribe a second antibiotic, culture and sensitivity testing is recommended and the efficacy of the combined antibiotic therapy should be re-evaluated when the results are known, provided the patient's condition does not worsen during this time. 3) If worsening of the infection or the patient's condition is observed, a consultation with an oral and maxillofacial surgeon is indicated. 4) Signs and symptoms of progressing infection include: impaired breathing and sounds of respiratory obstruction (crowing), difficulty swallowing, deviation of the uvula to one side of the pharynx, the spread of infection beyond the initial tissues affected, and the presence of lymphadenopathy. When warranted by the initial presentation of the infection (i.e., size and/or location of infection, and patient's condition), microbiological sampling for culture and sensitivity testing should be performed prior to beginning antibiotic therapy. 5) When it is necessary to administer a second antibiotic, a bacteriocidal drug should not be administered at the same time as a bacteriostatic drug. The slowing of an organism's growth with a bacteriostatic drug will inhibit the efficacy of a bacteriocidal drug.

VII. ANALGESICS FOR ORAL PAIN

An ideal agent for minimizing or eliminating oral pain should: resolve inflammation at the site of injury, abate pain, have no deleterious effects on hemostasis and not depress the central nervous system. No single analgesic preparation possesses all of these properties.

Studies have documented that nonsteroidal anti-inflammatory medications match or surpass the analgesic properties of narcotic preparations in alleviating oral pain. Nevertheless, narcotic medications continue to be prescribed for their euphoric effects. Although oral pain may not be completely controlled with either narcotics or non-narcotic analgesics, patients receiving narcotics may be less concerned if the pain persists and consequently may be more tolerant of residual discomfort. In general, mild to moderate pain can be effectively reduced with the use of a non-steroidal anti-inflammatory medication, while more severe pain may require the use of narcotic analgesics. When a narcotic is prescribed, it is recommended to use a preparation containing both a narcotic analgesic and a non-steroidal anti-inflammatory analgesic so that additive effects are realized. Many such preparations compound codeine or a semisynthetic narcotic with aspirin or acetominophen. In a hemorrhagic injury the use of a NSAID may be a relative contraindication. Acetaminophen, while a good analgesic, has little anti-inflammatory activity and is the NSAID of choice hemostasis is an important consideration. Table 1-10 describes commonly prescribed analgesic preparations and their dosages.

Table 1-10: Administration and Dosage of Analgesics for Oral Pain

Analgesic	Indication (pain intensity)	Dosage (PO)
Non-narcotic		
Non anti-inflammatory		
acetaminophen	mild	325-650 mg q 4 h
Anti-inflammatory agents		
acetylsalicyclic acid, aspirin	mild	325-650 mg q 4 h
diflunisal	mild to moderate	1 gram initially, then 500 mg q 8-12 h
fenoprofen	mild to moderate	200 mg q 4 h
ibuprofen	mild to moderate	400-800 mg q 8 h
ketorolac	moderate to severe	10 mg q 6 h
meclofenamate	mild to moderate	50 mg q 4-6 h
mefanamic acid	moderate	500 mg initially, then 250 mg q 6 h
naproxen	mild to moderate	500 mg initially, then 250 mg q 6-8 h
Narcotic analgesics		
codeine	moderate to severe	30 to 60 mg q 4 h
dihydrocodone	moderate to severe	16 mg, 1-2 tabs q 4 h
hydrocodone	moderate to severe	5 to 7 mg; 1 tab q 4 h
propoxyphene	mild to moderate	32 mg; 1-2 tabs q 4 h
Compounded anagesics		
aspirin with codeine	moderate to severe	aspirin 325 mg, codeine 16mg; 2 tabs q 4 h
acetaminophen with codeine	moderate to severe	acetaminophen 325 mg, codeine 16 mg;2 tabs q 4 h
aspirin with propoxyphene	mild to moderate	aspirin 325 mg, propoxyphene 25 mg; 2 tabs q 4 h
acetaminophen with propoxyphene	mild to moderate	acetaminophen 650 mg, propoxyphene 25 mg; 1 tab q 4 h
hydrocodone with acetaminophen	moderate to severe	hydrocodone 5 mg, acetaminophen 500 mg; 2 tabs q 6 h
hydrocodone with aspirin	moderate to severe	hydrocodone 5 mg, aspirin 500 mg; 2 tabs q 6 h
pentazocaine with aspirin acetaminophen	moderate to severe	pentazocaine 12.5 mg, aspirin 325 mg; 2 tabs q 4 h
pentazocaine with naloxone	moderate to severe	pentazocaine 50 mg, naloxone 0.5 mg; 1-2 tabs g 4 h

References

Basrani E., *Fractures of the Teeth*. Philadelphia: Lea & Febiger, 1985.

Bell W., *Orofacial Pains: Classification, Diagnosis, Management*. 4th ed, Boca Raton: Year Book Medical Publishers, Inc., 1989.

Brekke J.H., Olsen R.A., Scully J.R., Osbon D.B., "Influence of polylactic acid mesh on the incidence of localized osteitis." *Oral Surg* 29 (1983): 24.

Cameron C., "The cracked tooth syndrome: additional findings." *JADA*. 93 (1976):971.

Chatrian G.E., Fernandes de Lima V.M., Lettich E., Canfield R.C., Miller R.C., and Soso M.J. "Electrical stimulation of tooth pulp in humans. II. Qualities of Sensations." *Pain*. 14 (1982):233.

Chambers I.G., "The role and methods of pulp testing in oral diagnosis: a review." *Int Endo J*. 15 (1982):1.

Cooley R.L., Robinson S.F., "Variables associated with electric pulp testing." Oral Surg. 50 (Jul 1980):66.

Drinnan A.J., "Differential Diagnosis of Oral Pain." *Dent Clin North Am*. 22(1)(1978): 73.

Dubner R., Sessel B., Storey A., *The Neural Basis of Oral and Facial Function*. New York: Plenum Press, 1978.

Dummer P.M.H., Hicks R., Huws D., "Clinical signs and symptoms in pulp disease." *Int Endo J*. 13 (1980):27.

Fernandes de Lima V.M., et al., "Electrical stimulation of tooth pulp in humans. I. Relationships among physical stimulus intensities, psychological magnitude estimates and cerebral evoked potentials." *Pain*. 14 (1982):207.

Filipowicz F.J., "The lateral periodontal cyst and isolated periodontal defects." *J Periodontol*. 53 (3)(1982): 145.

Goldberg M.H., Nemarich A.N., Marco W.P., "Complications after third molar surgery: A statistical analysis of 500 consecutive procedures in private practice." *JADA*. 111(2)(1985): 277.

Graham L.L., Schinbeckler G.A., "Orofacial pain of cardiac origin." *JADA*. 104 (Jan 1982):47.

Grant D.A., Stern I.B., Everett F.G., *Periodontics in the Tradition of Gottlieb and Orban*. 8th ed, St. Louis: CV Mosby Co., 1988.

Johnson W.T., Leary J.M., "Vertical root fractures: diagnosis and treatment." *Gen Dent*. Sep-Oct 1984.

Jordan R.E., Suzuki M., Skinner D.H., Indirect pulp-capping of carious teeth with periapical lesions." *JADA*. 97 (July 1978):37.

Kahn C.S., "Dry Socket: Etiology and Management." *Compend Cont Dent Ed*. 10(1)(1989):48.

Kleinberg I., Sessel B., *Oro-facial Pain and Neuromuscular Dysfunction: Mechanisms and Clinical Correlations*. New York: Pergamon Press, 1985.

McGrath P., Gracely R., Dubner R., and Heft M., "Non-pain and pain sensations evoked by tooth pulp stimulation." *Pain*. 15 (1983):377.

Meechan J.G., MacGregor I.D.M., Rogers S.N., et al., "The effect of smoking on immediate post-extraction socket filling with blood and on the incidence of painful socket." *Br J of Oral Max Surg*. 26 (1988):402.

Melzack R., Terrence C., Fromm G., and Amsel R., "Trigeminal neuralgia and atypical facial pain: use of the McGill pain questionnaire for discrimination and diagnosis." *Pain*. 27 (1986):297.

Mjor I., *Reaction Patterns in Human Teeth*. Boca Raton: CRC Press, Inc., 1983.

Moss-Salentijn L., Hendricks-klyvert M., *Dental and Oral Tissues: an Introduction*. 3rd ed, Philadelphia: Lea & Febiger, 1990.

Mumford J.M., Bowsher D., "Pain and protopathic sensibility. A review with particular reference to the teeth." *Pain*. 2 (1976):223.

Petersen J., Milgrom P., *Pain Relief in the Orofacial Regions.* Copenhagen: Munksgaard, 1989.

Rood J.P., "The nerve supply of the mandibular incisor region." *Brit Dent J.* 143 (1977):227.

Russo M.C., Holland R., de Souza V., "Radiographic and histological evaluation of the treatment of inflamed dental pulps." *Intl Endo J.* 15 (1982):137.

Schuster G., *Oral Microbiology and Infectious Disease.* 3rd ed, Philadelphia: B.C. Decker, Inc., 1990.

Seltzer S., *Endodontology: Biologic Considerations in Endodontic Procedures.* 2nd ed, Philadelphia: Lea & Febiger, 1988.

Seltzer S., Bender I., *The Dental Pulp: Biologic Considerations in Endodontic Procedures.* 3rd ed, New York: J.B. Lippincott Company, 1984

Sessle B.J., Hu J.W., Amano N., and Zhong G., "Convergence of cutaneous, tooth pulp, visceral, neck and muscle afferents onto nociceptive and non-nociceptive neurons in trigeminal subnucleus caudalis (medullary dorsal horn) and its implications for referred pain." *Pain.* 27 (1986):219.

Sherrington C.S., *The Integrative Action of the Nervous System.* New York: C. Scribner's Sons, 1986.

Silvestri A.R., "The undiagnosed split-root syndrome." *JADA.* 92 (May 1976):930.

Simon D.E., Jacobs T.L., Senia E.S., and Walker W.A., "Intraligamentary anesthesia as an aid in endodontic diagnosis." *Oral Surg.* 77-78, July 1982.

Sorensen D.C., Preisch J.W., "The effect of tetracycline on the incidence of postextraction alveolar osteitis." *J Oral Max Surg.* 45 (1987):1029.

Swanson A.E., "A double-blind study on the effectiveness of tetracycline in reducing incidence of fibrinolytic alveolitis." *J Oral Max Surg.* 26 (1989):410.

Wilson S., Johns P., Fuller P.M., "The inferior alveolar and mylohyoid nerves: an anatomic study and relationship to local anesthesia of the anterior mandibular teeth." *JADA.* 108 (1984):350.

2 Orofacial Infections

Ronald C. King, D.D.S., M.S.

Infections of the oral and facial region can be the most difficult and distressing of all dental problems to manage. Fortunately most oral infections remain localized and can be successfully treated with routine surgical procedures and supportive therapy. However, the practitioner must always be alert to the importance of close observation of any swelling, until full resolution occurs. In a few hours a small, localized swelling can expand into a severe life threatening multiple space infection.

The intent of this chapter is to maximize the practitioner's insight into the prevention, causes, diagnosis and treatment of orofacial infections through compact visual presentations. The review of oral and facial infections will include information on etiologies, pathophysiology, responsible organisms, the anatomical relationship of progression, systemic manifestations, diagnostic techniques, treatment, pediatric considerations and less common non-odontogenic orofacial infections.

I. PATHOPHYSIOLOGY AND ASSOCIATED BACTERIA

Most oral and facial infections are dentoalveolar in origin, resulting from carious teeth with necrotic pulps or advanced periodontal disease. The organisms responsible for these infections are normally bacteria indigenous to the oral flora (i.e., organisms found in plaque, on oral mucosa and in gingival crevices).

Improvements in culturing techniques over the last decade (particularly in anaerobic culturing) have allowed for more accurate identification of the causative bacterial spectrum. Anatomically, supragingival bacteria are mainly gram positive facultative anaerobes or microaerophilic cocci or rods, while subgingival organisms consist mainly of anaerobic gram negative bacteria. However, the majority of orofacial infections (greater than 75%) result from a combination of aerobes and anaerobes. The obligate anaerobes cultured in orofacial infections range from 30 to 75%, while isolated aerobes range from 5 to 33%. This represents at least a 3:1 ratio of anaerobes to aerobes. Table 2-1 lists the major organisms and their relative frequency in dental and orofacial infections. In early cellulitis, aerobes dominate the culture, but as the local tissue oxygen is depleted anaerobes increase until the chronic abscess becomes almost completely anaerobic. Streptococci are the predominant causative organism(s) of the aerobic species and exist in 70% of all odontogenic orofacial infections. Staphylococcus is the next most common aerobic species, but has been cultured in only 6% of these infections. The predominant anaerobic microbes are gram-positive cocci such as *Streptococcus, Peptostreptococcus* and *Peptococcus* which are present in ½ of the infections cultured. The gram-negative anaerobic rods, principally *Bacteroides* and *Fusobacterium* organisms, are found in approximately half of all orofacial infections. The anaerobic gram-negative cocci and anaerobic gram-positive rods appear to be opportunistic and are of little significance in the etiology of odontogenic infections. It is essential to identify the predominant organisms and to recognize the relative changes in bacterial composition over time because these two factors determine appropriate antibiotic selection.

Table 2-1: Bacteria identified in odontogenic infections

Aerobic		Anaerobic	
	Gram + cocci		
Alpha hemolytic streptococcus	- very common	*Streptococcus* spp.	- common
Beta hemolytic streptococcus	- unusual	*Peptostreptococcus* spp.	- common
Group D	- rare	*Peptococcus* spp.	- common
Staphylococcus spp	- rare		
	Gram - cocci		
Neisseria spp.	- rare	*Veillonella* spp.	- unusual
	Gram + bacilli		
Corynebacterium spp.	- rare	*Eubacterium* spp.	- unusual
Lactobacillus spp.- unusual			
	Gram - bacilli		
Haemophilus influenzae	- rare	*Bacteroides*	
Eikenella corrodens	- rare	*oralis*	- very common
		melaninogenicus	- very common
		gingivalis	- very common
		fragilis	- rare
		Fusobacterium spp.	- very common

The *virulence* and *quantity* of the causative microbes combined with the local, humoral and cellular *defense mechanisms* of the host, determine the spread and extent of any infection. The mechanisms of the body which fight infection are evident in the cardinal signs of inflammation: rubor, tumor, calor and dolor. ***Rubor***, or *redness*, is the result of persistent vasodilation of arterioles and capillaries and increased venule permeability, which decrease venous blood flow. Exudate rich in plasma proteins, antibodies, nutrients and leukocytes permeate the insulted tissues. ***Tumor***, or *swelling*, results from this accumulating exudate and/or the production of pus, secondary to cellular and bacterial death. Bacterial products interact with plasma factors and cells to produce agents that attract neutrophils to the infected area, a process termed chemotaxis. The phagocytosis of bacteria, other organisms and dead cells occurs as macrophages migrate in and clean up the necrotic debris. ***Calor***, or *heat*, is produced by increased local blood flow, which also enhances the phagocytic activity of the PMNs (polymorphonuclear leukocytes). A fibrin network develops within the exudate and attempts to wall off the infected area. ***Dolor***, or *pain*, develops from the pressure of the swelling against sensory nerve endings, and from the liberation of pain producing substances such as serotonin, prostaglandins and bradykinin.

An odontogenic infection becomes a cellulitis when it spreads into the soft tissues. If the host response is aggressive, the infection can quickly localize into an abscess. A more sluggish reaction may appear as cellulitis alone, or as an abscess with a surrounding area of cellulitis. An ***abscess*** is a walled off area of disintegrating PMNs and microorganisms (pus), surrounded by viable leukocytes and lymphocytes and devoid of a central blood supply. Clinically an abscess appears as a discrete, usually indurated, intraoral or extraoral swelling without systemic manifestations. An abscess is more chronic and less aggressive a manifestation than cellulitis, indicating that the local host resistant mechanisms are performing adequately. Comparatively, a ***cellulitis*** is an indiscrete swelling characterized by doughiness to palpation in mild cases, and induration and "board-like" hardness to palpation in more severe infections. Patients commonly have systemic manifestations of fever and malaise with cellulitis, and the extent of the swelling is usually more widespread than with an abscess. Hence, a cellulitis represents a more aggressive infection, and as such is a greater threat to the host.

The aforementioned clinical manifestations of an infection are partially determined by the type of offending organism. Staphylococci are frequently implicated in abscesses because of their ability to produce the enzyme coagulase. This enzyme is thought to produce a fibrin protective film around bacteria or to form such a coat around the infection site. Streptococci, on the other hand, are more often associated with cellulitis because of their ability to produce enzymes such as streptokinase, hyaluronidase and streptodornase. These enzymes encourage the rapid spread of infection by breaking down fibrin and connective tissue ground substance. Some streptococcal strains also produce toxins that cause headaches and fever.

II. THE SPREAD OF ODONTOGENIC INFECTION

In the initial stage of odontogenic orofacial infections, the microbial invasion is localized to the teeth and periodontium. Bacteria infect the dental pulp through tooth decay, crown defects, or periodontal breakdown. Inflammation, vasodilation, edema and ischemia ensue, often followed by necrosis of the pulpal tissues. In the case of advanced periodontal disease or pericoronitis, bacteria and debris located in the gingival pocket crevice cause these inflammatory changes in the adjacent soft tissue. The active infection then spreads from the apex of the root or periodontal ligament into and along the medullary bony spaces in all directions. The infectious process seeks the path of least resistance until it encounters the cortical plate. Pressure then builds between the plates until a perforation appears at a weak and usually thin cortical region. The perforation occurs most frequently on the lateral (buccal) cortex of the maxilla or mandible (Figure 2-1a). As such, the periosteum represents the final barrier to occult infections.

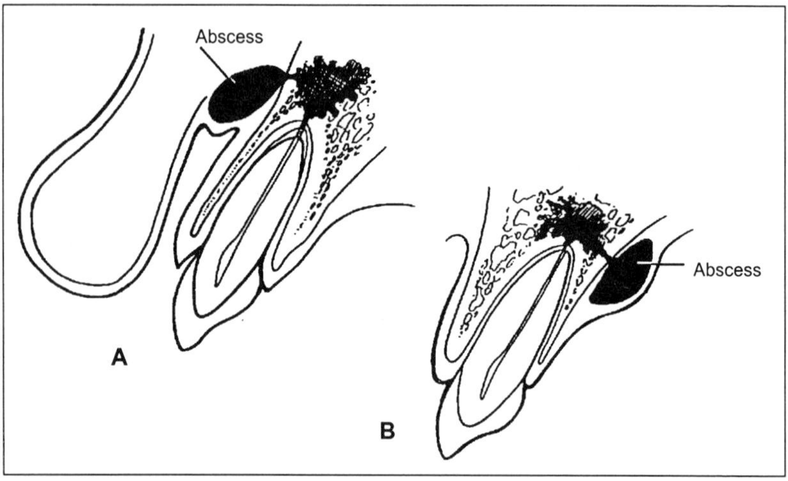

Figure 2-1: Perforation of labial and palatal cortex.

Once perforated, the process is clinically observed as a soft tissue swelling, and the very intense, localized pain of a toothache is replaced by the milder, pressure-like aching of soft tissue discomfort. Once in soft tissue, the direction of spread is usually established by the anatomical proximity of the perforation site to muscle and fascia (Figure 2-2). This relationship of soft tissue attachment to the perforation site, then determines which fascial planes will be involved in the developing cellulitis.

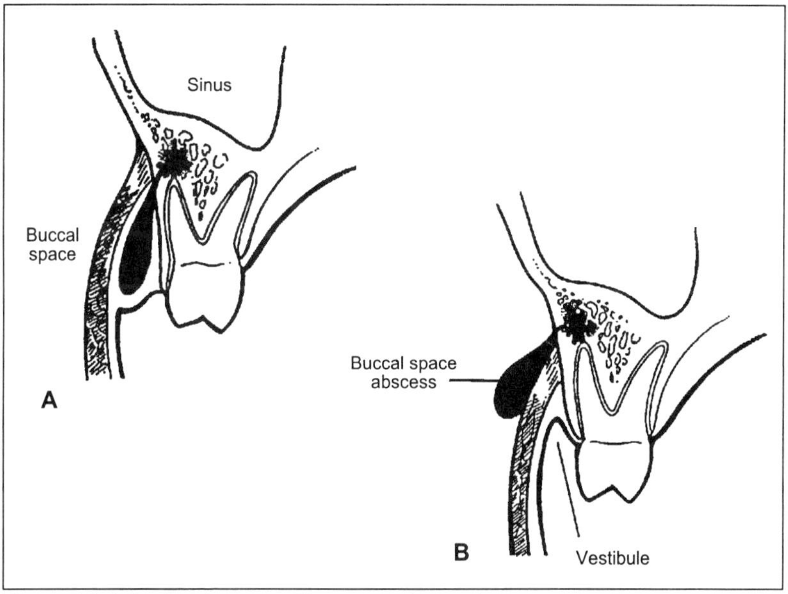

Figure 2-2: Infection from maxillary posterior teeth.

III. ANATOMICAL CONSIDERATIONS IN OROFACIAL INFECTIONS

Anatomically, localization and progression of a dentoalveolar infection depends on three factors: 1) the position of the involved tooth's root apex, 2) the thickness of the cortical plate and 3) the relationship of the cortical perforation site to regional muscle attachments. Familiarity with root locations is essential because acute dental abscesses or chronic fistulae are usually close to the affected root apex. Most infections from maxillary abscessed teeth erode through the thin lateral (labial-buccal) cortical bone below the maxillary muscle attachments (Figure 2-2a). Hence, abscessed maxillary teeth commonly show soft tissue vestibular swellings, although palatal abscesses periodically occur with lingually inclined maxillary incisors (usually lateral incisors) and also occur from the palatal roots of maxillary first molars (Figure 2-1b).

Infections involving the mandibular incisors, cuspids and bicuspids also commonly perforate the labial-buccal cortical plate above the associated musculature resulting in vestibular swellings. The lingual cortex is thinner around the mandibular molars and consequently, mandibular molar infections more frequently perforate the lingual side of the mandible and extend into either the sublingual or submandibular spaces. Third molar roots typically extend below the mylohyoid muscle attachment. Therefore, with lingual perforation, the infection spreads under the mylohyoid muscle into the submandibular space (Figure 2-3, 2-9).

The mandibular first molars, and less commonly the second molars, have roots that end above the level of the mylohyoid attachment. Therefore, infection from these teeth perforate above the mylohyoid muscle and infiltrate the sublingual space (Figures 2-3, 2-8). In summary, odontogenic infection in both dental arches are primarily found in the labial-buccal vestibules with the exception of the mandibular molars.

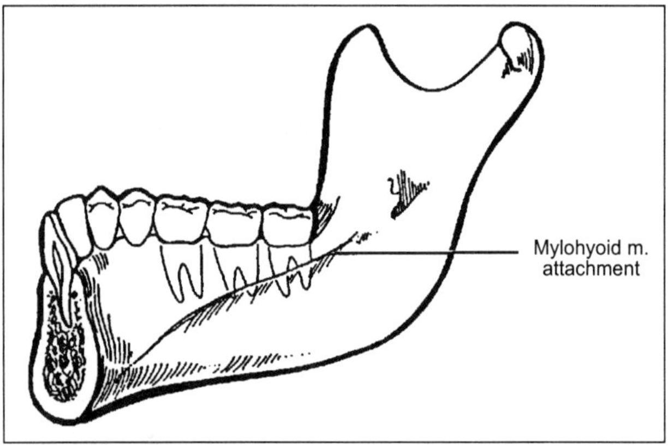

Figure 2-3: Mylohyoid attachment.

A. Primary Fascial Spaces

Although odontogenic infections are usually mild and easily controlled with the removal of the etiology, occasionally the infection perforates the alveolar bone and extends into the fascial spaces. The fascial planes are potential spaces of infection in the healthy patient and are formed by fascia that surrounds and separates muscles. When an infection courses the path of least resistance through loose connective tissue and along the fascial planes, the spaces are demarcated. The primary maxillary spaces are the canine, buccal and infratemporal. The major mandibular spaces are the submental, buccal, submandibular and sublingual.

Maxillary Fascial Spaces

The ***canine space*** is a small potential gap between the levator anguli oris and the levator labii superioris muscles. This space enlarges primarily with infections of the *maxillary canine*. The infection perforates the buccal bone superior to the origin of the levator anguli oris muscle and below the origin of the levator labii superioris muscle (Photo 2-1). Clinically the nasolabial fold is obliterated.

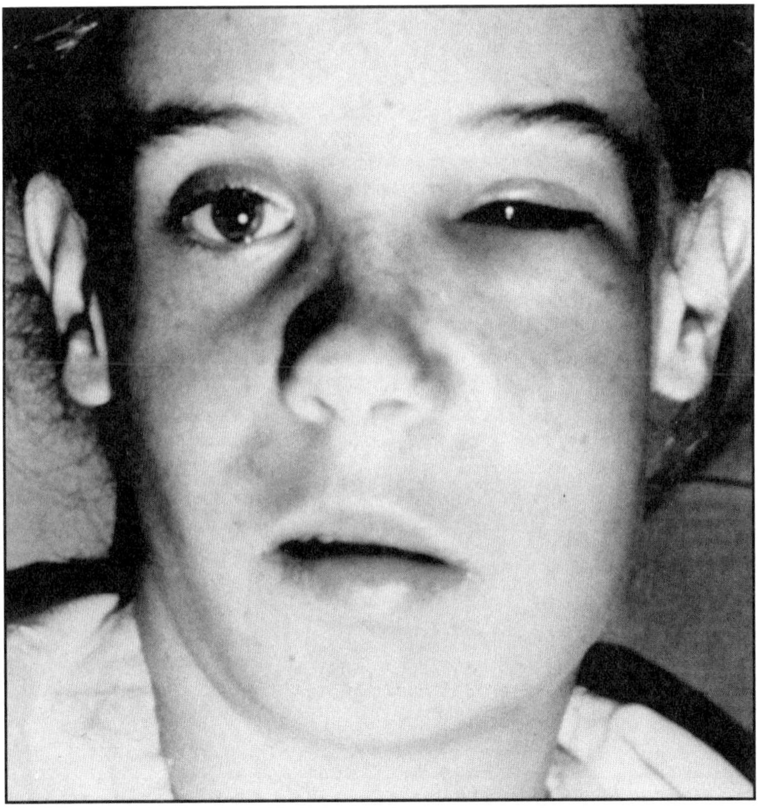

Photo 2-1: Canine space infection.

The potential ***buccal space*** is found between the skin of the cheek and the lateral surface of the buccinator muscle (Figure 2-4). This space enlarges when infections from the *maxillary posterior teeth* erode through the buccal cortex, superior to the origin of the buccinator muscle. Less frequently

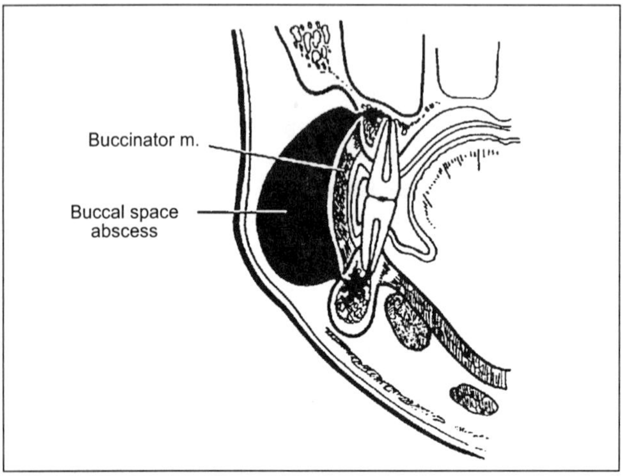

Figure 2-4: Buccal space.

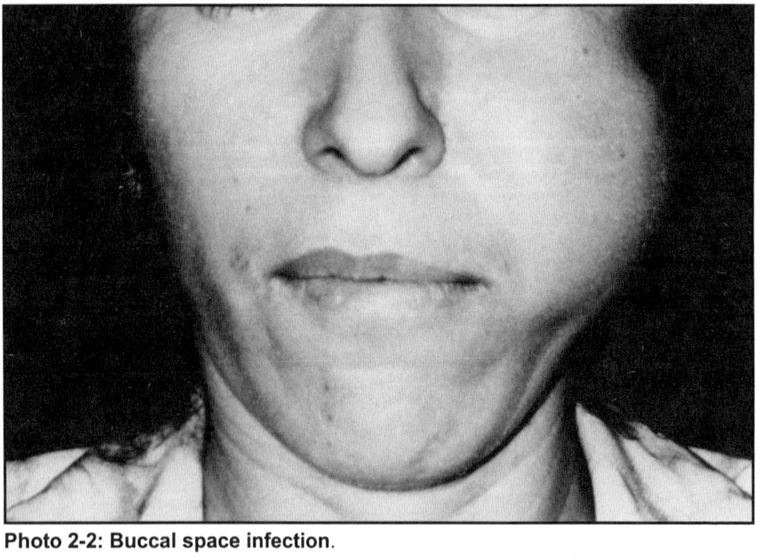

Photo 2-2: Buccal space infection.

this swelling arises from a mandibular posterior tooth infection that perforates the buccal cortex inferior to the attachment of the buccinator muscle; hence, this space is included in both maxillary and mandibular spaces. Clinically a buccal space swelling can extend superiorly to the zygomatic arch and inferiorly to the body of the mandible (Photo 2-2).

The ***infratemporal space*** is posterior to the maxilla, limited medially by the lateral pterygoid plate of the sphenoid bone and superiorly by the skull. The remaining boundaries of the infratemporal space are congruent with the deep temporal space (Figure 2-5). Therefore, the clinical manifestations of an infratemporal space infection are similar to those of the temporal spaces (trismus). An infratemporal space infection is rare and is usually associated with a *maxillary third molar* infection.

Odontogenic infections of the maxilla can spread hematogenously via the inferior or superior ophthalmic vein and rarely produce ***orbital cellulitis***. Characteristics of such infections include red, swollen eyelids, proptosis (bulging globe), impairment of vision and limited eye movement. Hematogenous spread of a maxillary infection can also infect the cavernous sinus via two routes. Bacteria can travel through the "valveless" angular and ophthalmic veins which permit bidirectional blood flow, or bacteria can travel posteriorly from the pterygoid plexus via emissary veins to the cavernous sinus (Figure 2-6). Bacterial contamination of the cavernous sinus

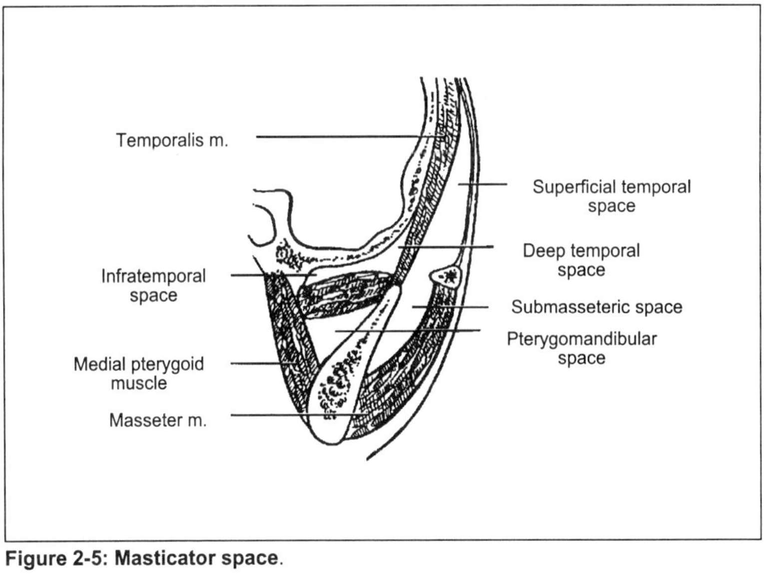

Figure 2-5: Masticator space.

can lead to the development of ***cavernous sinus thrombosis.*** Both orbital cellulitis and cavernous sinus thrombosis exhibit similar clinical findings including blindness, however, cavernous sinus thrombosis can also cause palsies of cranial nerves III, IV, and VI as well as paresthesias of the first and second divisions of the fifth cranial nerve. Although extremely rare, brain abscesses can occur as sequela of maxillary fascial space infections and require aggressive medical and surgical measures.

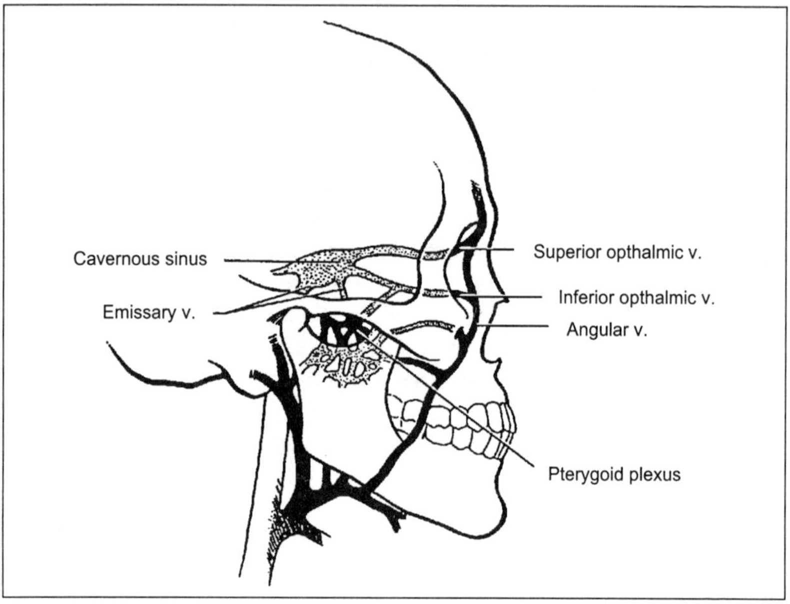

Figure 2-6: Venous drainage relationship to cavernous sinus.

Mandibular Fascial Spaces

Most infections related to the mandibular teeth are limited to the mandibular buccal vestibule, however, periodically an infection continues into one of the four primary mandibular spaces.

The ***submental space*** is commonly associated with infections from *mandibular incisors.* These infections can erode either through the anterior

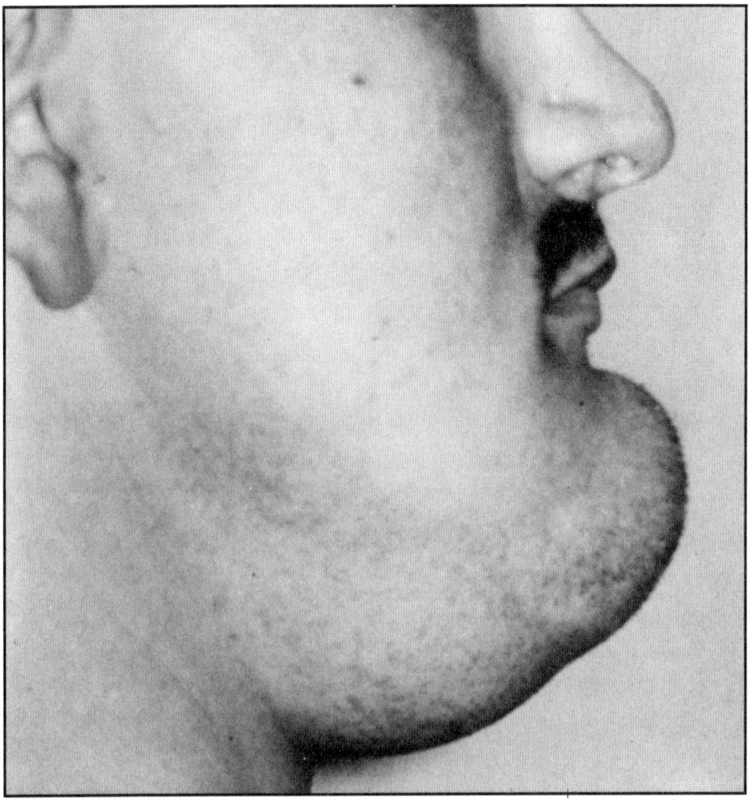

Photo 2-3: Submental space infection extending posteriorly into the submandibular space.

cortical plate inferior to the attachment of the mentalis muscle and proceed under the inferior border of the mandible into the submental space or lingually into the sublingual or submental spaces. Submental space infections may also occur from the spread of other space infections (i.e., from communications with the submandibular and sublingual spaces). These interspace communications are important because it is uncommon for submental space infections to occur alone. The submental space lies both between the anterior bellies of the digastric muscles and between the mylohyoid muscle and the overlying skin and platysma muscle (Figure 2-7). Clinically the chin appears swollen, firm, and erythematous, especially the inferior border (Photo 2-3).

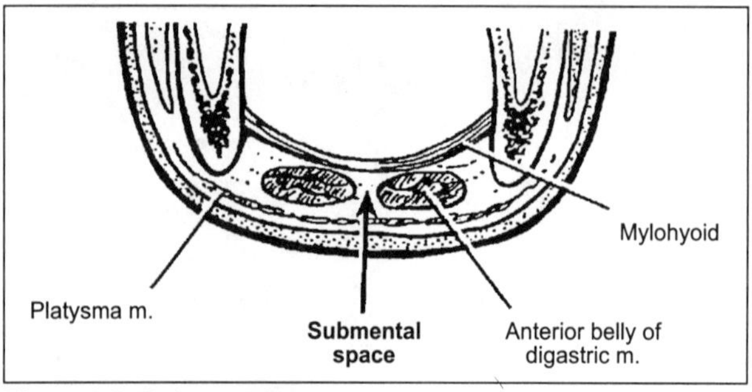

Figure 2-7: Submental space.

A ***buccal space*** swelling can result from infections of *mandibular posterior teeth* that perforate the buccal plate inferior to the attachment of the buccinator muscle. Impressive extraoral swelling is characteristic of buccal space infections since there is no musculature to limit lateral border expansion (Figure 2-4/Photo 2-2). The anatomical dimensions of this space have been previously described.

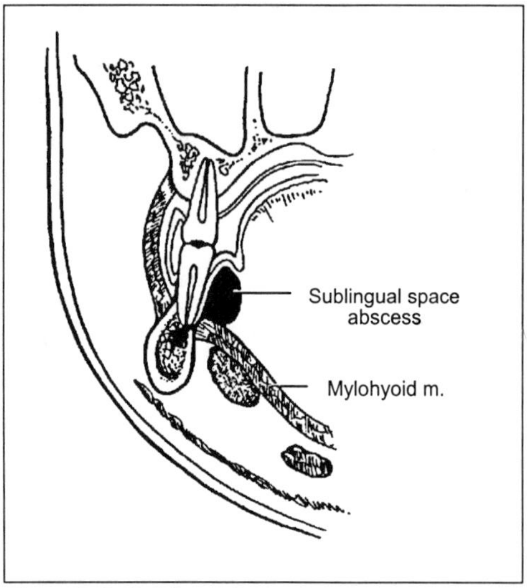

Figure 2-8: Sublingual space.

The ***sublingual space*** is primarily contaminated by infections from *mandibular bicuspids* and *first molars*. This space is bordered anteriorly and laterally by the medial border of the mandible, superiorly by sublingual mucosa and inferiorly by the mylohyoid muscle (Figure 2-8). The sublingual space communicates posteriorly with the submandibular space and with the secondary spaces of the mandible. The clinical presentation of a sublingual space infection is almost exclusively intraoral, with obvious floor swelling and associated elevation of the tongue. Bilateral sublingual space swelling is common because only loose connective tissue separates the two spaces.

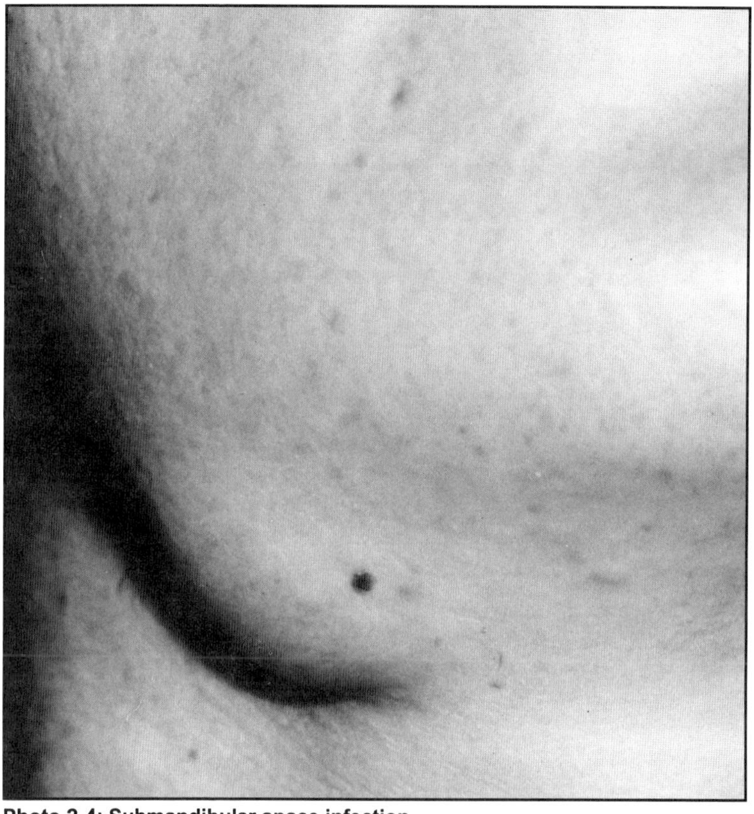

Photo 2-4: Submandibular space infection.

Involvement of the ***submandibular space***, the most frequently involved fascial space, is usually the result of odontogenic infections from *mandibular third molars*, and less frequently *second* and *first molars*. As mentioned earlier, the relationship of the root apices to the mylohyoid muscle attachment determines whether the sublingual or submandibular space will be infected (Figure 2-3). The submandibular space lies between the mylohyoid muscle, the medial surface of the mandible and the skin (including two fascia layers and the thin platysma muscle) (Figure 2-9/Photo 2-4). The digastric muscles form the medial border and the hyoid bone determines the posterior limit. Communication with the sublingual, submental, masticator and pharyngeal spaces is common. If the spread of infection extends bilaterally and involves all primary mandibular spaces (submandibular, sublingual and submental), the entity is known as ***Ludwig's angina***. This multiple space infection is a rapidly expanding cellulitis that commonly extends posteriorly into the masticator and parapharyngeal spaces. Clinically, there is marked elevation of the tongue, extensive firm submandibular and submental swelling, trismus (limited mandibular opening), drooling, difficulty swallowing and airway obstruction (Photo 2-5). Frequently the infection progresses at an alarming speed requiring hospitalization, vigorous surgical intervention, airway maintenance and intravenous antibiotic therapy for treatment.

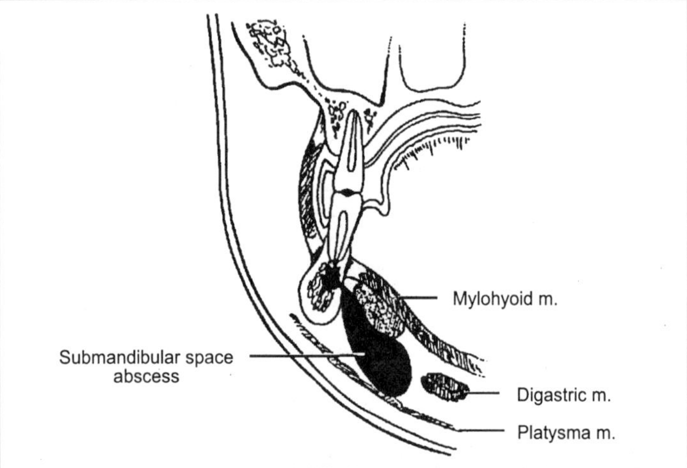

Figure 2-9: Submandibular space.

B. Secondary Fascial Spaces

Aggressive treatment of primary fascial space infections is not always sufficient to prevent their rapid posterior extension into the *secondary fascial spaces*. Once this occurs, complications, treatment, morbidity and mortality all escalate. The secondary fascial spaces consist of three masticator spaces and three cervical fascial spaces.

The ***masticator space*** includes the submasseteric, pterygomandibular and temporal spaces (Figure 2-5). Infection of one space generally involves all three because there is free communication among each, as well as with the parapharyngeal space. *Trismus* is the trademark of a masticator space

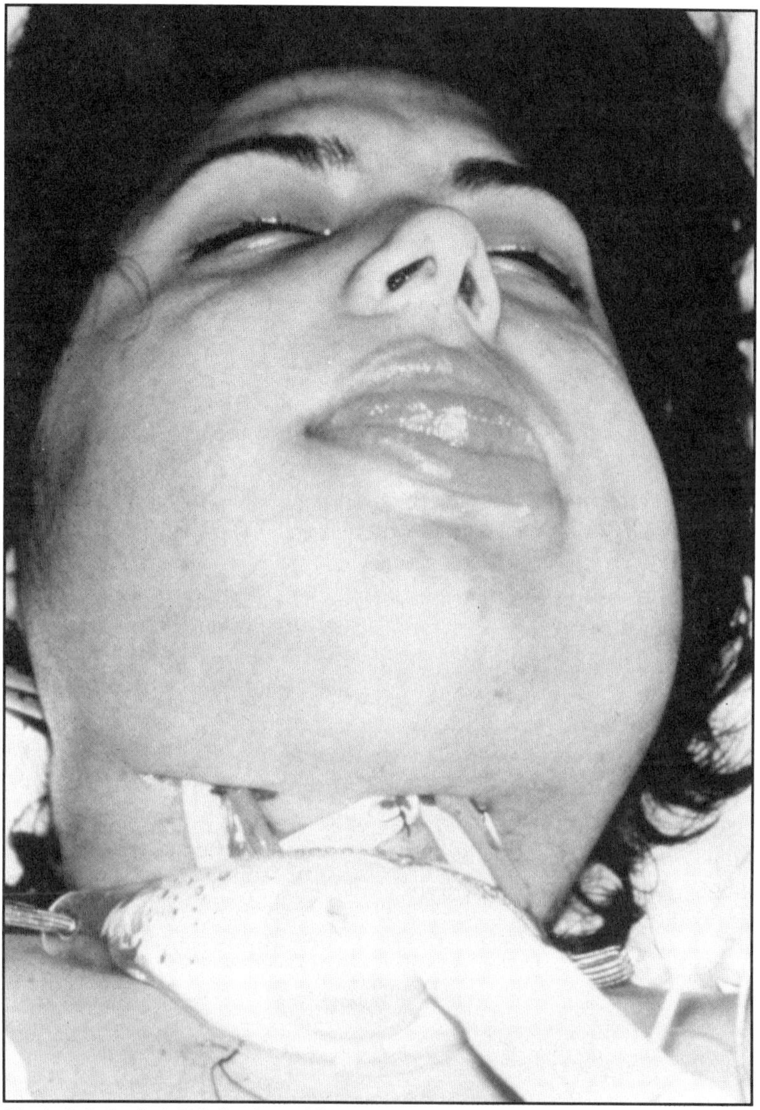

Photo 2-5: Ludwig's infection with tracheostomy and drains.

infection because the muscles of mastication are directly affected by the swelling and inflammation.

The ***submasseteric space*** lies between the lateral surface of the ramus of the mandible and the medial surface of the masseter muscle. Infection within the space usually develops from the spread of a buccal space infection or directly from a *pericoronitis of the third molar* (inflammation and swelling of the soft tissue around the tooth). Swelling beneath the masseter muscle is often clinically obscure, but trismus is usually evident. This is in contrast to a buccal space infection which displays obvious swelling but little trismus.

The ***pterygomandibular space*** is located medial to the ramus and lateral to the medial pterygoid muscle. Local anesthetic for inferior alveolar nerve blocks is routinely injected into this space. Infections of this space originate from *contaminated local anesthetic needles*, from third molar *pericoronitis* and secondary to the spread of submandibular or sublingual space infections. Trismus without extra- or intraoral swelling may indicate an isolated pterygomandibular space infection.

The ***temporal space*** lies posterior and superior to the submasseteric and pterygomandibular spaces and is divided into superficial and deep portions by the temporalis muscle. The deep portion extends medially into the infratemporal space. This space is the least commonly infected of the masticator spaces; involvement is usually secondary to other space infections. When infection is present, temporal space swelling is superior to the zygomatic arch and posterior to the lateral orbital rim.

The other group of secondary fascial spaces is the cervical fascial spaces. Fortunately the extension of infections beyond the primary and secondary masticator spaces is rare. However, when this occurs, life-threatening sequelae such as airway obstruction or mediastinitis are not unusual, even with hospitalization and maximum surgical and medical therapies. Infections that spread posteriorly from the pterygomandibular space first encounter the ***lateral pharyngeal space***. This space is in the lateral neck, extending inferiorly in the shape of an inverted cone from the base of the skull at the sphenoid bone to the hyoid bone inferiorly. The pharyngeal constrictor muscle and mucosa separate the pharynx from the lateral pharyngeal space medially (Figure 2-10). This space is medial

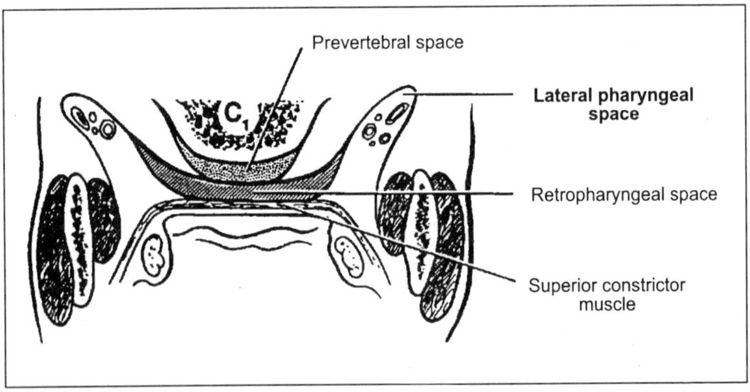

Figure 2-10: Lateral pharyngeal space.

to the medial pterygoid muscle and bounded anteriorly by the pterygomandibular raphe. The medial wall of the space is continuous with the carotid sheath and the styloid process. Associated muscles and fascia divide the space into *anterior* and *posterior* portions. Infections of the lateral pharyngeal space may result from *pharyngitis*, *tonsillitis*, *parotitis*, *otitis* and *mastoiditis*, in addition to *dental infections*. The clinical picture of an *anterior* compartment infection includes intraoral bulging of the lateral pharyngeal wall, extraoral swelling below the angle of the mandible and severe trismus from medial pterygoid muscle involvement. *Posterior* compartment involvement is characterized by minimal trismus or visible swelling; however, signs of airway obstruction are common. The most serious problems encountered with posterior compartment infections involve the structures located in the carotid sheath that pass through the space. These problems can include thrombosis of the internal jugular vein, erosion of the carotid artery or its branches and interruption of cranial nerves IX through XII. Patients with infection of either compartment have difficulty swallowing, usually exhibit a high fever and rapidly deteriorate.

The ***retropharyngeal space*** lies posterior to the pharynx and the superior pharyngeal constrictor muscle (Figure 2-10). The space extends inferiorly from the skull to the upper mediastinum and only alar fascia separates the retropharyngeal space from the prevertebral space (Figure 2-11). With few contents in the retropharyngeal space (unlike the lateral pharyngeal space), infection can rapidly spread inferiorly into the posterosuperior mediastinum. Difficulty swallowing (dysphagia), and difficulty breathing (dyspnea), marked neck stiffness (nuchal rigidity), burping (esophageal regurgitation) and fever characterize an infection of this space. If an intraoral exam is possible, bulging of the posterior pharyngeal wall may be observed.

Posterior to the retropharyngeal space lies the ***prevertebral space***, termed the "danger space" because it extends from the skull to the level of the diaphragm and can rapidly carry infection to the thorax and mediastinum (Figure 2-11). Some authors specify the retropharyngeal area as "danger space 3" and the prevertebral as "danger space 4." The prevertebral space becomes contaminated when an infection under pressure in the retropharyngeal space perforates the alar fascia posteriorly.

Infections involving either the retropharyngeal or prevertebral space can cause upper airway obstruction by displacing the posterior pharyngeal wall anteriorly. When the posterior pharyngeal wall ruptures, pus can be aspirated by the patient, plus the infection can spread into the mediastinum causing mediastinitis. Signs and symptoms of ***mediastinitis*** include chest pain, severe dyspnea, persistent fever and radiographic evidence of mediastinal widening. Substernal pain and fever following drainage of fascial space infections indicate possible

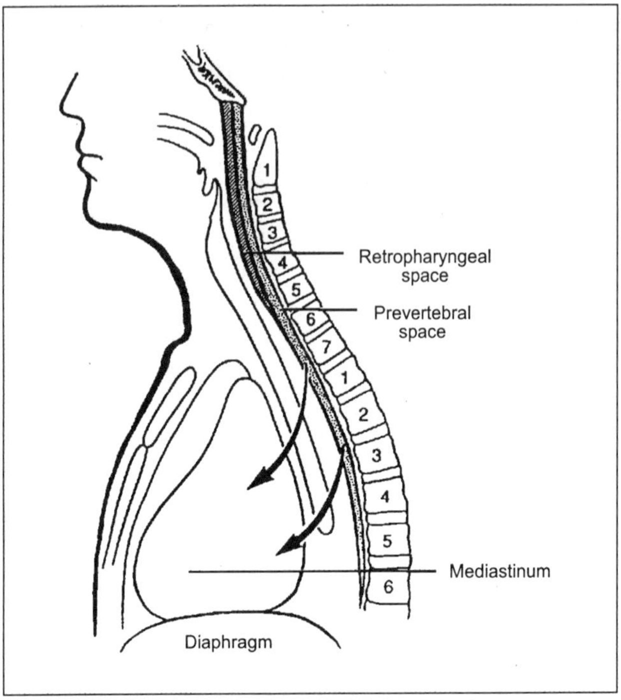

Figure 2-11: Retropharyngeal space/Prevertebral space.

mediastinal involvement. The dangerous sequela to mediastinitis can be a progression from septicemia to mediastinal and thoracic abscesses, and finally to pleural effusion, pericarditis, and death. The treatment of suppurative mediastinitis includes massive doses of long-term antibiotics and surgical drainage of the mediastinum.

IV. SYSTEMIC MANIFESTATIONS OF OROFACIAL INFECTIONS

Fever and lymphadenopathy commonly herald the systemic spread of infection. Fever is attributed to circulating bacterial endotoxins that act on monocytes, macrophages and Kupffer cells to produce the pyrogen, interleukin-1. This endogenous substance acts on lymphocytes to stimulate the immune system and activate the hypothalamic thermoregulating centers to increase body temperature and conserve body heat through peripheral vasoconstriction. Shivering follows decreased skin temperature and increased core temperature. ***Chills*** indicate that showers of bacteria (bacteremia) and their associated endotoxins are circulating in the vascular system. A low-grade fever (below 102°F) may be beneficial to the host because an elevation in body temperature inhibits many microorganisms and increases antibody production. Headaches commonly accompany a fever and are assumed to result from the dilation of intracranial arteries. ***Lymphadenopathy*** is frequently associated with head and neck infections. It is attributed to either the proliferation of intrinsic lymphocytes and histiocytes or to the invasion of circulating PMNs and macrophages into the respective lymph nodes. Lymph node enlargement is commonly palpable, especially in thin or young patients. With acute infection the enlarged nodes are usually soft and tender, while in chronic infection the nodes are typically firm and nontender. Often this nodal enlargement remains long after the etiology has been removed. Rarely does a node abscess, unless the infecting organism overpowers the node's defense mechanism, resulting in excessive cellular reaction and suppuration.

Determining the presence of an infection is more difficult when recent tissue insult has occurred, such as following surgery or trauma. Swelling, pain, redness and trismus are expected sequelae in the first three days following trauma. These sequelae result from disruption of cell membranes, activation of complement and white cells, and release of inflammatory products that cause thrombosis, vasoconstriction and tissue edema. When severe, a large number of lymphocytes release interleukins. These are polypeptides which not only affect body temperature but also activate multiple biologic effects including tachycardia and proteolysis. The results are malaise, fever and an elevated leukocyte count (greater than 10,000 cells per cubic millimeter) in the absence of true infection. Fever is often augmented by limited oral intake and developing dehydration. Close follow-up of such patients including observation, palpation for fluctuance, serial temperatures and careful scrutiny for signs of airway compromise is necessary until complete resolution of the swelling occurs. The late development (more than 3 days) of these symptoms is a reliable indicator that more than the expected post trauma edema is occurring and signals the need for more aggressive treatment (antibacterial).

V. DIAGNOSING OROFACIAL INFECTIONS

The classic "toxic appearance" associated with a serious infection includes *fatigue*, *fever* and *malaise*. The first step in the initial examination of a patient with an orofacial infection is to determine the location and severity of the problem. Obtaining the history of the current infectious process, assessing the physical status of the patient and performing a "hands on" examination should be completed on all patients. In the history, it is important to listen carefully to the patient's description of the symptoms (pain, swelling, trismus, dysphagia or dyspnea) and their onset, duration and progress. The patient should also be questioned regarding any received or self administered treatments. Finally the patient's medical history should be reviewed for diseases that would enhance patients' susceptibility to orofacial infections such as diabetes mellitus, AIDS, prior head-neck radiation therapy, chemotherapy, immunosuppressive medications, etc. Assessing a patient's innate ability to fight infection requires an understanding of the body's four basic defensive mechanisms. ***Mechanical defenses*** are body secretions, the intact skin and mucosa. When the barriers of skin and mucosa are violated by purposeful incisions, trauma, periodontal pockets or necrotic pulps, bacteria is given access to the submucosal and deep tissues. Body secretions act as protective mechanisms by carrying bacteria into the digestive tract where enzymes and a low pH can destroy the invading organisms. ***Normal microbial flora*** are a second host deterrent, exerting an antibiotic-like effect on foreign organisms. One example is streptococci which produce bacteriocin, an antibacterial substance that is active in the host's oral flora. Altering the normal oral flora with such things as chronic antibiotic administration can facilitate the development of pathogenic organisms and infection. ***Cellular*** or ***inflammatory protective mechanisms*** occur in deeper tissues and primarily include lymphocytes and phagocytic cells (PMNs, monocytes and macrophages). The action of T-lymphocytes is the mainstay of cell-mediated immunity. The final components of host defense are the ***immunoglobulins*** and ***complement*** which together comprise humoral immunity. The immunoglobulins produced from plasma cells are antibodies which can attach to invading bacteria (opsonization) rendering the bacteria more susceptible to leukocytes phagocytosis and can trigger complement activation. There are five immunoglobulins; IgG comprises about 75% and acts primarily against gram-positive bacteria. Complement is a complex protein produced in the liver, which when activated, encourages the migration of leukocytes from the bloodstream to the site of bacteria invasion (chemotaxis). This promotes opsonization and phagocytosis, and enhances the lysis of bacterial cells (bacteriolysis).

In the patient's medical history, the clinician must recognize possible compromises in host defenses. For instance, a facilitator of phagocytosis called tuftsin can not be released without a spleen producing enzyme. Therefore, patients such as children with *splenectomies* are more susceptible to infections caused by encapsulated organisms like *Pneumococci*. The stress of trauma causes an increase in endogenous epinephrine and steroids, which leads to both a decrease in insulin secretion and an increase in glucagon production and release. If the stress is persistent, a significant increase in susceptibility to infection can result. Deficiencies in leukocytic synthesis and function are often found in cancers such as *leukemias* and *lymphomas*, and in poorly controlled metabolic diseases such as *renal failure*, *diabetes*, *rheumatoid arthritis* and severe alcoholism with *malnutrition*. In poorly controlled diabetics, neutrophilic chemotaxis, phagocytosis and microbial killing are reduced. *Chemotherapeutic agents* induce severe leukopenia and exogenous *corticosteroids* inhibit chemotaxis and phagocytic activity. *Immunosuppressive agents* administered following organ transplantation impair lymphocyte function and immunoglobulin synthesis. Recurrent or frequent infections of the skin or respiratory tract may signify a patient's compromised antimicrobial defenses. This information should be solicited on all patients in an attempt to identify the reason for infection, to determine the need for therapy, to improve the underlying health problems and to treat the infection.

A *physical examination* includes the patient's vital signs: heart rate, blood pressure, temperature and respiratory rate. Prominent among the vital signs is temperature because fever is one of the most consistent signs of systemic infection. Most orofacial infections manifest low grade oral temperatures of less than 102°F, although there is significant interpersonal variation. For example, young patients can exhibit fever with very minor infections, while the elderly may fail to show temperature elevation even with severe infections. A pulse rate of greater than 100 beats per minute (tachycardia) and a rapid respiratory rate (more than 20 breaths/minute = tachypnea) are usually present in serious infections. The pulse rate can increase by 10 beats/minute for each degree (F) of temperature elevation. Although infection does not significantly affect blood pressure, pain and anxiety can elevate both the heart rate and the blood pressure.

The clinical examination should include a careful search for extraoral swelling and erythema, noting the presence of asymmetry and the extent of any swelling. An inspection of the airway and oral cavity is performed by carefully listening to and looking for indications of airway obstruction such as stridor, elevation of the tongue, decrease in pharyngeal diameter, deviation of the uvula and the use of accessory respiratory muscles to breath. Gentle palpation of any intraoral or extraoral swelling can provide information concerning the character and surface temperature which is indicative of the infection's stage. For example, firm (indurated), tender, warm swellings that lack border definition are characteristic of a *cellulitis*, while fluctuant (fluid filled) swellings that are less warm and tender with distinct borders, suggest an *abscess*. The intraoral and extraoral examinations must also include a search for the cause of infection, such as caries, periodontitis, pericoronitis, skin infections, parotitis, etc. Intraoral indicators of an infection's origin include gingival or mucosal swellings, carious teeth, gingival fistulas, dark colored teeth, excessive tooth mobility, suppuration, malodor and sensitive teeth on percussion. ***Regional lymph nodes*** must be palpated to determine the presence of lymphadenopathy. Knowledge of the direction of lymph drainage can also aid in locating areas of infection (Figure 2-12, Table 2-2). During acute infections the draining group of nodes may be enlarged, soft and tender while in chronic infections the enlarged nodes are usually firm and nontender.

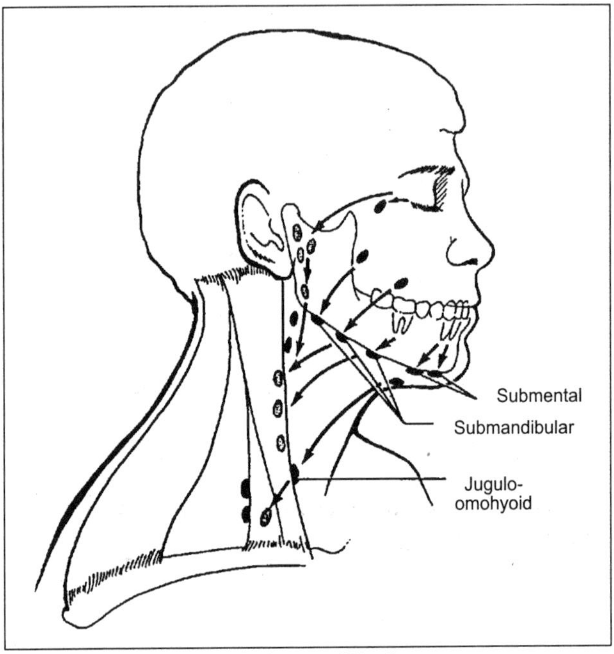

Figure 2-12: Lymphatic drainage of the face.

A. Laboratory Studies

Because most of the bacteria responsible for odontogenic infections have remained predictable and sensitive to available antibiotics for several years, culture and sensitivity testing for routine odontogenic infections is not considered cost effective. Hence, empirically prescribing antibiotics is acceptable unless: 1) clinical symptoms indicate that the infection is unchanged after 48 hours of therapy, 2) the infection is advancing at an alarming rate, 3) the patient's history suggests the host is infection prone, or 4) there is an advancing post operative infection without a history of preoperative infection. This last sequela suggests the presence of a nonindigenous bacterium strain. In addition, careful evaluation of antibiotic coverage is warranted if either osteomyelitis or actinomycosis is suspected.

Table 2-2: Lymph Node Drainage of the Orofacial Area

Responsible Nodes	Site
Anterior auricular (preauricular, parotid)	skin anterior to temple, external meatus, lateral eyelids, lateral forehead, posterior neck, outer ear, parotid gland
Infraorbital	skin of inner corner of eye, skin of anterior face, superficial aspect of nose
Buccal	skin over anterior face, mucous membrane of lips & cheeks, rarely mandibular & maxillary teeth & gingiva
Mandibular	skin over mandible, mucous membrane of lip, cheeks, rarely mandibular & maxillary teeth & gingiva
Submental	tip of tongue, mandibular lip, chin, mandibular incisors & gingiva
Submandibular	maxillary & mandibular teeth & gingiva except mandibular incisors, nasal cavity, palate, tongue body, maxillary lip, lateral mandibular lip, angle of mouth, medial angle of eye
Superficial cervical	pinna & adjacent skin
Deep cervical	submandibular, submental, inferior auricular, tonsillar, tongue nodes

Finally, culture and sensitivity testing is recommended with recurrent infections, because this may indicate a bacterial strain with altered antibiotic sensitivity.

Needle aspiration is the ideal method of specimen collection. This can be accomplished with an 18 gauge needle and a 3cc syringe. Aspiration provides verification of abscess formation, assists in locating the area of suppuration and produces a protected, uncontaminated specimen essential in accurate culturing. The proper preparation of the mucosa or skin is necessary to minimize contamination during the collection of the culture specimen. Repeated irrigation with sterile water or saline is the preferred method since the application of a topical antiseptic can contaminate and destroy bacteria prior to isolation. To aspirate, the needle is inserted into the most fluctuant area, one to 2ml of fluid is removed and the specimen is placed directly into aerobic and anaerobic media. Inserting the needle under negative pressure will maximize the likelihood of a positive result, especially when deep probing of multiple spaces is required. Remember that some infections will not have purulent material to culture (gas producing bacteria); hence, failure to acquire a specimen should not change your diagnosis.

The commercially prepackaged transport systems now available allow protection and easy transportation to a laboratory within a reasonable amount of time. These kits prevent specimen drying, provide nutrients that prevent disproportionate organism growth and protect anaerobic bacteria from oxygen. When the culture media is not available, all air bubbles should be tapped out of the syringe, the needle or syringe stoppered (with cap or wax) and the specimen taken directly to the laboratory for culturing. The culturing of orofacial infections should always include both aerobic and anaerobic testing. The use of swabs to obtain a culture is undesirable because organisms (especially fungi) and cells can become entrapped in the swab's fibers and not transferred to the culture media. Cotton swabs also contain fatty acids that are toxic to many bacteria.

Following a successful aspiration, a ***Gram stain*** can be prepared and immediately reviewed in the office. Gram staining provides the clinician with verification of the specimen's quality, thus identifying a satisfactory culture or the need for a better specimen. An abundance of neutrophils and the absence of squamous cells indicate a pure, uncontaminated exudate. This quick diagnostic procedure provides the clinician with an early impression of the predominant bacterial type. This information can be particularly important while waiting for culture and sensitivity results in a rapidly advancing infection. The steps involved in the preparation of a gram-stained specimen are listed in Table 2-3. *Commercial anaerobic transport kits* are available at a cost of approximately two dollars each and *aerobic kits* cost approximately fifty cents each. Laboratory techniques usually require at least 24 hours to grow aerobic organisms properly and another 24 to 48 hours for a sensitivity evaluation. Anaerobic bacteria require more time; at least 48 hours for growth and possibly up to five days before culture and sensitivity information becomes available. For the

Table 2-3: Gram-Stained direct smear preparation

1. Select flecks of the specimen that contains exudate.
2. Dip the slide in alcohol and wipe clean prior to use.
3. Spread the specimen on the slide as thin as possible.
4. Gently heat the slide over a flame to provide fixation.
5. Flood the specimen with an alcoholic solution of crystal violet for 5 to 10 seconds, rinse briefly with tap water.
6. Flood with iodine and potassium iodide for 5 to 10 seconds to fix the crystal violet to proteins in the bacteria's cell wall.
7. Rinse with tap water.
8. Wash slide briefly with acetone or acetone and alcohol and rinse with water within 2 to 3 seconds of exposure.
9. Counterstain with red dye safranin for 5 to 10 seconds and rinse with water.
10. Blot dry with a paper towel.

To examine a gram stain, **office laboratory equipment** should include a 97-100 X objective microscope (binocular type is not necessary) with illumination for oil immersion and a compound condenser.

identification of fungi, up to six weeks of incubation may be required. Two hours is the maximum allowable elapsed time between collection and microbiologic examination or culturing, irrespective of the technique employed.

The most commonly identified oral bacteria displayed by gram stain are listed in Table 2-4. Gram positive rods are listed last because they are seldom responsible for an oral infection. When reviewing bacteriology laboratory results, consider that one or two colonies of a possible pathogen may be ignored when there is another pathogen present in overwhelming numbers. Also, the identification of more than three isolates in a mixed culture is not usually clinically meaningful or cost effective when attempting to identify the appropriate antibiotic therapy.

Table 2-4: Gram stain organisms

Gram Stain Description	Species	Aerobic/Anaerobic
gram+ cocci, clumps, single	Staphylococcus	A
	Micrococcus	F
	Peptococcus	AN
gram+ cocci, pairs, chains	Streptococcus	F
	Peptostreptococcus	AN
gram- cocci, pairs	Neisseria	AN/F
gram- cocci	Veillonella	AN
large gram- rods	Enterobacteria	A
thin gram- rods	Pseudomonas	A
small gram- rods	Bacteroides	AN
	Fusobacterium	AN
	Haemophilus	A
large gram+ rods	Bacillus	
medium gram+ rods	Clostridium	AN
small gram+ rods	Lactobacillus	AN
	Corynebacterium	AN
	Propionibacterium	AN
small gram+ rods, branching	Actinomyces	AN/F

A = aerobic AN = anaerobic F = facultative

Conventional radiographs are of little value in the evaluation of early orofacial infections for two reasons. First, diagnostic soft tissue radiographs are difficult to obtain because the area must be free of surrounding bone, metal and other high density structures to be beneficial. Secondly, 40 to 60% of alveolar mineral content must be resorbed before bony lesions become radiographically visible; hence, clinical signs of infections are usually present long before infections are radiographically evident. In retropharyngeal space infections, however, a lateral soft tissue radiograph of the neck or a CT scan can be diagnostically beneficial. With these infections a widened retropharyngeal space of greater than 3 to 5mm suggests a compromised airway. Ultrasonography, magnetic resonance imaging, positron emission tomography and three dimension computed tomography are becoming excellent diagnostic tools in evaluating the location and extent of orofacial infections.

Intraoral periapical x-rays are important in helping to identify a dentoalveolar source. When patients are unable to open sufficiently or when the etiology is not apparent through intraoral x-rays, a panoramic radiograph may be helpful. Other extraoral x-rays are seldom of diagnostic benefit in locating dentoalveolar infections unless the involved area is so large that it is already clinically apparent.

VI. THE TREATMENT OF ODONTOGENIC OROFACIAL INFECTIONS

A. Surgical Therapies

The fundamental principles of managing any host infection are to provide *drainage of accumulated suppuration/pus and debris*, and to *remove the etiology*. With odontogenic infections, satisfying the latter principle commonly includes one or some combination of three treatment alternatives. These treatments include the *extirpation or removal of necrotic pulp tissue (root canal therapy)*, *deep periodontal scaling*, or the *extraction of the offending tooth*. When the tooth is beyond restorative capabilities or is nonfunctional, extraction is the most efficient and efficacious therapy. It usually fulfills both primary goals. Although extraction of a tooth is often considered a failure in dental treatment, there are many situations in which this procedure is the best means of preventing serious consequences (i.e., when the host is immunodeficient, or has a healing deficit following one of the aforementioned therapies).

If the swelling does not recede or adequate drainage is not obvious, incision and drainage (I & D) is indicated. I & D is also recommended in space infections and whenever the treatment will accelerate or improve host recovery. The clinician should understand that once an abscess develops, antibiotics and other nonsurgical procedures will not assist in the elimination of the suppuration. Draining the suppuration via extraction, endodontics, deep scaling, or incision are the only procedures that can adequately promote elimination. Among these techniques, only the drainage provided by incision will reliably allow the escape of a large fluid volume. Hence, attempts to drain large single space and multiple space infections via the sulcus or apical foramen are not recommended. Once drainage is established, tissue tension is relieved and the original blood supply returns.

These changes allow the resumption of host cellular defense mechanisms and effective penetration of antibiotics.

The extraction of teeth in the presence of acute infection is questioned by some clinicians, fearing the spread of infection during the manipulation. The majority of recent studies however, suggest that immediate extraction does not cause extension of the infection, and instead, results in fewer postoperative problems. Hence, allowing the etiology to remain while waiting for antibiotic benefit in tissue with a compromised blood supply is unsound. Administering antibiotics just prior to appropriate surgical intervention appears to be the most reasonable approach, especially in space infections and pericoronitis. Maximum blood levels for most antibiotics can be reached within an hour after oral administration and within minutes following an intravenous route. In cases where the etiology can not be removed in the presence of fluctuance (i.e., with severe trismus), I & D should be performed in combination with antibiotic therapy. The source of the infection should then be removed as soon as access allows.

Routine adjunctive therapeutic suggestions include the application of heat, both intra and extraorally, to aid host defenses by dilating small vessels and thereby increasing vascular flow and diffusion. However, there is no evidence that the use of heat can redirect a developing abscess either by intraoral rinsing or with the application of external heat. Because of the discomfort and general malaise associated with infection, adequate fluids and nutritional intake are often lacking. Therefore, postincision instructions should strongly emphasize improving fluid and nutritional intake, postoperative rest and the use of adequate analgesics to insure patient comfort.

B. Intraoral Incision and Drainage

To perform an I & D, a regional local anesthetic block (i.e., an inferior alveolar nerve block for mandibular areas or a posterior superior alveolar block for a maxillary second and third molar abscesses), is the preferred method used to obtain local anesthesia in the area of infection. Injections into the infected tissue are problematic because of the pain involved, the chance of spreading the infection and the fact that the acidic environment (around pH 5.7) will reduce the local anesthetic's effectiveness. Regional anesthesia allows the injection to be as independent of the area of suppuration as possible, although anesthetic infiltration may still be needed anterior and posterior to the abscess.

In the presence of significant trismus, a closed mouth injection technique (i.e., Akinosi) may be required to anesthetize the mandible. This procedure places the anesthetic at the region of the inferior alveolar, lingual and mylohyoid nerves, even with severe trismus. The needle is inserted in the soft tissue overlying the medial border of the mandibular ramus adjacent to the maxillary tuberosity and to the mucogingival junction of the maxillary third molar (Figure 2-13a). The barrel of the syringe is held parallel to the maxillary occlusal plane and the needle is advanced 25 to 30 mm into tissue. The needle tip, upon injection of the local anesthesia, should be lying in the midportion of the pterygomandibular space above the mandibular foramen and proximate to the nerves that exit inferiorly from the foramen ovale (Figure 2-13b).

The tissue nearest the abscess should be anesthetized last to reduce seeding adjacent tissue with offending bacteria. Complete anesthesia is unattainable at times, and in such cases patient sedation or general anesthesia is preferred. When neither of these adjunctive modalities are available, a quick and decisive initial incision is advised. This can be followed by more effective local anesthesia once drainage has commenced.

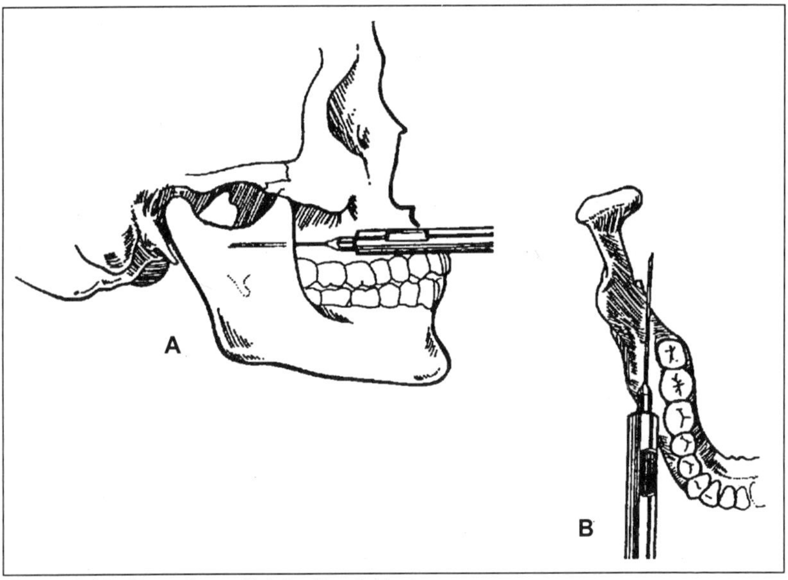

Figure 2-13: Closed mouth injection technique.

Following anesthesia, the I & D site should be selected. The desired site of the ***I and D incision*** is at the most dependent point of the swelling (the area most conducive to drainage with the help of gravity), and is usually no more than 1 cm in length. Incisions at the depth of the vestibule should be avoided if a denture flange will rest on the site. The frequent entrapment of pus under the associated periosteum requires that the depth of the incision extend through the periosteum. Following the initial incision, a small blunt instrument such as a closed hemostat is inserted through

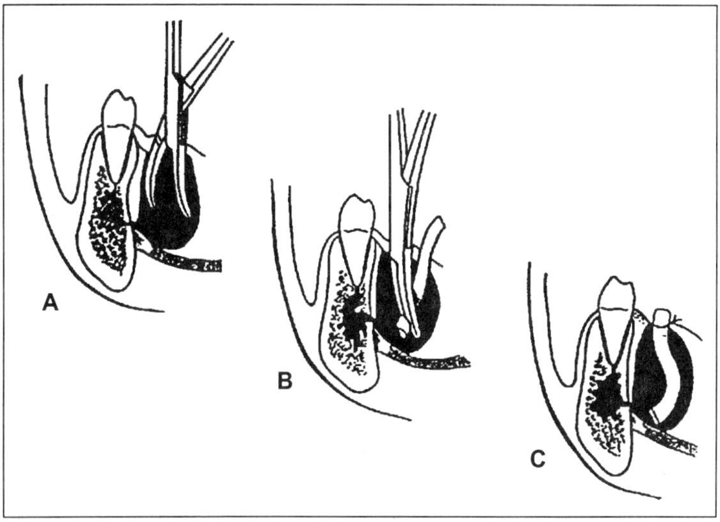

Figure 2-14: Blunt dissection and placement of intraoral drain.

the incision. The hemostat is used to probe for small undrained pockets or cavities of pus by blunt dissecting. This is accomplished by opening the hemostat after each advancement and spreading the tissue (Figure 2-14a). Blunt dissection is used to avoid damage to vital structures, which can occur with blind surgical dissection. Any released pus should be expediently suctioned from the oral cavity to avoid drainage into the patient's throat. Following thorough exploration with the hemostat, ***a drain*** is inserted to the *depth of the abscess* and sutured to the mucosal edge of the incision (Photo 2-6). Drain material is commonly a ¼ inch penrose drain or a sterilized piece of rubber dam. Fenestrated penrose drains are often fabricated by notching with scissors but probably offer little function and provide the possibility of leaving small portions of the drain in the tissue during drain removal. Hemostats may be used to place the drain, which should be accomplished in one motion since subsequent attempts to increase the depth of placement are clumsy (Figure 2-14b). Folding the drain material prior to placement may assist in correctly positioning the conduit on the first attempt. Placing a suture in the end of the drain material prior to placement may also facilitate suturing. Usually a 4-0 silk suture is used to secure the drain to mucosa or skin and thereby prevents exfoliation (Figure 2-14c). The drain should remain *in place until no evidence of exudate* is found around the drain and incision site. However, before removing the drain, an additional 24 to 48 hours is recommended. If pus is not located after an incision and exploration, insertion of a drain is still recommended to maintain an avenue for irrigation and drainage, which will usually prevent subsequent abscess formation in the area. Occasionally, to obtain pain relief and release of suppuration, it may be necessary to drill a small hole through the alveolar plate via the mucosal drainage incision at the level of the infected tooth apex (***Fenestration***). Infrequently, an infected tooth will remain extremely tender after maximum anesthesia injection attempts. Therefore, using a high speed dental drill and light pressure, the dental pulp can be exposed, and either drainage will occur or an inserted sedative or medicament cotton pellet will provide relief.

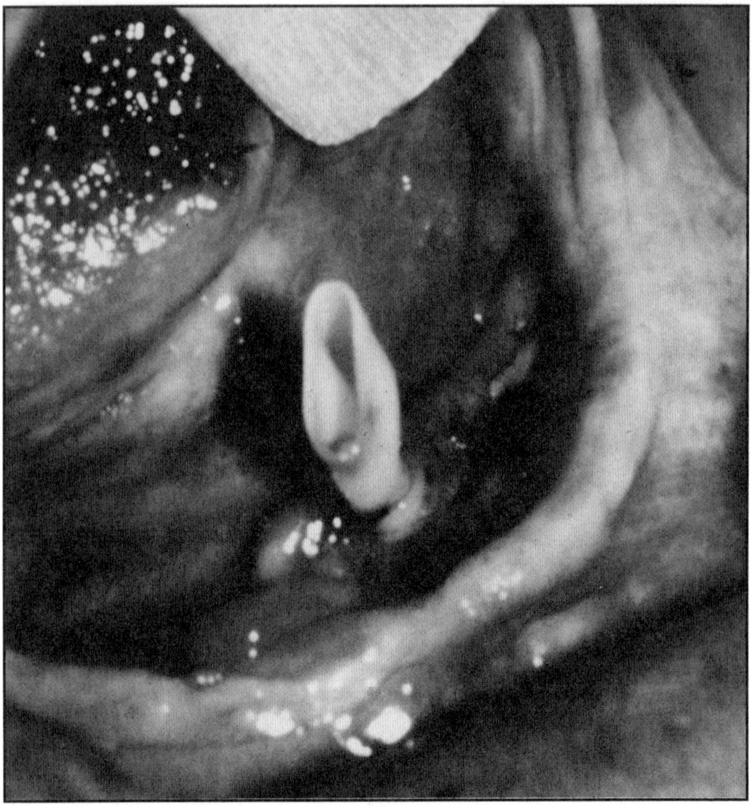

Photo 2-6: Intraoral drain sutured in place.

C. Extraoral Incision and Drainage

The incision and drainage of extraoral abscesses demands more attention be given to dissection technique and to the position of underlying vital structures. An extraoral I & D is indicated whenever an orofacial infection appears to be progressing toward spontaneous external drainage. In such cases the disparity between extraoral and intraoral swelling demands that an extraoral approach be used to provide the most effective management.

Preservation of underlying vital structures and good facial aesthetics will result if routine orofacial surgical principles are practiced.

Once an extraoral approach has been selected, the site of incision is the next concern. The site should be proximate to the area most prone to spontaneous breakdown (greatest erythema and most fluctuant) and in the most dependent portion of the infection. Generally this will place the incision below the inferior border of the mandible and hence, in an esthetically acceptable location. The three typical sites for extraoral I & D are shown (dark broken lines) in Figure 2-15. Dependency is important to facilitate the effect of gravity on drainage. Following site selection the patient should be draped with sterile towels to minimize the soiling of clothes. The skin is then prepped with an appropriate antiseptic solution (iodine or chlorhexidine) to disinfect the skin. The antiseptic solution should be applied in a spiral fashion beginning at the incision site and extending outward. This procedure should be repeated 2 to 3 times using a fresh applicator (gauze) each time.

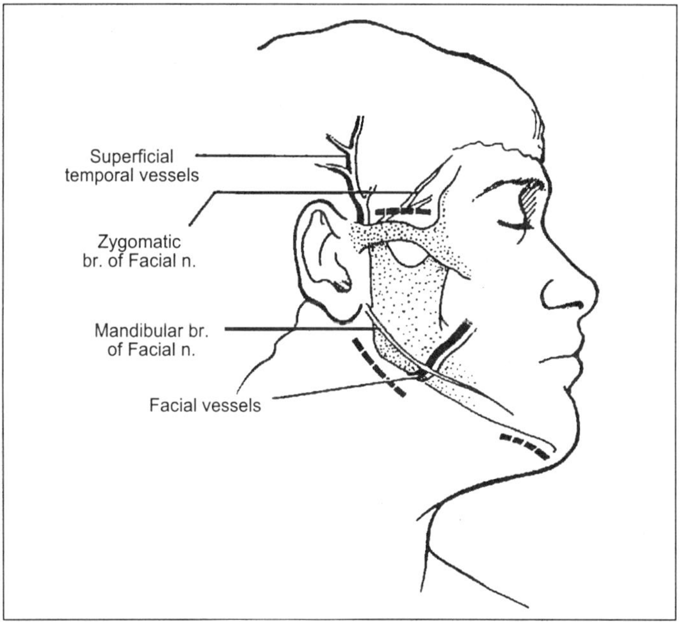

Figure 2-15: Extraoral incision and vital structures.

Local anesthesia is usually provided through regional blocks or by infiltrating around the periphery of the swelling. As with intraoral I and Ds, the resultant local anesthesia may be less than ideal; however, additional

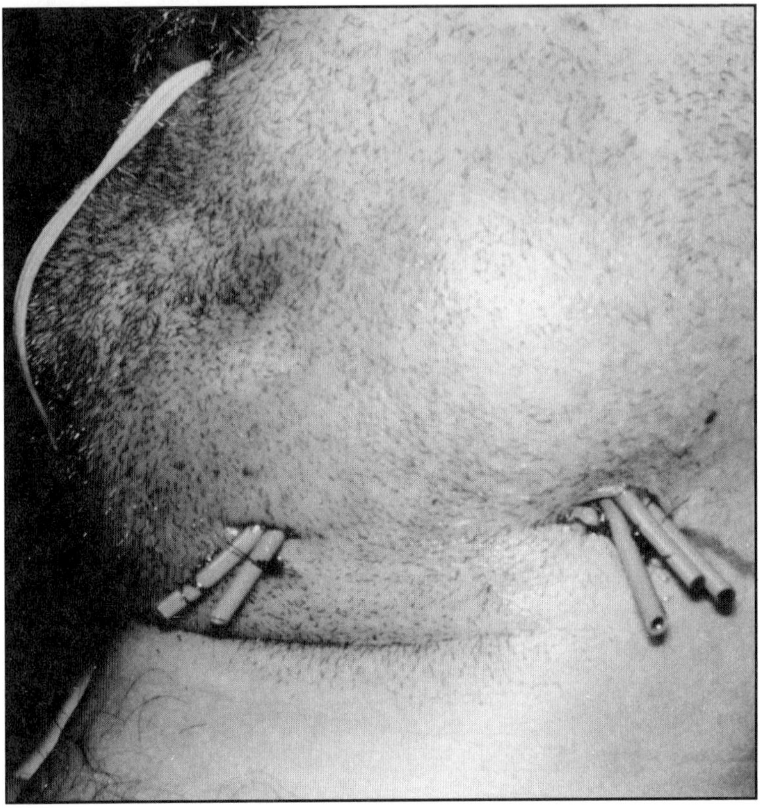

Photo 2-7: Extraoral drains in place.

local anesthesia can be provided following initial perforation of the abscess and prior to exploratory dissection. When possible conscious sedation is desirable to minimize patient discomfort. Preoperative information should be presented in a thorough, compassionate and reassuring manner.

Following local anesthesia, a needle aspiration at the center of the fluctuance can be taken to provide a representative culture specimen. A skin incision is usually made 3 to 5mm inferior to the abscess, and access is gained by subcutaneous blunt dissection using a hemostat. The incision should be approximately 1cm in length and should extend only into the subcutaneous tissue. If through-and-through drainage is desired, the incisions are made superior-inferior or anterior-posterior to the abscess and blunt dissection is carried from one incision site to the other. Because the bulk of the dissection is blunt, the risk of injury to underlying vital structures is minimal. The beak of the hemostat should never be completely closed while dissecting, and whenever possible the blunt dissection should be parallel to any vital structures in the area. Suction and an emesis basin should be positioned to collect the draining fluid. If the skin incision is made directly into the abscess through tense, vascularly compromised skin, post operative sloughing and more extensive scar formation are likely.

Culturing and exploration are performed in a fashion similar to the intraoral technique and are followed by thorough irrigation of the spaces with sterile saline. The drain is prepared, placed through the incision and sutured to the skin in a manner similar to that described for intraoral I & Ds. With through-and-through incisions, the drain extends from one incision to the other. Both ends of the drain may be sutured together or small safety pins can prevent extrusion. If vital structures are not near the incision site, noncollapsible drains such as the red Robinson catheter or the Jackson-Pratt drain are preferred for extraoral I & D's. Both methods offer additional patency for drainage and open avenues for irrigation (Photo 2-7). Irrigation through these drains should be accomplished several times daily until the drains are removed. A bandage to collect the drainage and prevent contamination of surrounding areas should be placed over the drain and incision site; sterile gauze and surgical tape are well suited for this purpose. Identification and removal of the etiology, odontogenic or otherwise, should be completed at the first opportunity.

Antibiotics are recommended with all fascial space infections and extraoral I & D's (see Tables 2-5, 2-6). The same criteria for determining the time to remove intraoral drains can be applied to extraoral drains. Generally patients are evaluated every 24 hours until no evidence of exudate is present. At each exam practitioners may wish to irrigate through the drain. After one to two days of no exudate, the drain is removed. For deep wounds with long drains, gradual removal of the drain (a few centimeters each day), will allow the preferred depth-to-skin closure. Remember that a drain is a foreign body and the tissue around the drain can become fibrosed over time; this reaction should not be confused with advancing infection. Once the drain is removed, this induration will gradually resolve. Sutures are not needed over the incision unless apposition of the flaps is poor.

Table 2-5: Indications for antibiotic therapy in orofacial infections

- cellulitis with signs of systemic involvement*
- persistent infection despite drainage/debridement of the etiology
- acute pericoronitis⁺
- fascial space infections
- infection or surgery in certain medically compromised patients (immunosuppressed patients or patients with poor healing capacity)
- osteomyelitis/actinomycosis

*A rapidly progressing cellulitis, with no evidence of containment, indicates that the patient's host defenses are not providing adequate containment.

⁺Acute pericoronitis refers to the infection of an erupting molar associated with a fever, trismus, and extraoral swelling.

Table 2-6: Common Antibiotics

drug	cidal/static	spectrum	infection severity	major side effects	average dosage	acquisition cost per day*
Penicillins						
Penicillin V (phenoxymethyl)	-cidal	Gr+, some Gr- aerobes, most anaerobes	mild	allergy	250-500mg q6h PO	$(.15) / 250mg $(.35).80 / 500mg
Aqueous crystalline Pen G	-cidal	Gr+, most Gr- aerobes, anaerobes	mod/severe	allergy	600,000 units to 5 mil units q 4h IV	$19.25 / 5mu
Pen G procaine	-cidal	same as aqueous Pen	mild/mod	allergy	600,000 units to 1.2 mil IM	$3.00 / 1.2mu
Pen G benzathine	-cidal	same as aqueous Pen	mild/mod	allergy	1.2 mil IM	$8.00 \ 1.2mu
Amoxicillin	-cidal	most Gr+, most Gr- aerobes	mild/mod	GI, rash	250-500mg q6h PO	$(.50).75 / 250mg $(.80) 1.25 / 500mg
Erythromycin	-static	Gram+ cocci	mild	nausea cramping diarrhea	500mg q6h PO	$(.50)1.80
Clindamycin	-static -cidal @ high doses	Gram+ cocci anaerobes	mod/severe	diarrhea colitis	150-300mg q6h PO 600mg q8h IV	$3.00 / 150mg $5.00 / 300mg $35.00
Cephalosporins						
Cephalexin (Keflex) (1st generation)	-cidal	Gr+ some Gr- aerobes	mod/severe	allergy	250-500mg q6h PO	$(1.04)3.50 / 250mg $(3.50)7.00 / 500mg
Cefazolin(Ancef) (1st generation)	-cidal	Gr+ some Gr- aerobes	mod/severe	allergy	1gm q6h IV	$15.00
Cefaclor(Ceclor) (2nd generation)	-cidal	Gr+ most Gr- aerobes, anaerobes	mild	allergy	250-500mg q8h PO	$4.50 / 250mg $6.50 / 500mg
Metronidazole (Flagyl)(usually w/pen)	-cidal	anaerobes only	mild/mod severe	nausea	500mg tid PO 500mg q6h IV	$(.75)4.95 $(25.00)45.0
Timentin (Ticarcillin) (clavulanate)	-cidal	most Gr+, most Gr- aerobes, most anaerobes b-lactamase resistant	severe	GI, rash	3.1gm q6-8h IV	$30-40
Augmentin (Amoxicillin) (clavulanate)	-cidal	similar to Timentin	moderate	GI, rash	250-500 q8h PO	$3.00 / 250mg $5.00 / 500mg

*Professional fee of approximately $3.50 should be added to each prescription. Cost to patient can vary 50% higher. Generic prices are in parenthesis.

*Hospital costs of parenteral drugs vary greatly; added costs of preparation, etc. can increase patient cost > 100%

D. Antibiotic Therapy

A misconception, shared particularly by the public, is that an antibiotic is always required in the treatment of an infection. Antibiotics assist in the isolation and destruction of bacteria, but it is the individual's antimicrobial defenses that ultimately eradicate the infection, not the antibiotics. Antibiotics also do not improve healing or reduce pain. A healthy individual (immunocompetent with normal healing) with an orofacial infection that is well localized, non-spreading and without multiple space or systemic involvement (fever, lymphadenopathy or malaise) requires drainage of the abscess, removal of the etiology, routine post operative care and close observation. Antibiotics provide little additional benefit in the localized abscess. The indications for using antibiotics in oral and facial infections are listed in Table 2-5.

Fortunately, the organisms responsible for most odontogenic infections are highly predictable. Despite a gradual increase in the number of orofacial penicillin resistant organisms appearing, there is presently no indication that the usual regimen requires modification. Hence, in the presence of a typical orofacial infection, empirical antibiotic therapy can be initiated with confidence. If the infection is *not responding to the initial antibiotic* after 48 hours, attempts to identify the responsible organisms and their sensitivity to antibiotics through gram staining and culturing should be initiated. It is important to remember that the success of antibiotic therapy does not depend on the drug's effectiveness against *all* organisms present, but relies on the successful elimination of the predominant pathogen. Also, the appearance of fluctuance and suppuration following a period of antibiotic therapy is not a sign of drug ineffectiveness, but an indication that the antibiotic has effectively aided the host in the resolution or isolation of the infection. The organisms normally responsible for orofacial infections (Table 2-1) have remained remarkably consistent and susceptible to a small number of antibiotics that include penicillin, erythromycin, clindamycin, cephalexin, cefaclor, metronidazole and tetracycline.

When selecting an appropriate antibiotic, there are several considerations, in addition to the sensitivity factor:

1. Antibiotic selection should be as specific as possible against the causative organisms. Penicillin, for instance, has a ***narrow antibacterial spectrum*** that is well-matched to common aerobic and anaerobic oral pathogens. In addition, penicillin does not alter the remaining oral flora and thereby maintains the highly important, normal synergistic oral environment. In contrast, a broader spectrum antibiotic, such as tetracycline, kills many nonpathogenic oral and skin flora while attempting to destroy the causative bacteria. This side effect can lead to the development of resistant organisms

and superinfections. Penicillinase resistant and beta-lactamase-producing organisms are infrequently isolated in odontogenic infections but are a growing concern. Fortunately, these organisms remain sensitive to antibiotics such as dicloxacillin and clavulanic acid combinations.

2. A second principle involves selecting an antibiotic with ***few side effects*** and ***low toxicity***. Fortunately, toxicity is not a prominent issue with the antibiotics normally prescribed for orofacial infections, assuming the antibiotics are prescribed in the recommended doses. *Nausea* and *mild abdominal cramping* may be seen at times with most oral antibiotics; however, these side-effects are most common with erythromycin and are less frequent with clindamycin and metronidazole. Prescribing enteric coated tablets or ingesting the medication with food can minimize this problem. Penicillin has remarkably few side effects, while the broader spectrum antibiotics are associated with more serious problems. With prolonged use clindamycin, ampicillin, cephalexin and cefaclor have been reported to eliminate so much anaerobic gut flora that an overgrowth of antibiotic-resistant bacteria, *Clostridia sp.,* develops. This organism can damage the gut wall causing *serious diarrhea* and *colitis*. Patients taking these drugs should be aware of this possibility and instructed to contact the practitioner immediately should diarrhea appear. These side-effects are unlikely with the short-term therapy that characterizes the treatment of orofacial infections.

3. ***Allergic reactions*** should always be verbally reviewed with the patient before any prescription is written. Even with its many years of use, penicillin still has a remarkably low incidence of allergic reactions (1 to 10%). Most reported reactions following oral intake are minor symptoms of hives and itching. The reported incidence of serious anaphylactic reactions is between 0.015 and 0.04%, with the majority following parenteral administration. In moderate to severe orofacial infections, cephalosporins and metronidazole have been recommended as substitutes for patients with penicillin hypersensitivity. There is a reported hypersensitive cross-reactivity incidence between cephalosporins and penicillin of 3 to 12%. Therefore, a suggested approach in administering a cephalosporin to a penicillin-allergic patient is to base the administration on the severity of the allergic reaction. If the allergic manifestations remain localized (limited to the skin) and not life threatening, cephalosporins may be prescribed after detailed patient instructions. If anaphylactic-like reactions to penicillin have occurred, cephalosporins should be avoided.

The interaction between certain antibiotics and ***birth control pills*** should be discussed with women of child bearing age. *Penicillin*, *ampicillin*, *amoxicillin*, *cephalexin*, the *tetracyclines* and *erythromycin* have been implicated in hepatic and intestinal systemic effects. This complication lowers plasma estrogen levels and renders women fertile during the time of antibiotic administration.

4. ***Bactericidal*** antibiotics interfere with young bacteria cell wall production allowing cell rupture from unequal osmotic pressures. The bactericidal antibiotic plays an active role in the bacterial destruction, leaving host defense mechanisms to perform a more passive, debridement role. In contrast, ***bacteriostatic*** antibiotics slow the reproduction and growth of the organism but depend on host defense mechanisms to migrate, phagocytize and destroy the bacteria. Therefore, when host defenses are compromised, bactericidal antibiotics offer much more effective therapy. A summary of the common oral and parenteral antibiotics prescribed for orofacial infections is listed in Table 2-6.

Penicillin continues to be the antibiotic of choice for routine orofacial infections. It is the least expensive and has the narrowest spectrum, yet it is effective against the predominant oral pathogens. In addition, the drug is bactericidal, the least toxic and has performed well over many years. A patient history of ***penicillin allergy*** commonly leads to the use of one of four antibiotics, each with particular disadvantages. *Erythromycin* effects a spectrum similar to penicillin but is only moderately effective against anaerobes. It is bacteriostatic with absorption as its major problem, although improved brands are becoming available. *Metronidazole* is only effective against strict anaerobes. *Cephalosporins* have a broader spectrum than penicillin and a hypersensitivity cross-reactivity incidence of 3 to 12%, as mentioned earlier. *Clindamycin* has an 8% average incidence of diarrhea in addition to cases of life threatening pseudomembranous colitis (6 deaths in the early 1970's). The incidence of colitis has declined substantially with increased clinician awareness and a successful treatment regimen (which includes vancomycin). Irrespective of these problems, if the infection does not respond to penicillin and culture and sensitivity test results are not available, one of these antibiotics is usually selected to replace penicillin or is added to the regimen.

The major goal of antibiotic therapy is to provide adequate blood levels to destroy the bacteria without harming the patient. Laboratory data have provided clinicians with recommendations concerning the *appropriate dosages* and *proper administration intervals* to achieve successful outcomes. For example, minimum inhibitory concentration analysis (MIC: the lowest concentration needed to inhibit microorganism growth) has shown that the dose needed for maximally effective ***therapeutic antibiotic plasma levels*** must be in the range of four to five times the MIC. With the commonly used antibiotics for orofacial infections, low toxicity related to effective therapeutic levels is normally a minor concern. It is extremely important that medications be administered frequently enough to maintain adequate plasma levels and prevent subtherapeutic treatment. ***Subtherapeutic drug levels*** can mask infection, suppress clinical manifestations, encourage resistant strains and lead to recurrent infections. Recommendations concerning antibiotic ***administration intervals*** relate to the plasma half-life of the drug (the plasma half-life is the period over which 50% of the absorbed dose is excreted). The administration interval normally needed to maintain adequate sustained blood levels is four times the plasma half-life of the drug. For example, penicillin V with a half life of 1 hour would then require a dosing every four hours. However, for some antibiotics such as penicillin, their relative nontoxicity can be used to advantage and the dosage placed much higher than therapeutic requirements. This allows a more convenient, extended dosing interval, six hours in the case of penicillin V.

Maintaining proper dosage intervals to carry adequate blood levels over the full 24 hours is important to prevent periods of subtherapeutic levels, which usually occur at night. QID instructions can lead to 8 to 10 night hours without dosing. It is particularly important that bacteriostatic drugs be taken at the recommended intervals because the bacteria can resume a normal growth rate as soon as the antibiotic is absent in the tissues. For bactericidal agents, this nocturnal delay in drug administration is less damaging. Oral administration is adequate for most routine dental infections, and taking the medication in the fasting state (½ hour before or 2 hours after a meal) assures maximum absorption. However, when managing an uncontrolled infection, higher antibiotic blood levels are required for more extended periods of time to obtain maximum tissue penetration and bacterial destruction. Intravenous delivery is preferred over intramuscular because it is less painful and provides quicker and higher blood levels. For the uncooperative or noncompliant outpatient, a deep, intramuscular injection of ***penicillin G benzathine*** can provide an average duration of detectable antimicrobial plasma activity for at least 14 days.

Rarely will the reversal or resolution of an infection be noticeable in the first 24 hours following antibiotic administration unless surgical drainage is included. Hence, a perceived antibiotic effect is not likely for 48 hours. However, after 24 hours of antibiotic therapy, there should be evidence that progression of the infection has been interrupted, even though resolution is not yet evident. Close interval and proper timing of patient follow-up is critical. If initial signs of resolution are not evident after 48 hours of antibiotic therapy, reasons for the lack of progress should be sought. Potential causes include failure to provide complete drainage, presence of a foreign body, an underlying systemic disease that is compromising host defenses, inadequate antibiotic dosing, inappropriate antibiotic selection, resistant organisms, viral involvement, laboratory error, noncompliance or failure to remove the etiology. When patient response is poor, the decision to change antibiotics should be guided by culture and sensitivity results. If this information is not available, agents that are effective against anaerobic organisms such as clindamycin, metronidazole, timentin and augmentin should be considered. The rationale for this direction is the predominance of anaerobes in late orofacial infections, hence, the need for the antibiotic most effective against anaerobes. These agents may be given in addition to or in place of the initial antibiotic (i.e., metronidazole plus or minus penicillin). The discontinuation of an antibiotic should be tailored to each individual's rate of recovery. Oral antibiotics should be continued for 2 to 3 days after the dissipation of fever, exudate and severe pain.

E. Indications for Referral and Hospitalization

Careful examination and accurate clinical judgement are essential in the initial treatment of any infection. The early recognition of developing fascial space infection is critical because aggressive infections can become life-threatening in a matter of hours. The patient exhibiting signs of a swiftly progressing cellulitis that is either beyond initial therapies or has failed to respond normally should be referred to a practitioner who can provide aggressive treatment in a hospital setting. Such treatment includes *parenteral administration of high dose antibiotics* and *steroids*, *hydration*, *close patient monitoring*, and *early*, *extensive surgical exploration* and *drainage*.

There are several clinical findings signaling the need for aggressive treatment; however, these signs are frequently not recognized until airway compromise and the need for emergency intubation or tracheotomy is present. A suggested rule of thumb is that the patient should be referred the moment the clinician questions the efficacy of the oral antibiotic in resolving of the cellulitis, or realizes that an airway problem may be developing. A combination of signs, symptoms, laboratory findings and associated problems listed in Table 2-7 indicate the need for patient referral.

Table 2-7: Signs and Symptoms of Orofacial Infections suggesting the need for Patient Hospitalization

- dehydration, malaise, chills, marked pain
- oral temperature > 101° F, WBC > 10,000
- compromised host: diabetes mellitus, immunosuppressive drugs
- *dyspnea, *dysphagia, *severe jaw trismus,
- rapidly spreading swelling
- lateral deviation of the uvula
- elevation of the tongue
- Ludwig's Angina
- extensive multiple space infection
- swelling into the neck, soft palate, lateral pharyngeal wall, or around the eyes (periocular)

With the exception of the first three lines of clinical findings, the remaining indicators are of such magnitude that if any one is diagnosed, immediate referral and probable hospitalization is necessary.

*With dyspnea and dysphagia, the patient may be unable to lie down, will have difficulty talking, and will display moderate to severe trismus. Severe trismus is considered to be a central interincisal opening of less than a 10 mm.

F. Treating a Major Infection

Following hospital admission, intravenous fluids, appropriate intravenous antibiotics and often intravenous steroids are administered to restore fluid volume and to supplement host factors that are either compromised or have been overwhelmed by the infection. A typical admitting regimen for a rapidly progressing infection may include the intravenous administration of either 2 million units of aqueous penicillin every 4 to 6 hours, 1 gram of cefazolin every 6 to 8 hours or 3.1 grams of ticarcillin clavulanate every 6 hours. If early surgical intervention is required to prevent airway compromise, 10 to 15mg of intravenous dexamethasone may also be administered. Intravenous antibiotics are usually continued until resolution of the infection is well under way and the patient has remained afebrile for 24 hours. Oral antibiotics are then prescribed and continued for several days following hospital discharge. Throughout the hospitalization, a thorough search for fluctuance/suppuration is routinely performed and airway patency is regularly assessed. If pus is located with palpation or needle aspiration, prompt incision and drainage is recommended. When the airway is restricted, intubation and/or tracheostomy may be necessary in addition to appropriate I & D. General anesthesia is most often used when the fascial spaces are explored and drained, although intubation is at times very difficult and dangerous. The potential for the aspiration of pus secondary to the perforation of an infected, bulging lateral pharyngeal or retropharyngeal space is a major concern. Hospitalization should continue until the majority of swelling and all danger of airway compromise has resolved, the patient has remained afebrile for 24 hours, and oral intake, hydration, and electrolytes are within normal limits.

VII. PEDIATRIC CONSIDERATIONS

The diagnosis and management of orofacial infections in children is very similar to the measures previously described for adult infections with the following exceptions:

1. The signs and symptoms of infection in children are more pronounced and tend to progress and resolve more rapidly. Normal body temperatures in children normally run ½ to 1 degree higher than in adults, and subsequent fevers are typically greater. As such, antipyretics and cooling techniques are more often necessary in children to prevent the febrile convulsions that often occur with temperatures greater than 104°F. Submandibular and cervical lymphadenopathy in children can also present in a much more alarming fashion. With pyogenic infections, lymph nodes often become large, warm, tender and even fluctuant. Should the nodes not regress once the infection has cleared, referral for possible biopsy is indicated. Children also tend to become dehydrated much quicker than adults. Hospitalization for rehydration may be required at an early stage of an infection.
2. Skin fistula formation from dental infections is more common in children.
3. The white cell blood count is more elevated in children, usually with a higher percentage of lymphocytes and monocytes than found in adults.
4. Children's blood pressures usually run 15 to 30 mm Hg lower than adults. The average blood pressures range from $^{90}/_{60}$ for 3 to 9 year old children to $^{106}/_{65}$ for teenagers.
5. Dentoalveolar abscesses may damage developing teeth, resulting in hypoplasia or delayed eruption.
6. Bone infections in children seem to spread more rapidly, possibly secondary to wider marrow spaces. Osteomyelitis and condylar growth problems are also more frequent complications in children.
7. The use of tetracycline causes discoloration (intrinsic staining) in developing teeth and should be avoided in children.

VIII. LESS COMMON OROFACIAL INFECTIONS

A. Osteomyelitis

Osteomyelitis is an inflammation of bone caused by pyogenic organisms. Osteomyelitis of the jaw commonly begins with bacterial invasion of the marrow from odontogenic or periodontal infections or from an untreated jaw fracture. The inflammation and edema compromise the microcirculation, leading to ischemia, loss of nutrients and oxygen. These changes retard resorptive and lytic host mechanisms, preventing the removal of necrotic bone and promoting the formation of sequestrum. Osteomyelitis is almost exclusively a mandibular disease because the maxilla has a more abundant blood supply.

Osteomyelitis is classified according to its clinical presentation. ***Acute suppurative osteomyelitis*** (ASO) appears shortly after a predisposing infection. It presents as deep, severe pain and tenderness of the jaw with swelling, occasional fever and malaise. The appearance of ***chronic suppurative osteomyelitis*** (CSO) does not appear for several weeks following a local infection. It is commonly characterized by loose, tender teeth associated with either a purulent, sulcular exudate or a cutaneous fistula. In addition, a fever may not be present with CSO. The primary bacteria responsible for both acute and chronic suppurative osteomyelitis are the *anaerobic cocci, gram-negative rods, streptococci* and *staphylococci* found in normal oral flora. Patients with mandibular osteomyelitis usually have compromised host defense mechanisms or a healing deficiency. *Alcoholism malnutrition syndrome*, *diabetes mellitus*, *IV drug abuse*, *myeloproliferative diseases*, *corticosteroid therapy*, *osteopetrosis*, *Paget's disease*, *chemotherapy*, and mandibular *irradiation* are examples of host conditions commonly associated with osteomyelitis. A thorough medical history and physical examination should be pursued if osteomyelitis is diagnosed in a patient without a history of such predisposing factors. Radiographs are of little value with ASO because the clinical signs and symptoms appear much sooner than radiographic changes. However, radiographs can reveal the classic patchy, moth-eaten, islands of bony sequestra associated with CSO.

The ***treatment*** for osteomyelitis is comprised of high dose antibiotics and the removal of the etiology, including wires, loose teeth and any bony sequestra. Intravenous *penicillin* is the antibiotic of choice with *clindamycin* as an alternative. If culture and sensitivity reveals an organism with penicillinase properties, appropriate penicillinase-resistant or b-lactamase-inhibitor drugs should be prescribed. Intravenous antibiotics are administered for one to two weeks, followed by at least 4 weeks of oral antibiotics for ASO and up to 6 months for CSO. In addition, areas of necrotic soft tissue and bone must be debrided (sequestrectomy) in CSO. This is usually accomplished by removing (decortication and saucerization) bone until areas of normal bleeding are revealed. Despite meticulous debridement and irrigation, parenteral antibiotics, sequestrectomy and supportive care, osteomyelitis can persist. It may require repeat therapies, hyperbaric oxygen and/or radical surgical resection to cure.

B. Actinomycosis

Actinomycosis is an infrequent infection of the oral tissues that was once thought to be a fungus, but has since been identified as an *anaerobic* bacteria (usually *Actinomyces israelii*, and infrequently, *A. naeslundii,* or *A.viscosus).* Because of low virulence, the organism must be introduced through a recent tooth extraction socket, a severely carious tooth, or the site of minor oral trauma to become a causative agent. Once established, the infection gradually develops in the soft tissue and spreads by burrowing through tissue planes, rather than between them, as is characteristic of other orofacial infections. ***Clinically***, a tumorlike soft tissue mass near the jaw may be seen, which slowly enlarges until it ruptures through the skin forming multiple sinus tracts. The exudate from the tracts classically contain "sulfur granules", which are a collection of bacterial microcolonies that exhibit clusters of gram-positive branching rods on direct smear. Following culture, actinomyces must be incubated for 4 to 6 days in a strict anaerobic environment for definitive identification. However, since 50% of all actinomyces infections will not grow when cultured, the recurrence of actinomyces is common because antibiotic therapy is often discontinued following a false negative culture. Hence, repeat culturing is important when actinomycosis is suspected. Bony involvement can be extensive as granulomatous tissue gradually replaces the adjacent osseous tissue. ***Treatment*** of actinomycosis includes intravenous antibiotics accompanied by surgical incision and drainage, and excision of all sinus tracts. The antibiotic of choice is intravenous *penicillin*, in doses of up to 10 million units per day for serious infections. This dosage is continued until clinical resolution is observed. Then oral penicillin is prescribed for at least 3 months to prevent recurrence. Tetracycline is the antibiotic alternative.

C. Peritonsillar Abscess

The peritonsillar abscess (PTA) is primarily a disease of young adults, with an average patient age of 22 years. The primary ***causative organism*** appears to be Streptococcus which grows in the crypts (the slit-like cavities) of the tonsillar fossa and then spreads into the peritonsillar space. This space is located between the tonsillar capsule and the fascia of the superior constrictor muscle (Figure 2-16b). Infection of the peritonsillar space often occurs during the course of acute tonsillitis in spite of antibiotic therapy. Clinically PTA usually begins with a sore throat that progresses into a very painful, unilateral tonsillar swelling. Deviation of the palate and uvula, trismus, and tonsillar exudate are common findings. Fever greater than 100°F is rare; unlike acute tonsillitis, which is frequently associated with temperatures greater than 102°F. As purulent accumulation increases, pain can become extreme, causing drooling, difficulty in swallowing, and increased trismus. As with most respiratory infections, PTA's usually occur between October and February. ***Major complications*** are rare but include rupture of the abscess and aspiration, thrombophlebitis of the large neck veins, and spread of the infection into the parapharyngeal spaces. When spontaneous drainage occurs, it is usually from the superior portion of the anterior pillar area.

A PTA usually contains mixed flora, predominately streptococci with Bacteroides and staphylococci occurring less frequently. Anaerobes are present in almost all PTA infections, with ß-lactamase-producing organisms most frequently identified. ***Treatment*** includes a combination of antibiotic therapy and I & D. Oral *penicillin* (1 gram daily) remains the antibiotic of choice, with *clindamycin*, *erythromycin* and *cephalexin* as alternatives. An amoxicillin-clavulonate acid combination is prescribed if ß-lactamase-producing bacteria are suspected or identified. Intravenous antibiotics given just prior to surgical drainage or intramuscular injection of penicillin G procaine is recommended by some clinicians. Current surgical treatment includes either transoral incision and drainage of the abscess or aspiration with a 16 or 18 gauge needle. Both techniques can be performed under local anesthesia and offer rapid relief of symptoms. However, because patient discomfort is commonly associated with these procedures, even with local anesthesia, pharmacosedation should be considered. General anesthesia is also an alternative, but the danger of abscess rupture and subsequent aspiration during intubation limits its use. Most peritonsillar abscesses are under so much tension at time of surgery that there is a sudden, and often dramatic, release of pus upon initial perforation of the swelling with either a needle or a scalpel. As such, it is essential to have *good operator vision* and a *strategically placed suction* before attempting the drainage. This will greatly reduce the possibility of aspirating the purulent material. Proponents of needle aspiration emphasize the advantages of a low incidence of tracheal aspiration, limited instrumentation requirements, improved specimen collection, and less intraoperative and postoperative pain. Recurrence and recovery time for both techniques appear similar.

The surgical drainage technique begins by applying a topical anesthesia and injecting a local anesthetic into the overlying mucosa and around the periphery of the abscess. Suction should be available for any exudate that may occur following the local injection. A curvilinear incision or needle aspiration is then made lateral to the superior tonsillar pole or at a point of obvious fluctuation (Figure 2-16a). Following the immediate release of pus, a hemostat is extended through the incision into distant areas of the abscess to disrupt any loculations. When needle aspiration is intended, three points of aspiration are suggested (solid dots in Figure 2-16b). Postoperative care includes analgesics, a ten day course of oral penicillin(2 grams daily) or an appropriate substitute (cephalexin or erythromycin), bed rest, hydration, hot intraoral rinses every hour and external heat. Hospitalization is indicated in cases of advanced trismus, dehydration, inability to swallow, significant pharyngeal obstruction, and when close patient monitoring is needed for bleeding or the reaccumulation of suppuration. The average period until patients are eating comfortably is 3.7 days following drainage and the reported recurrence rate is less than 10 percent.

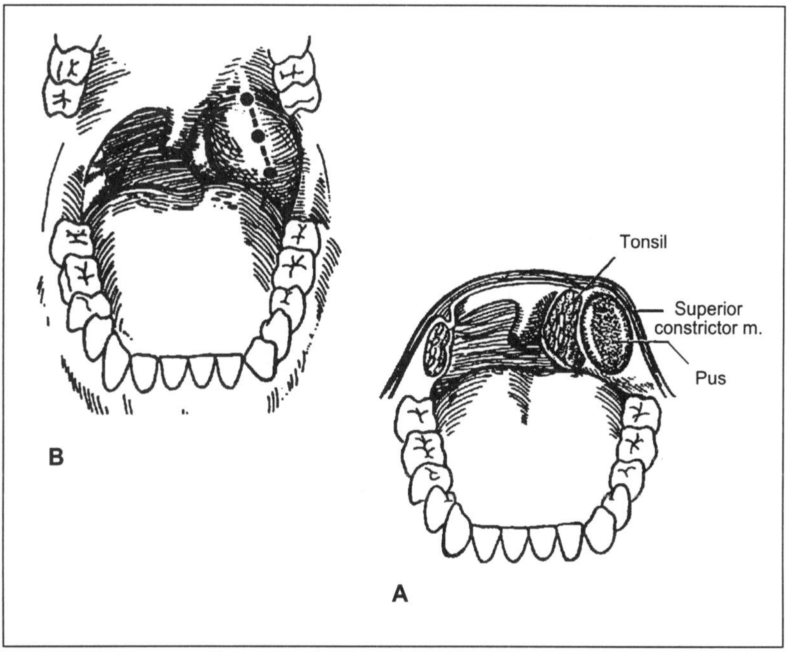

Figure 2-16: Peritonsillar abscess and surgical treatment.

IX. SALIVARY GLAND INFECTIONS

Infections of the major salivary glands are generally classified as acute or chronic, bacterial or viral, and obstructive or nonobstructive. Responsible organisms include aerobic and anaerobic bacteria, viruses, fungi and mycobacteria. The ***most common bacteria*** associated with salivary gland infections is *Staphylococcus aureus*, but opportunistic and gram-negative organisms have also been implicated, including *Bacteroides melaninogenicus*, Peptostreptococcus, Klebsiella, Proteus, diphtheroids, *E. Coli* and *H. influenzae*. The majority of bacterial salivary gland infections follow obstructive disorders such as sialolithiasis (salivary stones), mucous plugs or strictures. Other causes of bacterial infections include facial trauma, recent surgery, and the use of various drugs such as antisialogogues, chemotherapeutic agents, antibiotics, diuretics, antihistamines, tranquilizers, and anticholinergic agents.

Indications of bacterial salivary gland infections include the rapid onset of *swelling*, *tenderness*, and *erythema* in a major gland, concurrent with *facial pain* and *fever*. Acute swelling of a salivary gland at meal time that spontaneously recedes suggests a ductal obstruction is present.

Oral examinations should include bimanual palpation of the glands, ducts and ductal orifices, searching for stones, areas of inflammation, purulence, and the absence of salivary flow from duct orifices. Radiographs or sialography are recommended for the detection of strictures, foreign bodies, sialoliths, and parenchymal damage. However, sialography should not be attempted during acute infections since it is likely to increase symptoms. A history of allergy to contrast media or iodine compounds is a contraindication for sialography. Sialography has the therapeutic potential to dislodge mucus plugs and to destroy bacteria via the dye's bacteriostatic properties. Likewise, ductal probing with lacrimal probes can be helpful both diagnostically and therapeutically by revealing ductal stones, dislodging mucous plugs and dilating ductal strictures.

Antimicrobial therapy should be based on sensitivity and Gram stain studies completed on ductal exudate. Because *staphylococci* are the most common causative organisms, empirical antibiotic therapy should include a semisynthetic penicillin such as oxacillin, or a cephalosporin in the presence of mild penicillin hypersensitivity. Hospitalization, rehydration, and high doses of intravenous antibiotics are the usual routine for the seriously ill patient. Culture and sensitivity, as well as close observation of the progress, will dictate any necessary changes in therapy. Incision and drainage is infrequently required unless a mounting fever, rising white cell count, and rapid deterioration are evident.

Acute bacterial infections of the parotid gland, known as ***suppurative parotitis*** or ***surgical mumps***, occur primarily in the elderly, the malnourished, the chronically ill, the dehydrated, or in surgical patients. These patients are prone to acute bacterial infections secondary to diminished salivary flow that leads to stagnation and subsequent salivary gland infection. ***Chronic bacterial parotitis*** is characterized by intermittent swellings of the parotid gland lasting for days to months, interspersed with remissive periods. Cultures usually reveal *streptococci* or *mixed streptococcal-staphylococcal* organisms. Initial conservative therapy includes systemic antibiotics, ductal irrigation with antibiotics and "therapeutic" sialography. Long-term chronic parotitis often requires removal of the gland.

Viral parotitis, or *mumps*, is an acute and communicable disease. It appears as preauricular pain, fever, chills and headache, followed by rapid, painful swelling of one or both parotid glands. Complications include pancreatitis, orchitis (in approximately 20% of young men which can lead to sterility) and rarely meningoencephalitis. Mumps resolves in five to twelve days. Therapy consists of relieving pain, controlling fever and preventing dehydration.

The common causes of ***obstructive sialadenitis*** are stones, mucus plugs and ductal strictures. Stones are more common in adults and are usually located in the submandibular ducts. The clinical diagnosis of calculi is best confirmed by an intraoral occlusal radiograph. Ductal probing may provide enough dilation that simultaneous expulsion of the stone can occur. ***Treatment***, however, usually includes the surgical exposure and removal of the ductal calculi, followed by thorough irrigation of the duct. Repeated ductal stone formation can lead to chronic stasis and recurring gland infections, which usually indicate the need to remove the gland. Intraglandular calculi or stones lodged in the distal portion of the duct may also require removal of the gland.

References

Baillett, O'Keefe., "The Bacteriology of Perimandibular Space Infections." *J Oral Maxillofac Surg.* Vol 37 (1979): 407-409.

Dorlands Illustrated Medical Dictionary. 27th ed. WB Saunders Co., 1988.

Fonseca, R.J., Walker, R.V., ed. *Oral & Maxillofacial Trauma.* Philadelphia: WB Saunders Co., 1991.

Gilman, A. G.; Goodman, L. S.; Rall, T.W.; and Murad F., *Goodman and Gilman's The Pharmacological Basis of Therapeutics.* 7th Ed, New York: Macmillin, 1985.

Hurley, J.V., *Acute Inflammation.* 2d ed, Melbourne: Churchill Livingstone, 1983.

Moenning, J.E.; Nelson, C.L.; and Kohler, R.B., "The Microbiology & Chemotherapy of Odontogenic Infections." *J Oral Maxillofac Surg.* 47 (1989): 976-985.

Ogundiya, D.A.; Keith, D.A.; and Mirowski, J., "Cavernous Sinus Thrombosis & Blindness as Complications of an Odontogenic Infection: Report of a Case & Review of the Literature." *J Oral Maxillofac Surg* 47 (1989): 1317-1321.

Oral and Maxillofacial Surgery Clinics of North America Infections of the Head and Neck. Vol 3, No. 2, Philadelphia: W.B. Saunders Co 1991.

Peterson, L.J.; Ellis, E.; Hupp, J.R.; and Tucker, M.R., *Contemporary Oral and Maxillofacial Surgery.* St Louis: C.V. Mosby Co., 1988.

Spires, *Arch Otolaryngol Head Neck Surg.* Vol 113 (1987): 984-986.

Topazian, R.G., Goldberg, M.H., *Management of Infections of the Oral and Maxillofacial Regions.* 2d ed., Philadelphia: W.B. Saunders Co, 1986.

3 Dental Disease and Systemic Infections

Gloria G. Vaughan, D.D.S.

Diseases of the orofacial complex are not always localized and can play a role in causing or exacerbating certain systemic disorders. Conversely, systemic disease is frequently manifested in the oral cavity. The purpose of this chapter is to examine the relationship of orofacial disease to certain systemic illnesses. The following discussion will provide an overview of common situations in which the dentist may be consulted in order to rule out dental disorders as precipitators of or contributors to systemic diseases. Topics discussed include; fevers of unknown origin, aspiration pneumonia, immunosuppression and diabetic ketoacidosis. A discussion of oral manifestations of systemic disease is beyond the scope of this chapter and the interested reader is referred to other texts covering that material.†

I. FEVER OF UNKNOWN ORIGIN

Body temperature is maintained and regulated primarily by the hypothalamus via the activation of heat loss or gain mechanisms. The body's internal temperature varies with physical activity and external temperature. There is also an intrinsic diurnal fluctuation in body temperature of three degrees Fahrenheit. Basal body temperature is the result of heat produced by chemical reactions in the body which are necessary to sustain life. The temperature regulating center in the hypothalamus acts as a "thermostat" for the body to maintain a constant basal temperature. In order to accomplish this, the hypothalamus activates heat generation and heat loss processes which affect changes in internal and external temperature. The basal temperature may be altered by heat generating mechanisms such as vasoconstriction and shivering or by heat loss mechanisms that include radiation, conduction and water evaporation. Descending neuronal pathways from the hypothalamus control the output of somatic motor nerves to skeletal muscle and thereby activate shivering. In addition, sympathetic nerves to skin arterioles, sweat glands and the adrenal medulla are under hypothalamic

†See Suggested Reading at the end of this chapter.

control. Sympathetic stimulation results in peripheral vasoconstriction, sweating and the secretion of epinephrine from the adrenal medulla. In turn, epinephrine stimulates adrenergic alpha and beta receptors resulting in vasoconstriction, elevated heart rate and increased blood pressure.

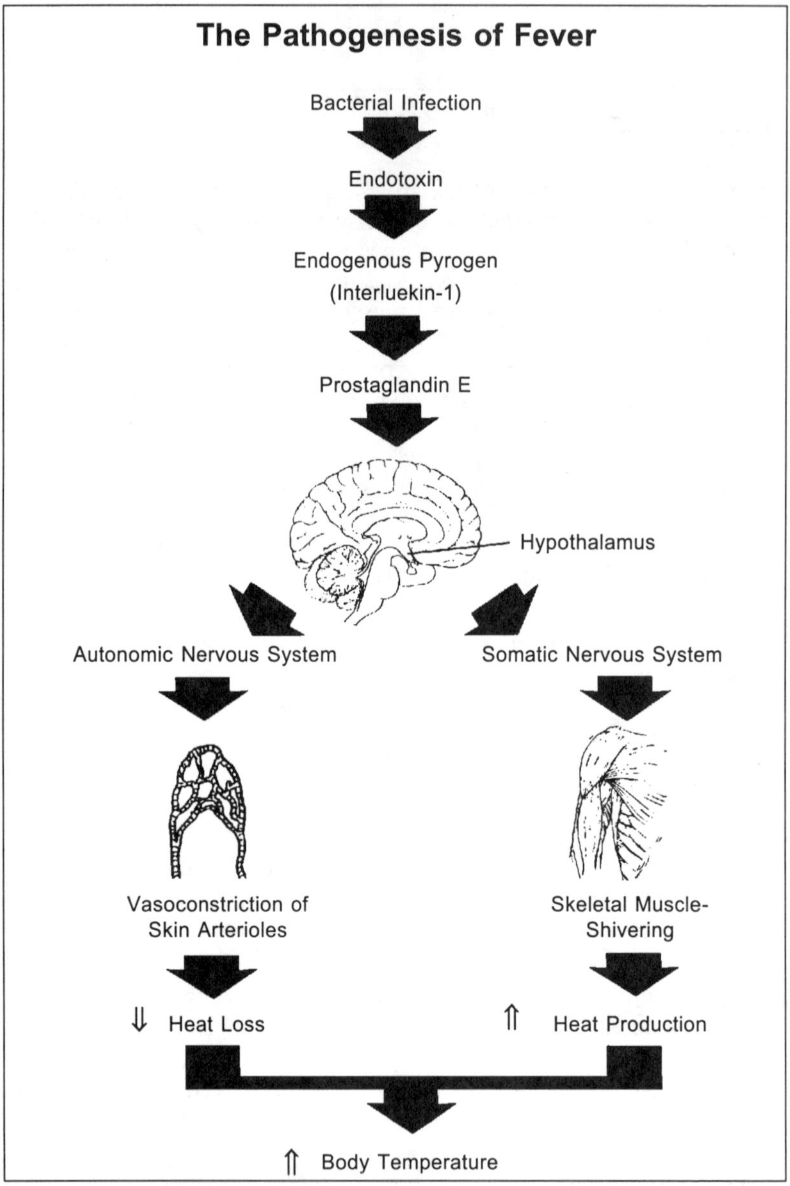

Figure 3-1: The Pathogenesis of Fever.

Fever, an abnormality in the body's thermoregulation system, may result from a variety of causes. The most frequent is bacterial infection; although fungi, viruses, steroids and non-microbial antigens may also act as pyrogens. Bacterial by-products known as endotoxins are responsible for the pyrogenic activity of bacteria. These endotoxins are large lipopolysaccharide molecules derived from the cell walls of gram negative bacteria. Once released into the body, bacterial pyrogens interact with leukocytes and other reticuloendothelial cells causing the release of an endogenous pyrogen identical to interleukin 1. This endogenous pyrogen initiates a cascade of processes ultimately producing prostaglandin E, which acts on the central nervous system resulting in fever. As such, fever represents a change in the thermoregulatory control mechanism because pyrogens cause the "setting" of the thermostat to rise. When this setting is increased, the mechanisms for raising the body's temperature are activated, including heat conservation via vasoconstriction and increased heat production from shivering (Figure 3-1).

When patients present with febrile illnesses, the cause is often quickly and easily diagnosed. If the etiology is not readily apparent, the fevers are termed fevers of unknown origin (FUO). FUOs have been defined as either a fever lasting more than three weeks, a temperature greater than 101°F on several occasions, or when the cause of a febrile illness is not readily apparent after one week of hospital study. In most cases the FUO results from a common illness. The most frequent cause of an FUO is infection, which is responsible for a third of the cases (Table 3-1). Of

Table 3-1: The Incidence of FUO Etiologies

CAUSE		INCIDENCE
Infection		33%
	Bacterial endocarditis	
	Tuberculosois	
	Abdominal abscess	
	Hepatobiliary	
	Urinary tract	
	Other	
Neoplastic disease		22%
	Lymphoma	
	Carcinoma	
Collagen vascular disease		16%
	Rheumatic fever	
	Lupus erythematosus	
	Other	
Miscellaneous		15%
	Myocardial infarction	
	Pulmonary embolism	
	Crohn's disease	
	Alcoholic hepatitis	
	Drugs	
Undiagnosed		14%

these infections, the most frequent offenders are bacterial endocarditis, intraabdominal abscesses and hepatobiliary infections. The next most frequent cause is neoplastic disease of which lymphoma is the most common. Less frequent causes include collagen vascular diseases such as rheumatoid arthritis and systemic lupus erythematosus. The remainder of the identifiable causes in FUO cases are attributable to rare illnesses. Undiagnosed cases represent roughly 10 to 15% of all FUOs.

Determining the cause of an FUO requires a careful and logical approach that focuses on the most common etiologic diseases. Patient history, physical findings and the results of screening tests should be used to formulate the diagnosis. Screening tests should begin with the non-invasive and proceed to more invasive procedures (i.e., biopsies) when warranted. A three tiered approach following such a sequence has been developed (Table 3-2). Level one screening tests include clinical laboratory studies such as complete blood count, urinalysis, blood urea nitrogen and creatinine levels. Blood, throat and sputum cultures may also be obtained in addition to these serologic studies. Level two testing involves non-invasive procedures such as the imaging of any clinically suspicious areas including chest, panoramic or sinus radiographs. Level three encompasses all invasive procedures such as liver, kidney and oral biopsies.

While seeking the cause of an FUO, practitioners should not overlook the oral cavity as a potential source. Although infrequent, dental disease has been identified as a cause of FUOs. Unfortunately, in several of these cases the dental problem was not identified in time to avoid a lengthy hospital stay and multiple, expensive laboratory procedures. Hence, in the investigation of an FUO, an early dental consultation may minimize patient discomfort, radiation exposure and the risks and expense of other diagnostic procedures.

TABLE 3-2: Stepwise Investigation of FUOs

LEVEL I.	**SCREENING TESTS**		
	General	Cultures	Serologies
	CBC	Blood	Viral
	Urinalysis	Throat	Fungal
	BUN/Creatinine	Sputum	
	Liver fuction tests	Urine	
LEVEL II.	**NON INVASIVE PROCEDURES**		
	Chest x-ray	Panoramic x-ray	
	Radiopaque dye imaging	Sinus series	
	Sonogram		
LEVEL III.	**INVASIVE PROCEDURES**		
	Tissue biopsies		
	Laparoscopy		
	Endoscopy		

A dental infection can present as anything from a low grade, well localized process to a severe, life-threatening, multiple fascial space infection. The associated swelling may be obvious or subtle depending on location, invasiveness and patient morphology. Trismus is also a common sign of an odontogenic infection. The associated pain may be poorly localized, and is often absent with a chronic and/or draining abscess. It is uncommon for an odontogenic infection to cause a significant fever (usually ≤101° F); however, with severe infections the temperature may reach 101 to 102° F. Pronounced leukocytosis is also uncommon as the white blood cell count typically increases to the high normal range, except with severe infections. Because pulse rate increases with rising body temperature, tachycardia commonly accompanies a systemic infection. In contrast, blood pressure does not vary significantly in the presence of fever unless there is an extreme degree of accompanying pain and/or anxiety. Fever may also elevate the respiratory rate to 18 to 20 breaths per minute, and with severe infections airway patency may be compromised.

Following the three tiered approach to determine the cause, Level I would consist of a thorough history and physical examination of the head, neck and oral structures. The general questions listed in Table 3-3 may help the practitioner determine the possibility of an occult dental infection as a fever's source. Infrequent visits to the dentist coupled with a positive response to any of the questions should alert the practitioner to a possible dental infection, especially if there are any positive physical findings. The presence of the physical findings presented in Table 3-4 should also be noted. Dentures or partial dentures must be removed and an adequate intraoral light source should be available to perform a thorough exam. Based on the history and clinical exam, if an orofacial infection is suspected, a dental consultation is recommended. Level II of the dental examination involves imaging studies that typically include a panoramic radiograph and/or selected periapical views. C-T scans and MRIs may be helpful in severe and unusual cases. Level III investigations would likely consist of a needle aspiration of the suspected area of infection. Less commonly, tissue biopsies or other invasive procedures may be indicated.

Table 3-3: Screening Questions for Orofacial Infection

1. Do you presently or in the recent past, have you had:
    - Toothaches?
    - Loose teeth?
    - Bleeding gums?
    - Oral or facial swelling?
    - Foul taste or bad odor in your mouth?
2. Have you noticed a change in the way your dentures fit?
3. When was your last dental visit?
4. How frequently have you gone to the dentist in the past?

Table 3-4: Physical Manifestations of an Orofacial Infection

Extraoral Findings	
	Enlarged lymph nodes in the head and/or neck
	Obvious facial swelling or facial asymmetry
	Trismus (Normal opening is 35 - 55 mm.)
	Fistulous tracts
	Erythematous and or warm regions of the skin
Intraoral Findings	
	Loose teeth
	Teeth tender to palpation or percussion
	Gingival swelling, erythema, or bleeding
	Carious teeth
	Mucosal ulcerations
	Fistulous tracts
	Halitosis

When an oral infection is identified, several criteria must be met to substantiate an etiological relationship with the fever. First, there must be signs and/or symptoms of oral disease whose bacteremia is temporally related to the febrile episode. Second, organisms cultured orally must match those determined by blood cultures. Third, there must be a negative correlation between blood cultures and other fluid cultures (i.e., urine, sputum, CSF). Finally, signs and symptoms of other concurrent disease processes must be ruled out as potential causes of the fever. In practice, rarely does the investigation of an FUO conclusively link the fever to an occult dental infection. Additionally, scientific investigations have been unable to illuminate the relationship between oral infections and systemic fever. As such, the true role of dental infections in FUOs remains unclear.

Empiric treatment of FUOs is not generally recommended unless there is strong clinical evidence indicating a specific diagnosis. For example, empiric antibiotic treatment may be initiated for patients with suspected endocarditis while awaiting culture results. Fever produced by tumors may respond to non-steriodal anti-inflammatory drugs. Anti-tuberculin regimens may be administered to patients suspected of having tuberculosis or granulomatous hepatitis. Empiric use of antibiotics, however, will obscure the cause, making diagnosis more difficult. When a dental etiology is suspected, potential therapies include extractions, incisions and drainage, root canal therapy, periodontal scaling and prophylaxis. Aggressive definitive therapies are indicated especially in hosts with prolonged fevers or with significant medical maladies (i.e., immunocompromised patients and insulin dependent diabetics).

II. ASPIRATION PNEUMONIA

The aspiration of small amounts of oropharyngeal secretions or gastric contents is common in healthy persons and rarely results in pathologic changes or clinical symptoms. In some patients, however, especially those with altered consciousness, dysphagia or a diminished cough reflex, aspiration pneumonia can ensue. Candidates for aspiration pneumonia include patients undergoing general anesthesia or deep pharmacosedation, persons with neurologic or seizure disorders, alcoholics, patients who have overdosed on drugs and patients suffering cerebrovascular accidents.

The pathologic picture of aspiration pneumonia is best described as a chemical burn of the lung which occurs when vomitus comes in contact with the pulmonary epithelium. Destruction of the respiratory lining causes pulmonary edema and collapse of the alveoli resulting in abnormal ventilation/perfusion ratios and intrapulmonary shunting. Hypoxemia from inadequate ventilation combined with hypovolemia from pulmonary edema may result in death if not corrected. In most cases the signs and symptoms of aspiration pneumonia are manifested within one hour of the insult. The clinical presentation can include fever, coughing, wheezing, tachypnea and cyanosis. Signs of infection are usually absent, but when present are secondary to an opportunistic infection of the damaged pulmonary epithelial lining. The diagnosis may be readily made if the aspiration of oropharyngeal contents is witnessed. When the event is not witnessed and the patient has unexplained cyanosis, tachypnea and tachycardia, a chest x-ray should be obtained. Radiographically, soft patchy mottling is usually visible throughout the lung fields without evidence of collapse. The right lower lobe is most frequently involved because of the anatomically favorable alignment of the right main bronchus to the trachea.

The severity of damage from aspirated vomitus depends on the aspirate's pH, and its composition, volume and distribution in the tracheobronchial tree. The critical pH below which severe lung damage occurs is 2.5. In addition, a minimum of .4 ml/kg of aspirate is necessary to produce the classic signs and symptoms. Particulate matter within the aspirate may mechanically cause airway obstruction in addition to epithelial lining damage. Even the aspiration of clear liquids or saline can result in epithelial damage, although the outcome is usually transient and less severe.

In a patient susceptible to aspiration with clinical and radiographic evidence of aspiration pneumonia, dentists are frequently called upon to rule out a dental etiology. The rationale is that because the predominant microorganisms in aspiration pneumonia are common to the oropharyngeal flora, a patient with poor oral health and/or hygiene may possess a more concentrated and perhaps virulent bacterial burden within their oropharyngeal secretions. As such, the oral health of patients at risk for aspiration may be an important predictive factor. In most cases, this relationship cannot be substantiated. However, in such patients, the extraction of potential sources of infection may benefit the patient's overall condition and have prophylactic value. Some authors have even suggested that the possibility of aspirating loose teeth, tooth fragments and/or calculus can cause a post obstructive pneumonia followed by necrosis and abscess formation. Because the risks and benefits of dental therapy cannot be accurately assessed when a patient is at risk to aspirate potentially pathologic saliva and/or oral material, the necessary dental therapy may be indicated prophylactically. To date, the scientific literature has not clarified the validity of this proposed relationship. To substantiate an etiologic relationship between salivary microorganisms and pneumonia, other potential sources of the infection must be ruled out and the causative organisms must be proven oral inhabitants.

III. IMMUNOCOMPROMISED PATIENTS

A variety of disorders may be treated with chemotherapy including aplastic anemia, leukemia, lymphomas and various solid tumors. The cellular toxicity of chemotherapy applies to all rapidly dividing cells. These include not only cancer cells but also non-cancerous host tissue such as mucosal cells, hemopoietic cells and hair follicles. Hence, side effects from chemotherapy commonly include inflammation of the mucosa lining the oral cavity and the gastrointestinal tract, that results in mucositis and gastritis. Hemopoietic bone marrow suppression produces anemia, leukopenia and thrombocytopenia, while destruction of the hair follicle causes alopecia. In the oral cavity, the complications can include odontogenic infections, hemorrhage, xerostomia, oral mucositis and opportunistic infections.

It is imperative, although often difficult, to determine the cause of fever in the immunocompromised patient. Because infections are a serious threat to life in this patient population, steps should be taken to prevent their occurrence. It has been shown that infection is the major cause of morbidity and mortality in patients with leukemia and that most of these infections are caused by organisms common to the host's normal flora.

In fact, among adult patients with acute leukemia, 54% of the microbiologically proven septicemias were caused by organisms that inhabit the oral flora. Similarly, in bone marrow transplant patients 41% of the microbiologically proven septicemias were caused by organisms that inhabit the oral cavity. Periapical, periodontal and pericoronal diseases are those most frequently associated with septicemia in immunocompromised patients. Among these three diseases, periodontal and pericoronal are most often implicated. A significant drop in the septicemia rate among these patients has been demonstrated when both a thorough dental evaluation and necessary treatment are completed prior to the initiation of chemotherapy. The goal of the pre-chemotherapy dental treatment is to remove all potential sources of infection from the oral cavity such as teeth suffering moderate to severe periodontitis, pulpitis, large carious lesions and those teeth prone to pericoronitis (Table 3-5). Treatment tends to be aggressive in nature and typical therapies include extraction, root canal therapy and/or prophylaxis. The uncertainty of conservative therapies on questionable teeth and the potentially deleterious systemic implications favor such an approach.

Table 3-5: Considerations for Tooth Extractions Prior to Chemotherapy

Gross carious lesions	Deep periodontal pocketing
Irreversible pulpitis	Severe bony defects
Significant mobility	Partially erupted third molars
Non-cleansable third molars	Periapical pathosis

When managing a febrile, neutropenic patient, physicians usually begin with empirical antibiotic treatment: Gentamycin 2 mg/kg as a loading dose followed by 1.6 mg/kg IV every 8 hours and Ticarcillin 200 to 400 mg/kg IV every 4 hours. Concommitantly, all suspected sites of infection are cultured including the throat, sputum, stool, urine, blood, IV access sites and cerebrospinal fluid. If the patient's fever is relapsing, blood cultures are taken with each febrile episode. All such patients should be evaluated by a dentist as early in the work-up as possible. The dental evaluation should include a thorough head and neck examination. Recognizing that the neutropenic patient may not exhibit the usual signs and symptoms of infection (i.e., swelling, pus and erythema), screening radiographs are also recommended.

If it is necessary to treat a patient who is already neutropenic (i.e., the absolute neutrophil count [ANC] is less than 500 mm^3), then the patient may require antibiotic prophylaxis prior to and following dental surgery. Pharmacotherapeutic agents commonly employed are a combination of a semi-synthetic penicillin, such as carbenicillin (400 to 500 mg/kg IV every 4 hours), and an aminoglycoside, such as gentamycin (2 mg/kg IV as a loading dose, then 1.6 mg/kg IV every 8 hours). The patient's physician should be consulted regarding both the antibiotic selection and the timing of treatment. Recently it has been recommended that additional prophylactic agents such as ticarcillin plus clavulanic acid (3.1 g q4h) be used to cover microorganisms such as beta-lactamase-producing capnophilic and anaerobic bacteria. These organisms have been increasingly associated with septicemia in immunocompromised hosts.

Oral mucosal ulcerations can result from chemotherapy either as a direct effect of the chemotherapeutic agent on the mucosa or as an indirect result of the drug's immunosuppressive effect (opportunistic infection). These ulcerations frequently have a generalized distribution, attain a large size and are exquisitely painful to the patient. In addition, the ulcerated tissue provides a portal for bacterial, fungal and viral organisms to secondarily infect the lesions and potentially lead to septicemia.

When evaluating an oral ulceration in the immunocompromised host, care must be taken to differentiate between those lesions that have resulted from the chemotherapeutic agent and those that represent opportunistic infections. The physical appearance of the lesions are usually indistinguishable; hence, physical examination alone is unreliable. A gram stain or a KOH prep performed on a cytologic scraping of the ulcerated area is recommended to detect a *Candida albicans* infection. Antifungal therapies can include nystatin, clotrimazole, ketaconazole, fluconazole or amphotericin B. Chlorhexidene has also been shown to be beneficial in the resolution and prevention of candidiasis in immunocompromised patients. Oral hygiene should be reinforced and, if significant discomfort is present, a topical anesthetic should be prescribed (i.e., viscous xylocaine or dyclone with or without milk of magnesia). The diagnosis of a herpes simplex viral lesion may be made by HSV culture of the lesion, direct immunoflurescence, indirect immunoperoxidase, ELISA or cytology. HSV lesions may be resolved with the use of intravenous or oral acyclovir (Table 4-6).

For pericoronitis, extraction of the offending tooth is recommended when possible, accompanied by antibiotic therapy (i.e., penicillin V 500 mg. every 6 hours for ten days post-surgery). Primary closure is desired when possible, and it is important to remove all potential sources of post-operative infection, such as a bony sequestrum. If it is not possible to extract the tooth, antibiotic therapy may be accompanied by a custom, soft, occlusal mouthguard fabricated to prevent further trauma to the area. In addition, frequent irrigation of the area with saline or chlorhexidine may help resolve the bacterial infection. Surgical procedures are generally not recommended unless the ANC is greater than 500 mm^3 and the platelet count is above 50,000 mm^3.

For the neutropenic patient with periodontitis, scaling and/or extractions may be indicated. Again, procedures likely to cause bleeding should be avoided in patients with inadequate platelet and/or neutrophil counts. Antibiotic therapy directed towards the offending organism should be employed, and oral hygeine should be reinforced. Chlorhexidene rinses may also be helpful in suppressing the bacterial counts associated with the periodontal disease process.

Table 3-6: Common Therapy for Patients with Oral Complications of Immunosuppression

Anti-viral Medications
Acyclovir IV 5 mg/kg every 8 hours for 7 days
Acyclovir 200 mg capsules 1 capsule five times daily for 7 days
Anti-fungal Medications
Nystatin oral suspension 100,000 U/ml Rinse with 4 ml for 2 minutes and swallow 4 times daily
Clotrimazole 10 mg troches Dissolve 1 troche in mouth 5 times daily for 14 days
Ketaconazole 200 mg tablets One tablet daily for 14 days
Fluconazole 100 mg tablets Two tablets on Day One then 1 tablet once daily for a minimum of 3 weeks and at least 2 weeks following the resolution of symptoms.
Amphotercin B - Intravenous Test dose 1 mg IV slowly. Then 0.25 mg/kg/day and advance to maximum dose of 1-1.5 mg/kg/day
Topical Anesthetics
Lidocaine - viscous 2% Rinse with 5 ml and expectorate every 2 hours as needed for oral pain
Dyclonine 1% with Milk of Magnesia / 50% mixture by volume Rinse with 5 ml and expectorate every 2 hours as needed for oral pain
Antimicrobial Rinses
Chlorhexidene 0.12% rinse Rinse with 15 ml for 1 minute and expectorate three times daily after meals

IV. DIABETIC KETOACIDOSIS

The most serious complication of diabetes mellitus is hyperglycemia which can result from multiple causes. Potential precipitators include: 1) patient noncompliance with diabetic medications (insulin or oral hypoglycemics), 2) poor regulation of nutritional intake and 3) increased stress secondary to infections or surgery. Of these, the most common precipitator is bacterial infections. A potentially fatal manifestation of hyperglycemia is diabetic ketoacidosis (DKA) which results from a relative or absolute insulin deficiency. DKA is characterized by accelerated gluconeogenesis, the production of ketogenic acids and electrolyte imbalances such as potassium depletion. The build up of the ketogenic acids results in a metabolic acidosis because the body is unable to break down the ketones as rapidly as they are produced. In addition, the body cannot compensate for the decreased pH via renal and respiratory buffering systems.

Research has shown that diabetic patients are more prone to infection than non-diabetic patients, and poorly controlled diabetics have a greater risk of infection than well controlled patients. Additionally, there is a positive relationship between the degree of hyperglycemia and the severity of the resulting infections. Many factors have been purported to be responsible for this increased susceptibility to, and severity of, infections in diabetics. Among these are impairments of phagocytosis, chemotaxis, and the bactericidal function of leukocytes in diabetics. Leukocyte impairment is thought to result from the small vessel disease that characterizes the pathophysiology of end-organ disease in diabetes. Thickening of the basement membrane may deter diapedesis and thereby account for chemotactic dysfunction. In addition, vessel narrowing may cause a decrease in blood flow and oxygen to peripheral tissues. The resulting hypoxia may promote anaerobic bacterial growth and impair leukocyte function. Cortisol and glucagon production are also increased during periods of stress or infection. This can antagonize the action of insulin, furthering the hyperglycemic state.

The diagnosis of DKA is made based on presenting signs and symptoms, the medical history and laboratory tests. Classic symptoms include the triad of polydipsia, polyuria and polyphagia (Table 3-7). Frequently patients exhibit rapid, shallow breathing, known as Kussmaul's respirations, which represents the body's attempt to compensate for the underlying metabolic acidosis by "blowing off carbon dioxide." Also the patient's breath may have a fruity odor caused by the build up of ketones in the body. Typical laboratory findings include: 1) an increase in urine and blood glucose, 2) elevated serum ketones, 3) a low arterial pH and 4) low serum bicarbonate. A patient suspected of being in DKA should be referred immediately for medical treatment because of the associated 10 to 20% mortality rate.

The treatment of DKA involves correction of the hyperglycemia through insulin administration, restoring electrolytic balance, and rehydration. While attempting to correct the patient's hyperglycemia, the cause precipitating the DKA event should be determined. When a patient in DKA presents, body fluid cultures (i.e., blood, urine, stool, etc.) should be taken to rule out infection. If infection is determined to be the precipitating event and a source is not readily apparent, the three tiered approach to determining the source of the infection should be followed. As a part of this investigation, a dentist should be consulted to rule out an oral source of infection.

Specific infections commonly associated with diabetes mellitus include candidiasis, mucormycosis, nonclostridial gas infection and periodontal disease. Aggressive periodontitis has been attributed to microangiopathies within the periodontal tissues, an increase in the glucose content of the crevicular fluid, and the aforementioned leukocyte impairment. This enhanced periodontal destruction has been correlated with the duration of known diabetes, the severity of diabetic complications, and blood sugar levels above 200 mg/dl (poor metabolic control). Conversely, periapical and periodontal infections have been shown to increase the insulin requirements of diabetic patients secondary to the "anti-insulin" effects of the infection. If the increased insulin requirement is not met, hyperglycemia and even DKA can result, even in previously stable diabetic patients. In light of the relationship between periodontal disease and diabetes, a goal in the treatment of all diabetic patients is the elimination of potential sources of infection including oral diseases. Attention to the presence of oral disease and patient education concerning the interplay of the systemic disease with oral health are recommended. Dental consultation followed by the control or elimination of potential sources of oral infection (i.e., periodontal therapies, extractions, root canal therapy or caries control) may improve the patients' medical management. For example, the incidence of hyperglycemic episodes may be reduced, the insulin dose may be lowered, and insulin regulation may be facilitated by improving the patients' oral health. Likewise, an improvement in the oral health of diabetics may be achieved through correction of the underlying metabolic disturbance. Finally, when an infectious etiology is suspected, dental disease should be considered as a potential cause for fever or hyperglycemic episodes (including diabetic coma, DKA, non-ketotic hyperosmolar coma and brittle diabetics).

Table 3-7: Signs and Symptoms Associated with DKA

Signs	Symptoms
Polyuria	Kussmaul's respirations
Polidypsia	"Fruity breath"
Weight loss	Tachycardia
Abdominal pain	Hypotension
Nausea	Decreased skin turgor
Vomiting	Dry mucous membranes

References

Baquero F., et al., "Capnophilic and anaerobic bacteremia in neutropenic patients: an oral source." *Rev Infect Disease*. 12 (1990): 157.
Bartlett J.G., Gorbach S.L., Finegold S.M., "The bacteriology of aspiration pneumonia." *Am J Med*. 56 (1974): 202.
Berry E., Silver J., "Pyorrhoea as a cause of pyrexia." *Brit Med J*. 2 (1976): 1289.
Brusch J., Weinstein L., "Fever of Unknown Origin." *Med Clin North Am*. 72 (1988): 1247.
Feretti G.A., et al., "Chlorhexidene for prophylaxis against oral infections and associated complications in patients receiving bone marrow transplantations." *J Am Dent Assoc*. 114 (1987): 461.
Finestone A.J., Boorujy S.R., "Diabetes mellitus and periodontal disease." *Diabetes*. 16 (1967): 336.
Greenberg M.S., et al., "The oral flora as a source of septicemia in patients with acute leukemia." *Oral Surg*. 53 (1982): 32.
Guyton A.C., *Basic Human Physiology*. Philadelphia: W.B. Saunders, 1971.
Heimdahl A., et al., "The oral cavity as a port of entry for early infections treated with bone marrow transplantation." *Oral Surg Oral Med Oral Pathol*. 68 (1989): 711.
Huebner G.R., Grout D., "The role of dental disease in fever of unknown origin." *Postgrad Med*. 79 (1986): 275.
Hurley D.L., "Fever in adults." *Postgrad Med* 74 (1983): 232.
Jackson R.M., Rice D.H., "Acute bacterial sinusitus and diabetes mellitus." *Otolaryngol*. 97 (1987): 469.
Levinson S.L., Barondess J.A., "Occult dental infection as a cause of fever of obscure origin." *Am J Med*. 66 (1979): 463.
Morgan J.G., "Pathophysiology of gastric aspiration." *Int Anesth Clin*. 15 (1977): 1.
Petersdorf R.G., Beeson P.B., "Fever of unexplained origin: report on 100 cases." *Medicine*. 40 (1960): 1.
Peterson L.J., et al., *Contemporary Oral and Maxillofacial Surgery*. St. Louis: C.V. Mosby Co., 1986.
Rayfield, et al., "Infection and diabetes: The case for glucose control." *Am J Med*. 72 (1982): 439.
Redding S.W., Montgomery M.T., *Dentistry in Systemic Disease*. Portland: JBK Publishing, 1990.
Rose L.F., Kaye D., *Internal Medicine for Dentistry*. St. Louis: C.V. Mosby, 1983.
Stein J.H., *Internal Medicine*. Boston: Little Brown, 1987.
Stein J.H., *Internal Medicine; Diagnosis and Therapy*. East Norwalk: Appleton & Lange, 1989.
Vander A.J.; Sherman J.H.; Luciano D.S., *Human Physiology*. New York: McGraw-Hill, 1980.
Williford S.K., et al., "The safety of dental extractions in patients with hematologic emergencies." *J Clin Oncol*. 7 (1989): 798.
Wynne J.W., Modell J.H., "Respiratory aspiration of stomach contents." *Ann Int Med*. 87 (1977): 466.

Suggested Reading

Coleman, G.C., Nelson, J.F., *Principles of Oral Diagnosis*. St. Louis: C.V. Mosby, 1993.
Eversole, L.R., *Clinical Outline of Oral Pathology - Diagnosis and Treatment*. 3rd Ed., Philadelphia: Lea and Febiger, 1992.
Regezi, J.A., Sciubba, J.J., *Oral Pathology Clinical - Pathologic Correlations*. Philadelphia: Saunders, 1989.

4 Oral Bleeding

Spencer W. Redding, D.D.S., M.Ed.

Acute oral bleeding is a diverse condition ranging from minor oozing secondary to a tooth extraction, to life-threatening bleeding in patients with severe hemostatic defects. The oral cavity is a common site for hemorrhagic problems because of its rich blood supply and susceptibility to trauma from such normal activities as speaking and eating. Also, commonly performed dental manipulations such as extractions, periodontal surgery, biopsies and scaling expose the oral soft tissues to significant iatrogenic insults. Of these, tooth extraction is one of the most severe insults to normal hemostasis, because primary closure is rarely achieved. As a result, patients with occult bleeding defects can be initially diagnosed following a dental procedure. In this chapter the most common causes of acute oral bleeding and their management will be discussed.

I. NORMAL PHYSIOLOGY OF HEMOSTASIS

Any defect in the normal hemostatic mechanism can lead to abnormal and potentially serious oral bleeding. Adequate evaluation and management of abnormal bleeding requires a basic understanding of normal hemostasis. Normal hemostasis is composed of three separate but interrelated phases, including the vascular phase, the platelet phase, and the coagulation phase. All three phases are initiated by vascular injury.

The ***vascular phase*** is initiated immediately following injury to a blood vessel. There is a direct vasoconstrictive response of the injured vessel which is mediated by the autonomic nervous system. The adjacent vessels are also reflexively stimulated. Vasoconstriction slows blood flow to the area of the injury and is critical in preventing massive bleeding following severance of large vessels.

The ***platelet phase*** is also initiated after injury to a blood vessel. Circulating platelets attach to the subendothelium through a process termed platelet adhesion. Subendothelial collagen, platelet receptors, fibronectin, thrombospondin and factor 8 Von Willebrand's all contribute to this process. More circulating platelets then stick to the initial group in a process termed platelet aggregation which requires substances both internal and external to the platelet including thromboxane A_2, ADP and thrombin. The clot mass formed in the platelet phase can occlude vessels up to 50 microns in diameter.

The third and final phase, the ***coagulation phase***, is also initiated by the vascular injury. Through a series of intricate biochemical processes, initial blood proteins (factors) are activated and subsequently activate other blood proteins in a sequence called the coagulation cascade. This cascade of activation eventually leads to the formation of thrombin. Then thrombin promotes the formation of fibrin from fibrinogen. Fibrin makes up the stabilized clot. There are two recognized pathways that activate factor 10 which converts prothrombin to thrombin. The intrinsic pathway, so named because all components are in the blood itself, contains factors 12, 11, 9 and 8. In contrast the extrinsic pathway relies on activation from substances, tissue thromboplastins, that are external to the blood and are in many cellular tissues. This pathway includes factor 7. Both pathways are necessary for normal hemostasis. Figure 4-1 provides a schematic diagram of the interrelated processes in the formation of the clot. Fibrinolysis, clot breakdown, is initiated while the clot is being formed. Tissue plasminogen activator derived from endothelium then stimulates release of plasmin which dissolves the clot. Both circulating factors and plasmin are inactivated by proteins and removed from circulation by the reticuloendothelial system. This limits clot formation and lysis to the site of injury.

Although these three phases are presented separately to facilitate understanding of their mechanisms, it is important to realize that there is significant interaction among them and that they occur simultaneously. For example, phospholipids released from the platelet phase are necessary for the normal activation of factors in the coagulation phase. Also thrombin is required for smooth functioning of platelet aggregation. The interaction of all three phases is required for clot formation and dissolution in a controlled fashion. Any disruption of the three phases or their interaction can result in a significant bleeding disorder. Due to the rich blood supply in the oral cavity, deficits in any of the three phases often result in abnormal oral bleeding.

II. DISORDERS OF HEMOSTASIS

Platelet defects resulting in abnormal bleeding may be either primary or secondary. Primary diseases include idiopathic thrombocytopenic purpura (ITP), thrombotic thrombocytopenic purpura (TTP) and thrombasthenia.

ITP is an autoimmune process that targets platelets resulting in lowered platelet counts. No source for the thrombocytopenia can be determined. The acute form which occurs primarily in children, usually responds to

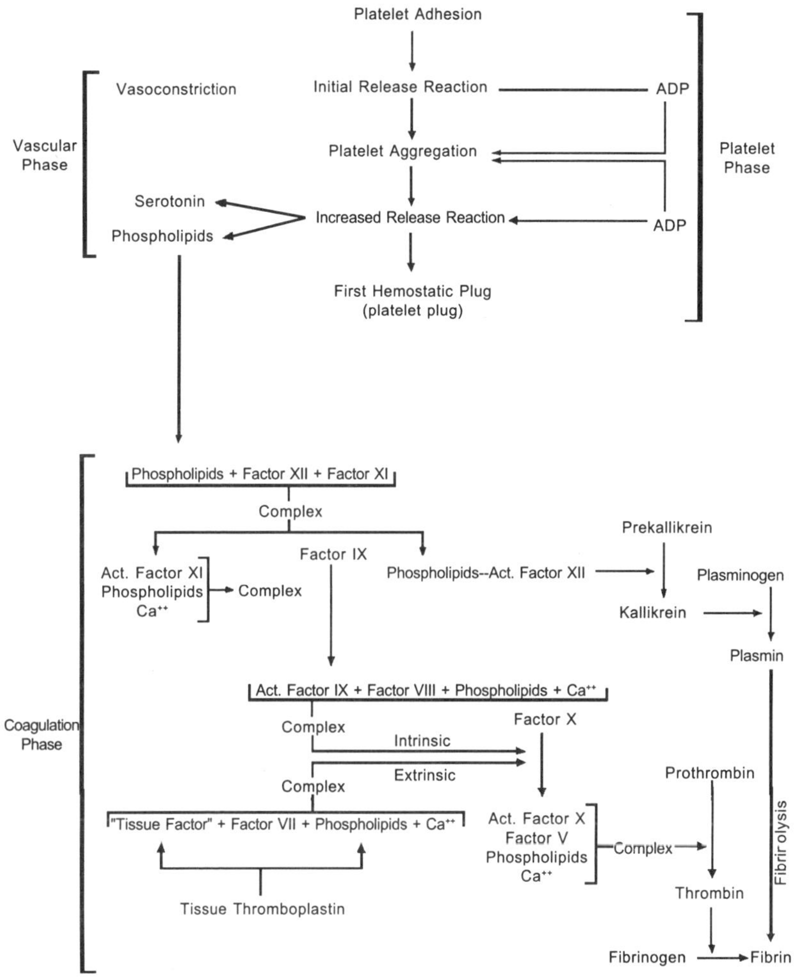

Figure 4-1: Diagram of Phases of Hemostasis.

steroid therapy and the prognosis is excellent. However, the chronic form in adults usually has a more protracted course. Splenectomy is commonly performed in an attempt to improve platelet counts.

TTP, also thought to be an autoimmune process, results in a lowered platelet count but paradoxically leads to formation of thrombi in the microcirculation. TTP is seen in all ages and is treated with high dose steroids and plasma transfusions. Unlike ITP, the prognosis for TTP is poor with up to a 50% disease mortality.

Thrombasthenia, Glanzmann Disease, is a rare genetic disorder resulting in a lifelong bleeding tendency. Platelet numbers are normal but platelet aggregation is compromised. Thrombocytopenia secondary to other causes is much more common than the above. These causes include leukemia, antineoplastic chemotherapy and other drug therapies. Since most patients with leukemia are ultimately treated with chemotherapy, these patients probably have the highest risk of platelet related bleeding problems.

Hemophilia A, factor 8 deficiency, is the most common of the coagulopathies and is characterized by bleeding into deep fascial planes and joints (hemarthrosis). Following dental extractions these patients will initially form a clot that can dissolve at a later time resulting in delayed bleeding. Therefore, classic hemophiliacs may present with post operative bleeding hours or even days following an extraction. Severity of bleeding is usually directly associated with factor 8 level — the lower the level the higher the potential for bleeding. Generally, severe hemophiliacs have less than 1% of normal factor 8, moderate hemophiliacs have between 1 and 5%, and mild hemophiliacs have between 5 and 30%. The factor level can be determined by a factor assay. Hemophiliacs will have an elevated partial thromboplastin time (PTT) and a depressed factor 8 level. Hemophilia B or Christmas Disease, factor 9 deficiency, is a slightly less severe disease than hemophilia A. However, severe bleeding episodes do commonly occur and are of the delayed type. Patients with hemophilia B will have an elevated PTT and a depressed factor 9 level. Generally, other factor deficiencies are very rare and when present are less problematic.

Von Willebrand's disease is characterized by a factor 8 deficiency and a qualitative platelet defect. As mentioned earlier a portion of the factor 8 molecule, factor 8 Von Willebrands, is necessary for normal platelet adhesion to endothelial surfaces following an injury. The bleeding tendency usually waxes and wanes over time and is usually less severe than with hemophilia A or B. There is a greater potential for these patients to be undiagnosed when they report with abnormal bleeding because this disease is less symptomatic. Patients will have an elevated PTT, an elevated bleeding time and a reduced factor 8 level.

Patients on anticoagulation (those with prosthetic heart valves, atrial fibrillation, deep vein thrombosis, transient ischemic attacks, strokes), especially warfarin, will commonly present with postoperative bleeding secondary to oral surgical procedures. With supra-therapeutic dosing, patients can present with spontaneous intraoral bleeding from gingival sites. This bleeding can be among the most difficult to stop and may continue in the presence of a slightly elevated prothrombin time (PT). Warfarin acts by inhibiting the Vitamin K dependent carboxylation of factors 2, 7, 9 and 10 (the so-called Vitamin K dependent factors). Carboxylation of these factors is needed because without this "activation" these factors are left out of the coagulation process. An elevation of the PT patients taking warfarin. Anticoagulants such as aspirin and ot can also induce abnormal intraoral bleeding, though these are not commonly responsible for severe postoperative bleeding. However, in combination with a mild coagulation or platelet defect, NSAID therapy may result in abnormal bleeding. The NSAIDS block the conversion of arachidonic acid to thromboxane. In turn, thromboxane accelerates the platelet's release of adenosinediphosphate (ADP) which is needed for platelet aggregation. NSAIDS will prolong the bleeding time.

Patients with severe liver disease will often develop abnormal bleeding problems. Acute and chronic hepatitis will compromise the synthesis of coagulation factors resulting in an increased PT and PTT. Chronic alcoholics will suffer from platelet deficits as well. Finally, patients with abnormal intraoral bleeding following a surgical procedure may be suffering from the inadvertent laceration of a small artery during the procedure rather than a hemostatic defect. This type of bleeding is generally pulsatile and rapid, forcing the patient to seek more immediate care.

III. PATIENT EVALUATION

A. History

The most critical factor in evaluating a patient's potential for abnormal intraoral bleeding is their past medical history. The vast majority of patients presenting with acute oral bleeding secondary to a defect in the hemostatic mechanism will have positive information in their past history. Therefore, a thorough bleeding history is essential to detect bleeding tendencies. Important questions to be asked are listed in Table 4-1 and are discussed in the following paragraphs.

Table 4-1: Hemostasis Questionnaire

1. Have any of the following members of your family ever had a problem with prolonged or unusual bleeding (parents, brothers and sisters, children, grandparents, great grandparents)?
2. Have you ever had marked bleeding for up to 24 hours after a surgical procedure (i.e., tooth extraction or tonsillectomy)?
3. Have you ever required a blood transfusion after surgery?
4. Females: Do you feel that you have abnormal bleeding during menstruation?
5. Do you get bruises larger than the size of a quarter for which you cannot remember the injury?
6. Do you experience numerous and severe nose bleeds for up to several hours?
7. Do your gums often bleed when not related to trauma or tooth brushing?
8. Are you taking any blood thinner (anticoagulant)?
9. Have you taken any medication, such as pills, powders or liquids in the last week?
10. Have you had or do you have any liver disease?

1. Have any members of your family ever had a problem with prolonged or unusual bleeding? This includes parents, brothers, sisters, grandchildren, grandparents, and great grandparents.

This question will assist in identifying patients with inherited bleeding disorders. It is essential to trace the patient's relatives beyond their parents at least to their grandparents since some inherited bleeding disorders, such as classic hemophilia, skip generations. Hemophilia is a sex-linked recessive disorder carried on the X chromosome (x^r gene). If a hemophiliac (x^r y) has a daughter, she will be carrier (x^r x) and be asymptomatic. If the daughter then has a son, he will be a hemophiliac (x^r y) and manifest clinical disease. If a hemophiliac marries a carrier then the possibility exists of producing a female hemophiliac (x^r x^r). This is very rare.

2. Have you ever had marked bleeding for up to 24 hours after a surgical procedure, such as a tooth extraction or tonsillectomy?

Even though bleeding following a tooth extraction is common, post-operative surgical bleeding for longer than 24 hours is unusual. It is suggested to ask about abnormal bleeding following either a tooth extraction or tonsillectomy because these surgical procedures are very common. Both the amount of bleeding and the bleeding duration after these procedures are important factors.

3. Have you ever required a blood transfusion after surgery?

This question will identify patients who have had excessive blood loss with a surgical procedure. It is important to determine how many units of blood were needed — the more blood transfused, the greater the likelihood of a bleeding disorder. Also important is the type of surgical procedure requiring transfusion — the more minor the surgery (such as tonsillectomy or tooth extraction) the higher the suspicion of a bleeding deficit. A patient requiring a transfusion with a hysterectomy would be less alarming. This question has become even more important in recent years, since blood transfusions are used more conservatively today secondary to increased fears of infectious disease transmission (AIDS, Hepatitis B, etc.).

4. Women: Do you feel that you have abnormal bleeding during menstruation?

This sign is common to women with bleeding disorders and as with surgical bleeding it is important to determine the length and amount of blood loss.

5. Do you get bruises larger than the size of a quarter for which you cannot remember the injury?

Many patients present with bruising from acute or chronic trauma. However, this sign is significant if the bruise is larger than the size of a quarter, and the patient cannot remember any traumatic event. Elderly patients, especially women, tend to bruise easily. Therefore this question may not be as significant in the elderly female population.

6. Do you experience numerous and severe nose bleeds for up to several hours?

Although epistaxis occurs commonly in children and adolescents, most will grow out of this problem. However, frequent nose bleeding in an adult patient is unusual and significant. This type of bleeding usually indicates a platelet disorder, or nasal vasculature that predisposes the patient to bleeding following trauma.

7. Do your gums bleed related to trauma or tooth brushing?

Gingival bleeding, although a common sign of periodontal disease, is significant if the patient repeatedly suffers spontaneous bleeding from the gingival tissue. As with nose bleeds, gingival bleeding usually signifies a platelet disorder such as Von Willebrand's Disease, ITP, or leukemia.

8. Are you taking any blood thinner (anticoagulant)?

Many patients are not familiar with the term anticoagulant, therefore, the term blood thinner should be used. Whenever a patient is taking an anticoagulant, (i.e., warfarin, NSAIDS, etc.) postoperative bleeding after dental surgical procedures is more likely.

9. Have you taken any medications such as pills, powders or liquids in the last week?

Many patients take over the counter medications and do not consider them drugs. One must ask specifically the form in which these medications are taken, such as pills, powders or liquids, because many preparations, especially aspirin, can be found in all three forms.

10. Have you had or do you have any liver disease?

Patients with chronic liver disease, including viral hepatitis and alcoholic liver disease, have a tendency for prolonged bleeding because most of the coagulation factors are synthesized by the liver. In fact, patients with viral hepatitis are often evaluated according to their bleeding status. When bleeding studies are abnormal, the disease is considered more severe than if the results are within the normal range. In chronic alcoholics platelet function may also be impaired secondary to decreased hepatic thrombin production (which hinders platelet aggregation) and platelet sequestration from accompanying splenomegaly.

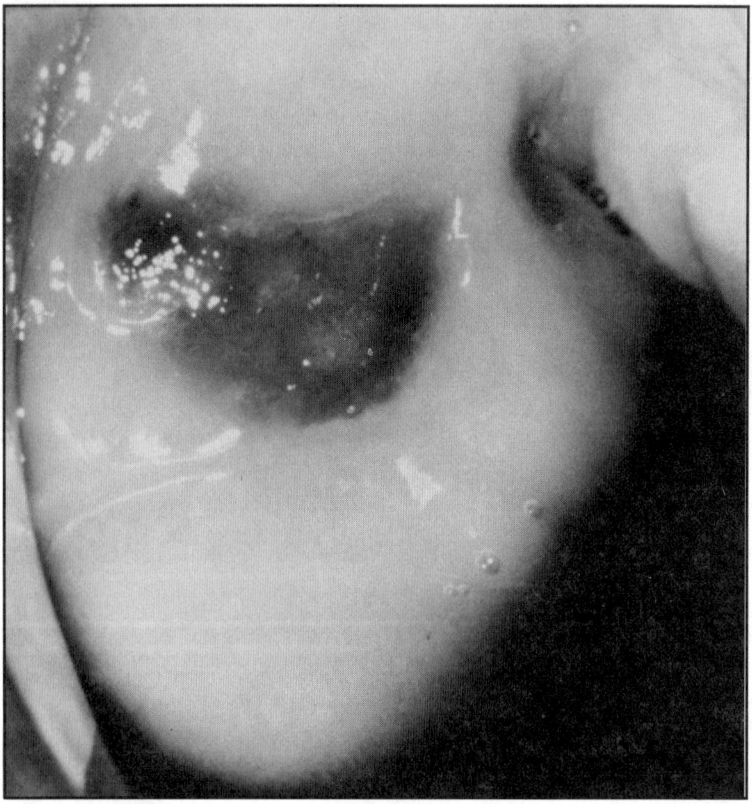

Figure 4-2: Hematoma of the buccal mucosa in a patient taking cancer chemotherapy who is thrombocytopenic.

B. Physical Findings

The vast majority of patients who report to the emergency setting with intraoral bleeding have had recent tooth extractions. Many of these patients have simply failed to follow postoperative instructions such as applying pressure on the extraction site or avoiding rinsing and spitting. Therefore,

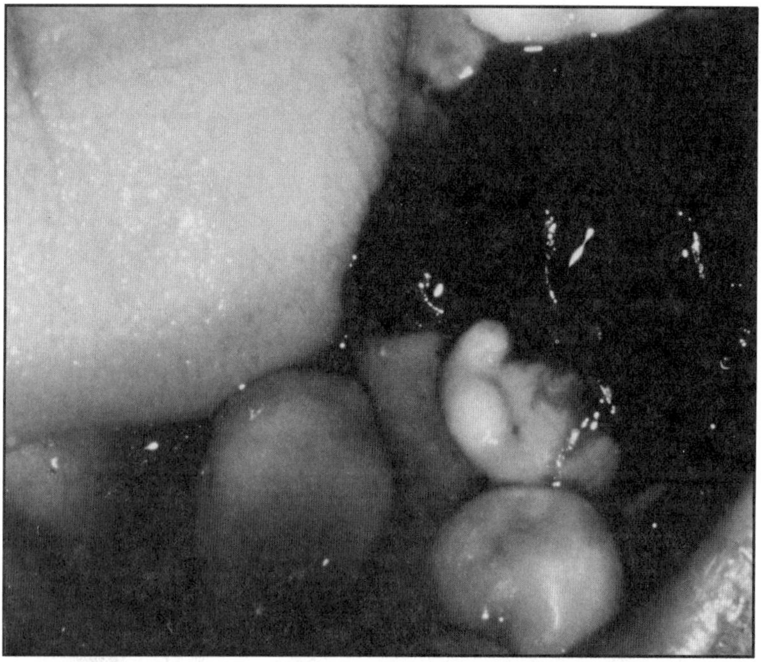

Figure 4-3: Intraoral liver clot after an extraction in a patient with hemophilia A.

minor intraoral bleeding within hours of a tooth extraction is common and usually results from noncompliance. A small quantity of blood mixed with saliva gives the appearance of significant bleeding. However, if a patient reports with postoperative extraction bleeding of up to 24 hours or longer, one's suspicion of an underlying bleeding defect should increase. Patients presenting with abnormal oral bleeding should be considered for any disease that can compromise the hemostatic system. A thorough medical history must be taken initially (Table 4-1).

This history should be combined with the physical findings. The signs manifested by the patient can be helpful in pinpointing the underlying deficit. For example, a platelet disorder is characterized by acute gingival bleeding because the small size of the vasculature can usually be occluded by the platelet phase alone. Other physical findings suggesting a platelet disorder include petechiae of the oral cavity or skin and bruising in areas of chronic trauma such as the extremities (Figure 4-2).

Pure coagulation disorders are characterized by delayed bleeding as intact platelet and vascular phases will initially stop the hemorrhage immediately following the insult. Hemarthrosis, ecchymosis and intraoral liver clots are additional physical findings with coagulation deficits (Figure

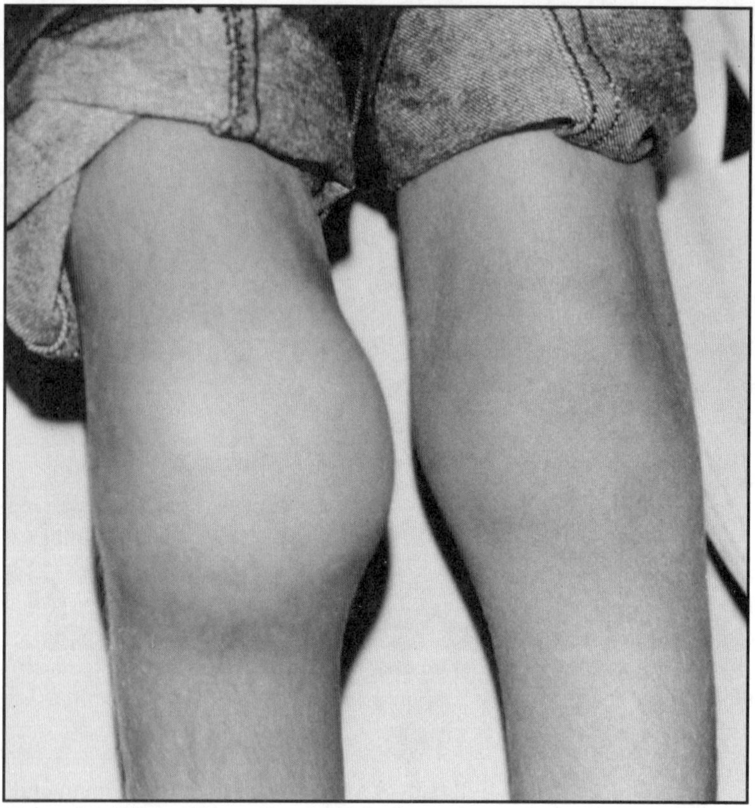

Figure 4-4: Bilateral hemarthrosis of the knees in a patient with hemophilia A.

4-3, 4). Patients with significant coagulation deficits (severe hemophilia A or Von Willebrand's Disease) will most likely have been diagnosed prior to experiencing an acute bleed, (i.e., from prior trauma, tooth extraction, tooth exfoliation, circumcusion or menstruation). Hence, patients with severe bleeding tendencies will normally have a medical history to research. In contrast, patients with mild to moderate coagulation defects may be undiagnosed requiring patient work-up and medical consultation.

C. Laboratory Evaluation

When a patient presents with intraoral bleeding and has a history of prolonged bleeding in the past, certain laboratory tests may be indicated. There are four basic tests that screen for hemostatic deficits which include: 1) the platelet count, 2) the prothrombin time (PT), 3) the partial thromboplastin

Table 4-2: Normal Coagulation Laboratory Values

· PTT	11-14 seconds
· PTT	25-35 seconds
· Platelet count	150-400 thousand/mm^3
· Bleeding Time	3-9 minutes

time (PTT) and 4) the bleeding time. These tests and the normal values are listed in Table 4-2. The platelet count evaluates the platelet phase of coagulation, and indicates the number of platelets present. The test must be requested individually as the complete blood count only includes an estimate of platelets. The normal platelet count is usually between 150,000 and 400,000/mm^3.

When the platelet count drops to 50,000 patients are considered to be at increased risk for prolonged oral bleeding following trauma. When the platelet count dips below 20,000 spontaneous oral bleeding may be observed. It is important to realize that the platelet count only yields information regarding cell number, hence, problems with platelet function will not be discovered by this test.

The bleeding time test evaluates the platelet phase of hemostasis and to a lesser extent the vascular phase. This test grossly evaluates platelet function and thereby provides some indication of platelet number. Hence, when this test is combined with the platelet count, questions concerning the platelet phase of hemostasis can be answered (i.e., does a problem exist and if so is the cause inadequate platelet number or platelet dysfunction?). The bleeding time test is performed by making standardized incisions (1 mm deep and 9 mm long) on the flexor surface of the forearm distal to a blood pressure cuff on the arm inflated to 40 mmHg. Due to the shallow depth of the incisions, only vessels smaller than 50 microns are affected. The incisions are blotted every 30 seconds until no blood is absorbed. The normal range is 3 to 9 minutes, and the test is usually stopped at 20 minutes if bleeding persists. A bleeding time between 9 and 20 minutes would be prolonged though functional. Beyond 20 minutes the platelet phase of hemostasis would be incompetent.

The PT and the PTT are usually ordered together since both evaluate the coagulation phase of hemostasis, and can be determined from a single blood sample. The PT evaluates the extrinsic pathway and is commonly elevated in patients taking oral anticoagulants. Platelet phospholipid is added to the patient's blood and time is recorded until clotting occurs. The normal value for this test is from 11 to 14 seconds and is usually compared to a standard control. The PTT assesses the intrinsic pathway and is elevated with classical hemophilia and Von Willebrand's Disease since Factor 8 falls within the intrinsic pathway of coagulation. Tissue phospholipid is added to the patient's blood and time is recorded until clotting occurs. The normal range for this test is between 25 to 35 seconds and the results are also reported in comparison to a standard control.

When any of these tests are abnormal, more specific tests should be performed to accurately diagnose the patient. If a patient has a coagulation defect, then individual factor assays can be performed to determine which factor is responsible. The normal range of individual factor assays is 50 to 150% of normal and the most commonly ordered factor assay is Factor 8. If the quantity of blood lost is unknown or significant, serial hemoglobins and hematocrits should be ordered to monitor and quantify the problem (Table 4-3 summarizes the characteristics of bleeding disorders).

D. Treatment

Fortunately, most intraoral bleeds that present in an emergency setting can be controlled by local measures alone, hence, the first therapy should always be the application of firm direct pressure to the bleeding site (Figure 4-5).

Prior to any therapy, however, it is mandatory to visualize the site of the bleed in a clean field with a good intraoral light source. The field can be cleaned with evacuation (preferably) or with gauze. Visualization

Evacuate Blood and Saliva (Use Good Light Source)
↓
Apply Firm Manual Pressure Directly to the Sight of Bleeding with Moist Cotton Gauze for 5 Minutes
↓
Repeat above with Topical Thrombin Soaked Cotton Gauze

Extraction Site Bleeding	Generalized Gingival Bleeding
↓	↓
Pack Extraction Socket with Oxidized Cellulose Sponge or Gelatin Sponge Soaked in Topical Thrombin and Suture	Construct Soft Acrylic Carrier, Line with Microfibrillar Collagen, and Place on Bleeding Arch
or	
Pack Extraction Socket with Microfibrillar Collagen and Suture	
↓ consider	
Construct Soft Acrylic Carrier and Place on Bleeding Arch	

Figure 4-5: Flow Diagram to Manage Oral Bleeding Using Local Measures.

Table 4-3: Characteristics of Bleeding Disorders

Disorders	Dysfunction				Signs & Symptoms					Laboratory Tests			
	Platelets		Coagulation		Petechiae	Ecchymosis	Epistaxis	Gingival bleeding	Hemarthrosis	BT	PC	PT	PTT
	number	function	intrinsic	extrinsic									
Platelets													
ITP	+	-	-	-	+	+	+	+	-	+	+	-	-
TTP	+	-	-	-	+	+	+	+	-	+	+	-	-
Thrombasthenia	-	+	-	-	+	+	+	+	-	+	-	-	-
NSAID/Aspirin	-	+	-	-	+	+ -	+	+	-	+	-	-	-
SecondaryTP	+	-	-	-	+	+	+	+	-	+	+	-	-
Coagulation													
Hem A	-	-	+	-	-	+	+ -	+ -	+	-	-	-	+
Hem B	-	-	+	-	-	+	+ -	+ -	+	-	-	-	+
Coumadin	-	-	-	+	-	+	+ -	+ -	-	-	-	+	-
Heparin	-	-	+	-	-	+	+ -	+ -	-	-	-	-	+
Coagulation & Platelets													
Von Will	-	+	+	-	+	+	+	+	-	+	-	-	+
Alcoholism	+	+	+	+	+	+	+	+	-	+	+	+	+

is essential to determine the location and rate of the hemorrhage. Vigorous bleeding from a small arteriole may warrant different treatment than a slow ooze from a single extraction site.

Initially, firm manual pressure should be applied with moist cotton sponges for a period of at least five minutes. It is important to match the size of the sponge with the size of the bleeding site and to insure that the placement of the gauze focuses the pressure on the bleeding site itself. Frequently, patients fail to perform these measures electing to place the gauze in an indiscriminate fashion (between the teeth) which accounts for the lack of success in hemorrhage control. If the bleeding is controlled with this technique, it is prudent to watch the patient for several minutes longer to assure that bleeding will not resume. The patient should be instructed to: 1) avoid manipulating the area, 2) to avoid masticating on that side of the mouth, 3) to avoid spitting and rinsing, and 4) to consume a soft diet for several days. Patients should be given extra gauze to reapply pressure if bleeding resumes.

When local pressure is inadequate, topical hemostatic agents may be employed to supplement the pressure. An absorbable gelatin sponge soaked in topical thrombin may be applied to the area of bleeding with direct pressure or packed in extraction sockets (Figure 4-6). Topical

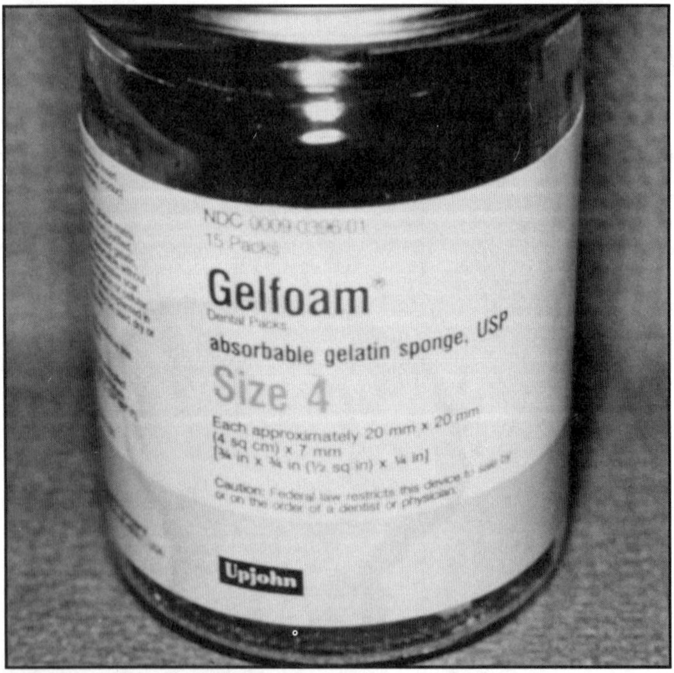

Figure 4-6: Absorbable gelatin sponge.

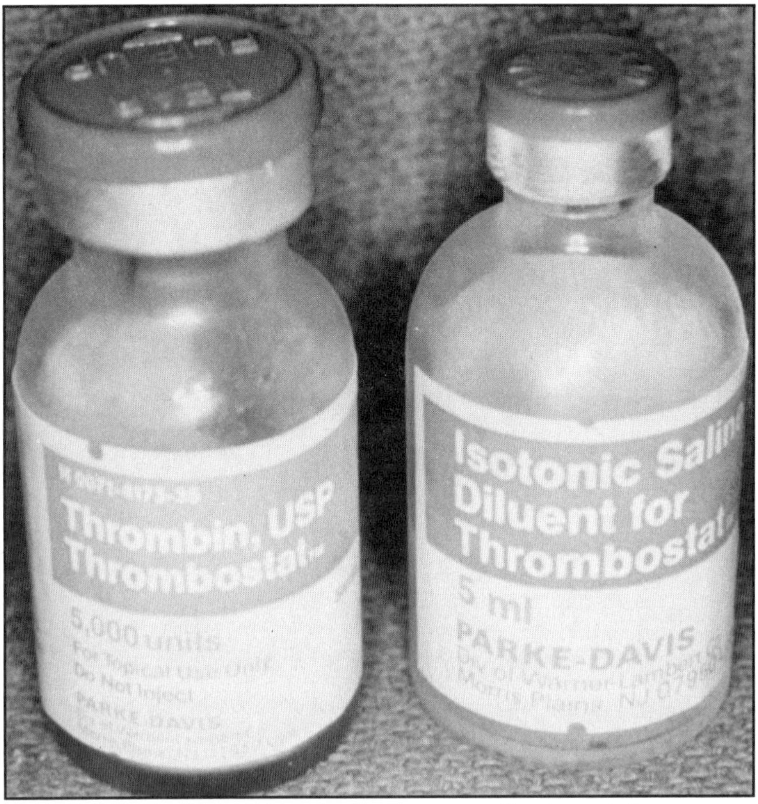

Figure 4-7: Topical Thrombin and saline for preparation to apply to absorbable gelatin sponge.

thrombin comes as a powder to which sterile saline or water must be added. The desired minimal strength is 1000 units per cc (Figure 4-7). Once whetted the sponge is difficult to pack, hence, the material should be placed in a single motion on the first attempt using curved hemostats or cotton pliers. Suturing can also be performed using resorbable suture material to augment and maintain the dressing. Other topical hemostatic agents, such as oxidized cellulose, may also be used to pack extraction sockets (Figure 4-8). However, oxidized cellulose should not be used in combination with topical thrombin since the acidity of the oxidized cellulose will render the topical thrombin ineffective. A third option, microfibrillar collagen powder or sponges, can be applied to localized areas of gingival bleeding in addition to extraction sockets (Figure 4-9).

If bleeding is generalized within the oral cavity, the microfibrillar collagen powder can be placed in a custom made oral carrier. These carriers (trays) are made of soft acrylic and require an alginate impression for

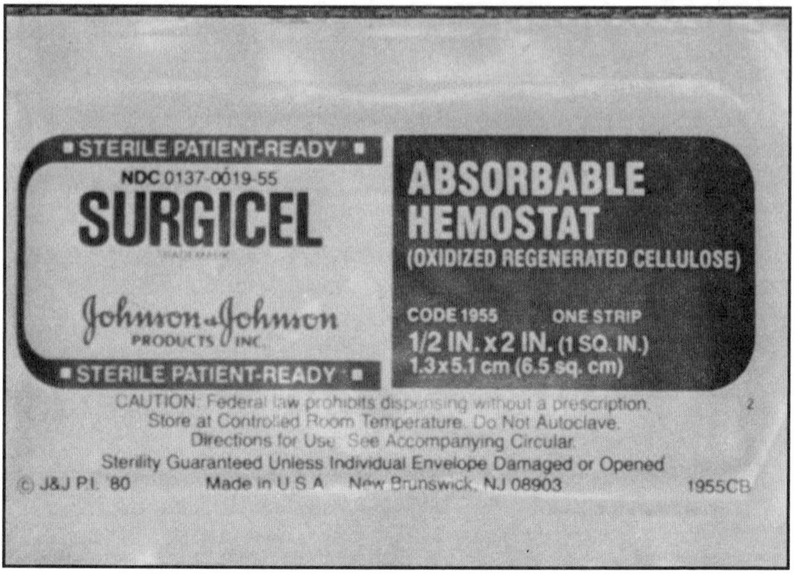

Figure 4-8: Oxidized cellulose.

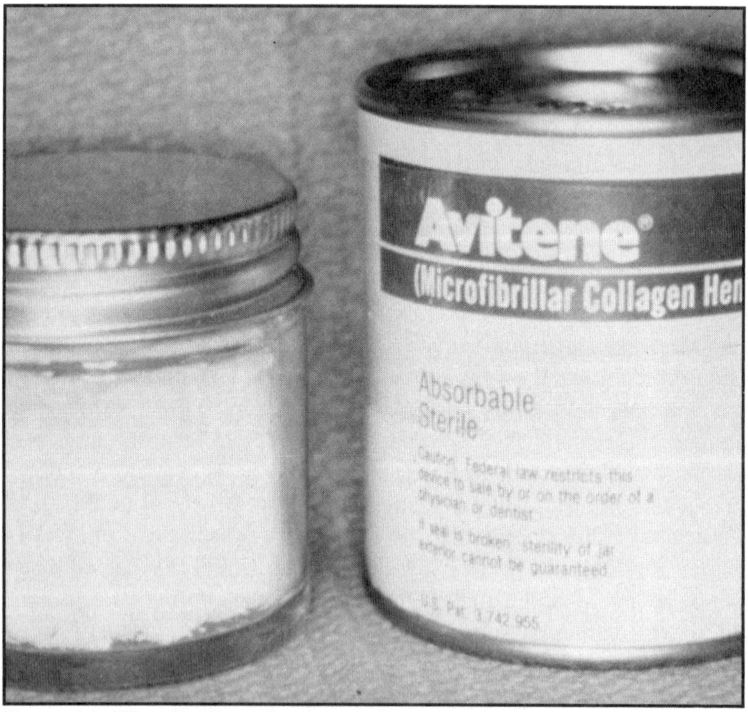

Figure 4-9: Microfibrillar collagen powder.

construction. The time required for fabrication is approximately 45 minutes (Figure 4-10). This technique combines the hemostatic effects of the microfibrillar collagen with the pressure of the custom made carrier. The carriers can also be used to protect extraction sockets after packing with hemostatic agents. Finally, injection of a local anesthetic with a vasoconstrictor such as lidocaine 2% with 1:100,000 or 1:50,000 epinephrine can be employed to slow blood flow to the area of the bleeding. However, caution must be used with this technique as bleeding may resume when the effects of the vasoconstrictor end.

If the aforementioned methods are unsuccessful in hemorrhage control, an occult systemic hemostatic deficit should be suspected and the appropriate screening laboratory tests ordered. Patients receiving anticoagulant therapy commonly present with intraoral bleeding secondary to trauma and/or supratherapeutic drug levels. The most commonly used outpatient anticoagulant, warfarin, is given orally and appears to inhibit the action of coagulation factors 2, 7, 9 and 10. These are the vitamin K dependent factors which require vitamin K for activation. Warfarin blocks this activation process and creates a hemostatic deficit. This anticoagulation is usually measured by the PT, although some believe that the PTT should be included because factor 9 inhibition is not assessed by the PT. Generally,

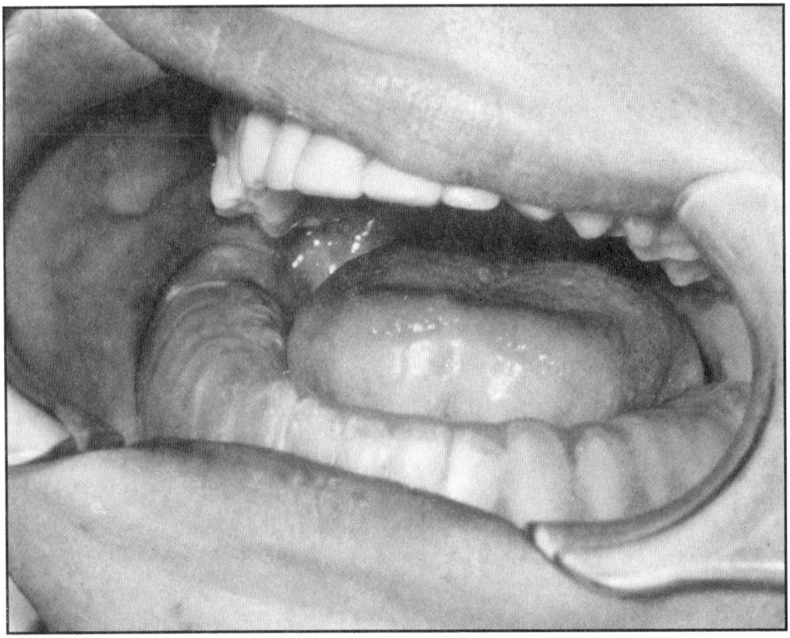

Figure 4-10: Custon made soft acrylic tray (carrier).

the anticoagulant is adjusted to maintain the PT at approximately 1½ to 2 times the control value. When patients taking warfarin report with intraoral bleeding, a PT should be ordered to determine if the patient is within the therapeutic range. Irrespective of the PT value, the local measures of hemostasis listed above should be attempted to control the bleeding.

If the patient lies outside the therapeutic range and the bleeding is not controlled with local measures, then systemic measures should be considered. Such measures can include stopping the warfarin, transfusing the patient with fresh frozen plasma or administering vitamin K. Warfarin therapy is cumbersome because of a prolonged latency period of 36 to 72 hours prior to therapeutic effects and a protracted duration of action (4 to 5 days). Vitamin K will reverse the action of warfarin; however, after this therapy the patient will be refractory to subsequent warfarin administration. Therefore, treatment with fresh frozen plasma (1000 ml) and stopping the warfarin therapy is preferred initially, followed by vitamin K if necessary. Warfarin therapy can be resumed when bleeding has stopped and the clot appears stable (1 to 2 hours). 10 mg of vitamin K may be administered either orally (slow reversal requiring days) or intravenously (fast reversal requiring hours).

In the unusual situation in which a patient presents with acute oral bleeding while on heparin anticoagulation, medication adjustment can be accomplished much more expeditiously. Heparin acts by accelerating anti-thrombin 3 and can only be administered parenterally. Anti-thrombin 3 inhibits coagulation factors throughout the cascade in both pathways. The therapy is usually monitored by the PTT and the dosage is adjusted to maintain the PTT between 1½ to 2 times the control. Since the half life of heparin is relatively short (between 2 and 4 hours) its effects will be diminished shortly after the drug is discontinued. When patients are taking heparin, a PTT should be ordered to determine the patient's level of anticoagulation. The aforementioned local measures should be attempted and if unsuccessful, the patient should be taken off their heparin anticoagulation. When bleeding is not life threatening, local measures should be continued until the bleeding stops. The patient should be followed to assure that adequate hemostasis occurs, then restarted on heparin anticoagulation shortly thereafter.

When emergency cessation of bleeding is necessary the action of heparin can be reversed by the parenteral administration of protamine. The protamine can be titrated according to the PTT until a desirable level of hemostatic competency is attained. As mentioned earlier, many patients are now on anticoagulation with aspirin because of its antiplatelet effects. This is especially true in patients who have suffered heart attacks or strokes. Although this therapy alone is not typically responsible for abnormal oral bleeding, in combination with a minor hemostatic deficit, serious oral bleeding may occur following trauma. In the vast majority of cases, this bleeding will be controlled with local factors. However, if bleeding continues, the aspirin should be stopped and the patient should be worked up for an occult hemostatic disorder. Patients with inherited coagulopathies may require factor replacement when presenting with acute oral bleeding, especially secondary to tooth extraction. As with all bleeding patients, local measures should be attempted initially, and if unsuccessful, systemic therapies considered. The type of replacement therapy employed will depend on the type and severity of the factor deficiency. Hence, the information must be obtained either historically or via a factor assay.

Severe coagulopathies require factor replacement in concentrated forms (i.e., factor 8 concentrate or cryoprecipitate for hemophilia A) to achieve hemostasis. The therapeutic goal following factor 8 replacement is 50% of the normal factor level. Hence, the needed factor replacement may be determined once the patient's factor level is determined.

A formula for determining the needed quantity of replacement factor 8 is as follows: # of units needed = (Desired factor level in units/cc of blood minus Patient's present factor level in units/cc of blood) times Patient's plasma volume. In computing this formula it should be understood that 1 unit/cc of blood is the normal level (100%); hence, if the goal was 50%, then the desired factor 8 level would be .5 units/cc. Also plasma volume is approximately 41 ml/kg of body weight (Table 4-4).

Factor concentrates represent the most concentrated form of factor 8 replacement, and this therapy has a 12 hour half life. The more concentrated the source of factor 8 replacement, the smaller the transfused fluid volume and the less the chance for fluid overload. However, this concentration requires blood from thousands of donors and exposes the recipient to risk of blood born infectious diseases (Hepatitis B and AIDS). This risk has been lessened in recent years with heat treating of factor concentrates.

Table 4-4: Therapies to Reduce Bleeding in Hemophilia A

Factor 8 Units Needed = (Desired Factor 8 Level-Initial Factor 8 level) x Plasma Volume (41 ml/kg body weight)

Factor 8 Concentrate - infuse appropriate number of units as estimated above

- Cryoprecipitate - 80 to 100 units/bag, estimate number of units as above
- Desmopressin - 0.3 μg/kg in 50 ml saline infused over 30 minutes
- EACA - 8 gm orally three times daily for 7 to 10 days after surgery

(Factor 8 levels should be drawn after infusion to determine accurate levels for all therapies. One unit of Factor 8 is the activity in 1 ml of normal plasma)

A second form of replacement therapy for moderate to severe factor 8 deficiencies is cryoprecipitate, which is the precipitate formed when plasma from multiple donors is frozen. Cryoprecipitate is high in factor 8 activity with approximately 80-100 units per bag. Because cryoprecipitate is a less concentrated source of factor 8, a larger fluid volume must be transfused compared to factor concentrates to reach the same endpoint. However, the risk of infectious disease transmission is less with cryoprecipitate, because the donor number is much smaller. Both factor concentrates and cryoprecipitate are administered slowly (5 cc per minute) as an intravenous infusion.

Regarding mild to moderate hemophilia A or Von Willibrand's Disease, desmopressin or DDAVP (1-desamino-8-*D*-arginine vasopressin) can increase factor 8 levels by 4 to 6 fold. The drug is administered intravenously and produces peak blood levels at 90 minutes tapering to baseline at 24 hours. To administer, .3 mcg/kg are infused slowly over a 15 to 30 minute period, and the most common side effect is blood pressure elevation (Table 4-4).

In addition to restoring coagulation competency, the maintenance of clot stability following formation is critical to prevent re-bleeding. Epsilon-aminocaproic acid (EACA) inhibits plasmin formation and is helpful in preventing clot breakdown. The half-life is 4 hours and the drug can be given as tablets or elixir. The elixir is preferred for oral bleeding because of potential topical effects (plasmin has been found in saliva) and is given as 8 gm three times per day for 7 to 10 days (Table 4-4).

Patients who have hemophilia A with intraoral bleeding are handled according to their residual factor level as previously discussed. While local measures may suffice for mild factor 8 deficiencies, local measures, transfusions (factor 8 concentrates or cryoprecipitate) and EACA are generally required for severe factor deficiencies. The combination of DDAVP, local measures and EACA would be indicated for mild to moderate disease. Moderate to severe deficiencies of factor 9 (Hemophilia B) are treated with factor 9 complex transfusions, local measures and EACA.

Table 4-5: Relative Costs of Products to treat patients with factor 8 deficiency

Product	Cost per Dose
· Factor 8 Concentrate	$ 1260
· Cryoprecipitate	$ 672
· DDAVP	$ 209
· EACA	$ 323
· Topical Thrombin	$ 22
· Microfibrillar Collagen	$ 97

Mild factor 9 deficiencies can be managed with local measures alone or in combination with fresh frozen plasma. Factor 9 levels of 25% normal are desirable and can be accomplished by administering an initial dose of 50 units/kg of factor 9 complex intravenously followed by 20 units/kg every 12 to 24 hours. Treatment of Von Willibrand's Disease attempts to normalize the factor 8 level and correct the qualitative platelet defect. Cryprecipitate, local measures and EACA are the treatment of choice in patients with moderate to severe deficiencies. DDAVP, local measures, and EACA can be used on moderate cases and local measures alone with mild deficits.

Some patients with hemophilia A (as high as 10%) will develop significant antibodies (inhibitors) against factor 8 rendering this therapy ineffective. Patients with high antibody titers should be treated with factor 9 complex whereas those with low titers can be managed with high doses of factor 8 (Caution: patients with high antibody titers may not respond to any transfusion therapy). Therefore, it is important to determine from history the presence of antibodies to factor 8. Products used to treat patients with factor deficiencies tend to be very expensive, but have enabled these patients to be treated on an outpatient basis. However due to their cost and potential for transmission of infectious disease, it is imperative that these products be used only when needed after the proper diagnosis is made (Table 4-5).

Table 4-6: Management of Bleeding Disorders

Disorders	Therapeutic Management
Platelets	
I T P	Local measures, platelet transfusion
T T P	Local measures, platelet transfusion
Thrombasthenia	Local measures, DDAVP
NSAID/Aspirin	Local measures, cessation of drug
Secondary T P	Local measures, platelet transfusion
Coagulation	
Hem A	Local measures, DDAVP, Cryoprecipitate, Factor 8 concentrate, EACA
Hem B	Local measures, fresh frozen plasma, Factor 9 complex, EACA
Coumadin	Local measures, fresh frozen plasma, vitamin K
Heparin	Local measures, cessation of drug, protamine
Coagulation & Platelets	
Von Will	Local measures, DDAVP, cryoprecipitate, Factor 8 concentrate, EACA
Alcoholism	Local measures

Patients who are mild to moderately thrombocytopenic can commonly be treated with local measures alone to control acute bleeding. However with very low platelet counts (below 20,000), platelet replacement therapy must be considered in addition to local measures. Replacement therapy for oral bleeding should attempt to raise the platelet count to at least 50,000 for a period of time to enable adequate hemostasis and clot formation. The transfusion of 1 unit of platelets should raise the platelet count by 10,000 mm^3. The development of platelet antibodies is high (75%) in patients receiving repeat platelet transfusions. Therefore, platelet transfusions should be given judiciously. In addition to platelet transfusions, local measures should always be employed. With any acute bleeding the transfusion of red blood cells (RBCs) should be performed when 750 cc of blood has been lost or the patient shows signs and symptoms of anemia. Such manifestations would include pallor, tachycardia (an increase of 20 beats per minute above baseline in the heart rate) and hypotension (a 10mm Hg decrease in diastolic pressure). Signs and symptoms are generally manifested when 15 to 30% of the blood volume is lost. Changes in the patient's hematocrit are not helpful with acute bleeding, because extravascular compensation for the lost fluid volume occurs over a 24 to 48 hour period. Until this equalization takes place, the relationship of RBCs to the plasma will be maintained, since whole blood is being lost. When RBC transfusion is indicated, one unit of packed red blood cells (PRBCs) can be expected to elevate the hematocrit by 3%. When the need for transfusion is uncertain, 2 liters of a crystalloid solution can be infused over a 5 to 10 minute period and the patient observed. If signs and symptoms fail to improve, then RBC transfusion is warranted. The transfusion of a crystalloid solution is also indicated until blood crossmatching results are available (requires approximately 1 hour) in the patient needing a RBC transfusion (Table 4-6 summarizes the management of bleeding disorders).

References

Biggs R., *The Treatment of Hemophilia A and B and Von Willebrand's Disease.* Oxford: Blackwell Scientific Publications, 1978.

Evans B.E., Aledort L.M., "Hemophilia and Dental Treatment." *J Am Dent Assoc.* 96 (1978): 827.

Evans B.E., Irving S.P., Aledort L.M., "Use of microcrystalline collagen for hemostasis after oral surgery in a hemophiliac." *J Oral Surg.* 37 (1979): 126.

Larson C.E., et al., "Anesthetic considerations for the oral surgery patient with hemophilia." *J Oral Surg.* 38 (1980): 516.

Lucas O.N., Prescott G.H., "Hemophilia and other hemorrhagic disorders." *Dent Clin North Am.* 19 (1975): 63.

Needleman H.L., Kaban L.B., Kevy S.V., "The use of epsilon aminocaproic acid for the management of hemophilia in dental and oral surgery patients." *J Am Dent Assoc.* 93 (1976): 586.

Olive J.A., "Disorders of hemostasis." In Tullman M., Redding S. (eds). *Systemic Disease in Dental Treatment*. New York: Appleton Century Crafts, 1982.
Redding S.W., Montgomery M.T., *Dentistry in Systemic Disease*. Portland: JBK Publishing, 1990.
Redding S.W., "Evaluation of Bleeding Disorders." *Compen of Cont Ed in Dent*. 5 (1984): 25-30.
Sacks S.A., Lipton R., Frank R., "Management of ambulatory oral surgical patients with hemophilia." *J Oral Surg*. 36 (1978): 25.
Stein J.H., *Internal Medicine - Diagnosis and Therapy*. East Norwalk: Appleton & Lange, 1988.
Thompson A.R., Harker L.A., *Manual of Hemostasis and Thrombosis*. 3rd Ed., Philadelphia: FA Davis Company, 1983.

5 Acute Mucogingival Inflammatory Conditions

Robert M. Craig, Jr., D.D.S.

Mucogingival inflammatory conditions are probably the most common presenting complaint of patients excluding toothache. Despite the wide spectrum of pathosis included in this group, the clinical presentation for many of these lesions is surprisingly limited. Erythema, swelling and ulceration are frequently the mucosal changes noted; as such, the diagnosis can often present a challenge to the clinician. Because of the similar presentation but differing clinical management of some of these lesions, it is imperative that an accurate diagnosis be established from a thorough medical/dental history, a complete head and neck examination and appropriate laboratory studies. The following discussion of these entities will start with the most common lesions and proceed to the less common.

I. RECURRENT APHTHOUS STOMATITIS

Although the lesions of recurrent aphthous stomatitis (RAS), also known as canker sores, are well known to practitioners, the etiology of these lesions remains unclear. Current theory favors an immunologic defect in the humoral immune system, but other factors including nutritional status, stress, food allergies and microbiologic organisms have been considered. Excluding trauma, RAS is the most common etiology of oral ulcers. RAS is seen in a wide age spectrum but most frequently occurs between the ages of 10 and 30. It is more prevalent in professionals and individuals in a higher socio-economic level. Recurrence is common, although frequency of recurrent episodes varies greatly between individuals.

RAS has three recognized forms: minor, major and herpetiform aphthous ulcers. Minor aphthous ulcers are by far the most common and usually consist of one of two painful ulcers less than 1.0 cm in diameter. The ulcerations are superficial with a grey/white center and prominent erythematous periphery. They occur on movable mucosa including the vestibule, tongue, buccal mucosa and soft palate, and heal in 7 to 10 days without scarring. Major aphthous ulcers are also known as periadenitis mucosa necrotica recurrens or Sutton's disease. Compared to minor RAS, the ulcers are larger than 1.0 cm, are more painful, have a longer duration (up to 6 weeks), occur more frequently and tend to heal with scarring (Figure 5-1). Major aphthae occur in the same mucosal areas as minor aphthae, whereas herpetiform aphthous ulcers, the third variant, may also involve the gingiva and hard palate. As the name implies, herpetiform ulcers resemble those of recurrent herpetic stomatitis. Both lesions occur in small crops and in similar locations. In contrast, however, herpetiform ulcers are not preceded by a vesicle and viral cultures for herpes will be negative. Aphthous ulcers can also occur in association with HIV infection, in which their presentation may be atypical with respect to size, location, frequency of episodes and duration.

The diagnosis of RAS is based on clinical identification since the histologic changes are nonspecific and there is no known microbiologic organism to culture. Differential diagnosis includes: 1) trauma, which

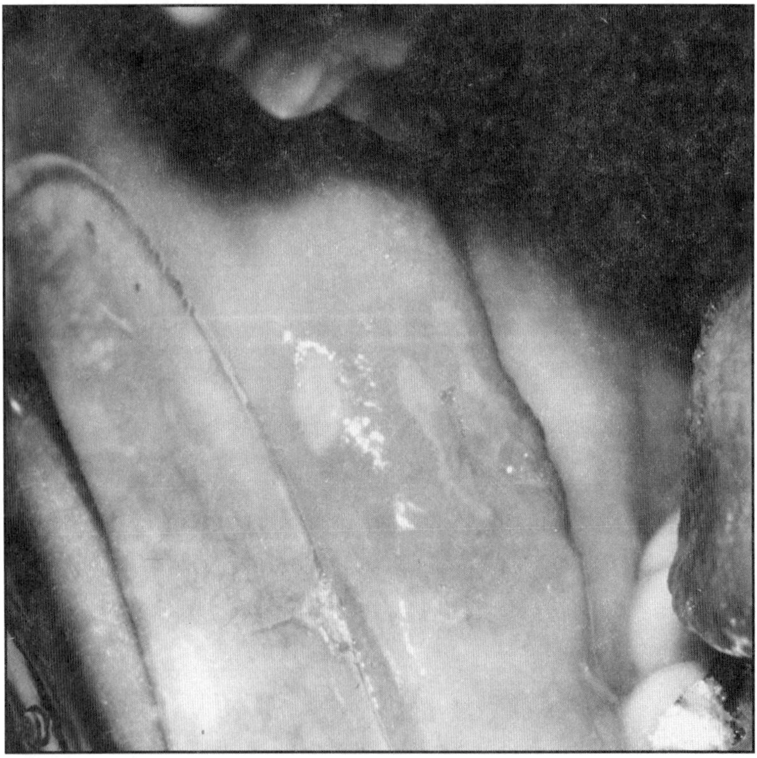

Figure 5-1: Major aphthae - These ulcers are similar to those of minor aphthae but they tend to be larger, last longer and heal with scarring.

can usually be determined by the history, 2) recurrent herpes simplex, which unlike aphthous ulcers has a vesicular stage and herpes virus cultures are positive, 3) pemphigus vulgaris, which has a distinct histologic appearance and clinically demonstrates the formation of vesicles or bullae, and 4) one of the aphthous-like ulcers associated with systemic conditions such Bechet's syndrome, Crohn's disease, neutropenia and ulcerative colitis.

Treatment of aphthous ulcers is primarily based on relief of symptoms. For minor aphthae topical steroids such as fluocinonide or tetracycline suspension have been used with some success. 0.12% chlorhexidine gluconate mouthrinse has also provided relief for some patients with minor aphthae. Major aphthae and herpetiform aphthae, however, are less likely to respond to fluocinonide and often require the use of systemic corticosteroids (usually prednisone) in severe cases (See Table of Medications).

II. HERPES SIMPLEX VIRUS

Oral lesions resulting from infection by herpes simplex virus (HSV) are classified as primary or recurrent (secondary). The oral cavity may be infected by either HSV I or HSV II variants and the clinical manifestations are identical. The primary infection is the initial attack by the virus following contact with an infected person, and most commonly occurs in children and young adults. Primary HSV infections consist of an acute gingivostomatitis with a vesicular eruption involving any area of the oral mucosa, lips or perioral skin. The lesions are often accompanied by fever, malaise, painful lymphadenopathy and arthralgia (Figure 5-2). The infection usually runs its course in one to two weeks and the lesions heal without scarring. Many patients apparently experience a subclinical infection following the initial exposure to HSV as there are a large number of people who have serum antibodies to HSV but who have never manifested the clinical signs or symptoms of a primary infection. It is also of interest to note that viral shedding may occur in the saliva of an asymptomatic person previously infected with HSV. The potential for transmission from such an individual is unknown.

A hallmark of HSV infection is a latency period following the primary exposure, with later recurrent or secondary infections. Approximately 40% of the population, primarily adults, suffer from recurrent HSV infections. After the initial exposure, the virus migrates to the trigeminal ganglion where it remains latent until reactivated by any of a number of factors including stress, trauma, sunlight or cold. Prodromal symptoms consisting of a burning sensation, mild pain or pruritis may occur after viral reactivation. Presumably these symptoms result from the virus traveling along the trigeminal nerve to the mucosa where a focal eruption of small

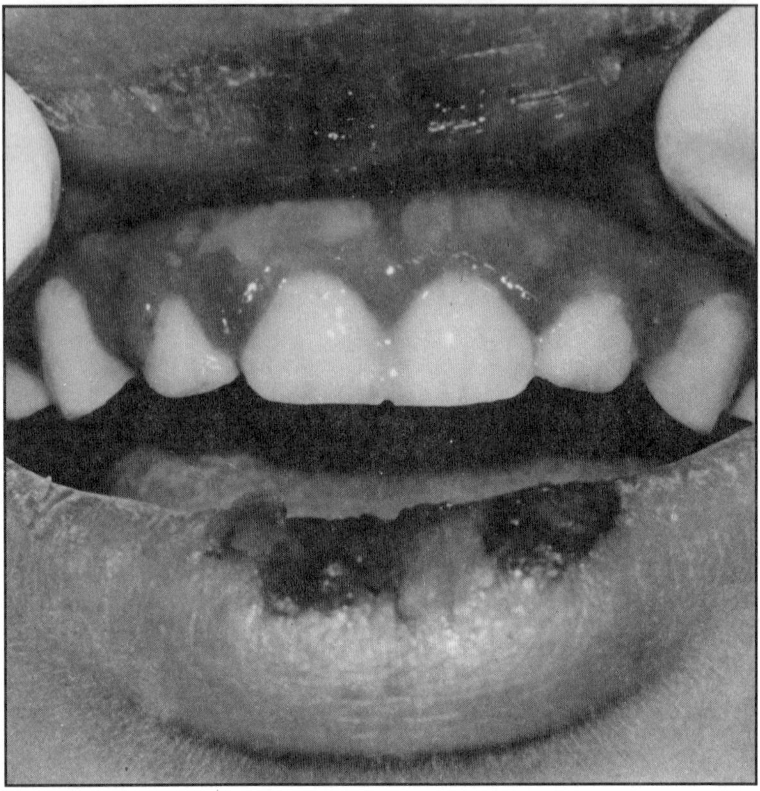

Figure 5-2: Primary herpetic gingivostomatitis - These painful oral-labial lesions are accompanied by fever, malaise and lymphadenopathy (Courtesy of Dr. Craig Miller).

vesicles is the first clinical sign of a secondary infection. The vesicles occur on the lip, gingiva or hard palate and quickly rupture to form small, shallow, painful ulcers which coalesce to produce a larger ulcerated lesion. The secondary infection will resolve in one to two weeks when the virus returns to the trigeminal ganglion where it remains latent until reactivated again. It is during the vesicular stage that HSV lesions have the greatest potential for transmission.

The diagnosis of an HSV infection is based on the clinical appearance of the lesions and the patient's history of previous exposures (past signs and symptoms) in combination with certain laboratory tests for confirmation. In evaluating the patient's history, it is important to investigate the frequency, location, duration, appearance and associated etiologies of intraoral and extraoral ulcerations. The terms "fever blister" and "cold sores" are more commonly recognized by patients.

Regarding laboratory tests, cytologic smears are rapid and inexpensive but nonspecific for HSV unless stained with fluorescent antisera. The smears are best obtained from the base of vesicles, although samples can also be obtained at the base of ulcers and beneath crusted lip lesions. A sterile swab or cotton tipped applicator can be used to obtain the specimen which is immediately transferred to a laboratory slide. Crusted lesions can be "unroofed" with a moistened gauze prior to obtaining a sample. The specimen is stained with Wright-Giemsa or Papanicolaou stain, and if positive shows epithelial changes typically associated with viral infections. These histologic findings include the presence of multinucleated giant cells and ballooning degeneration of epithelial cells with eosinophilic intranuclear inclusions displacing the nuclear chromatin and nucleolus to the periphery. A biopsy of HSV lesions is also nonspecific and positive specimens shows similar changes in epithelial cells associated with intraepithelial vesicles containing inflammatory cells and exudate. Viral culture is the most sensitive of the diagnostic tests, especially during the early stage of the infection, and can establish the diagnosis within 48 hours. Samples are obtained as previously described and transported in an appropriate medium which is generally provided by the laboratory. The medium usually contains an antifungal agent and an antibiotic to minimize the overgrowth of nonviral organisms. The medium should be kept cold during transportation (i.e., placed in the refrigerator or in a cup of ice).

Less specific but more rapid than culture is detection of HSV antigens by enzyme immunoassay, immunofluorescence or immunoperoxidase staining, which will yield results in less than 24 hours. Serologic antibody assays may also be used in the diagnosis of HSV infections, but because of the length of time involved (two to three weeks) are less useful for making therapeutic decisions.

Other entities included in the differential diagnosis of primary HSV infection include acute necrotizing ulcerative gingivitis (ANUG), streptococcal pharyngitis and erythema multiforme. In ANUG, the lesions are limited to the gingiva and the ulcers do not go through a vesicular stage. Also, necrosis of the interdental papillae, characteristic of ANUG, is not a feature of HSV. Streptococcal pharyngitis does not feature vesicular eruptions or involve lip lesions. Erythema multiforme forms larger ulcers, usually without vesicles, and the lesions uncommonly involve the gingiva. Aphthous ulcers which were described previously, traumatic ulcers and lesions associated with allergic reactions may resemble secondary HSV infections. Herpes zoster also resembles HSV clinically but usually has a characteristic distribution that ends abruptly at anatomical midlines and the lesions have a longer duration than HSV. Distinguishing HSV from zoster can be made by antigen typing of the virus. As with aphthous ulcers,

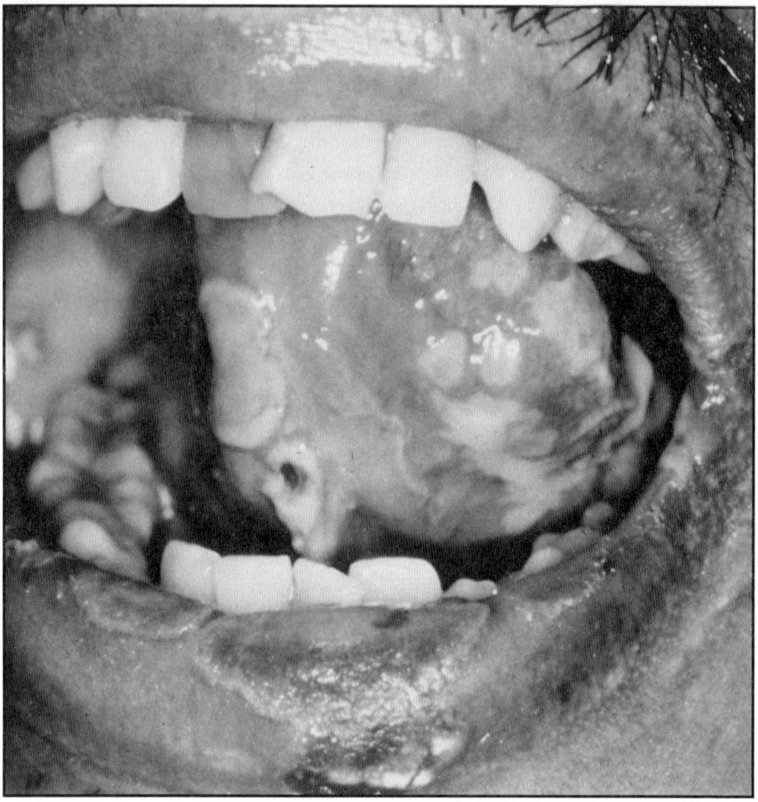

Figure 5-3: Recurrent herpes simplex in an HIV- infected patient - The vesicular eruptions are larger, more widespread, and have a different distribution than in the immunocompetent patient.

HSV infection in the immunocompromised patient may be confusing to the clinician. Atypical presentations occur in which the appearance, distribution and duration of the lesions, either primary or secondary, do not conform to the expected clinical pattern for the disease (Figure 5-3). HSV etiology should be considered in immunocompromised patients to include HIV positive, chemotherapy, bone marrow transplant or organ transplant patients with oral ulcers. In such cases, and in all cases when lesion identification cannot be made based on historical and clinical data, laboratory testing is recommended. HSV lesions lasting more than one month in an HIV positive patient qualify as an opportunistic infection defining Acquired Immunodeficiency Syndrome (AIDS).

Many forms of treatment have been used for HSV infection with varying results. The primary anti-viral drug currently used for HSV infection is acyclovir. It is important that therapy be instituted as soon as possible to maximize the drug's effectiveness. However, the efficacy of acyclovir therapy has yet to be proven in non-immunocompromised patients. Although patients empirically report therapeutic benefit, scientific validation is lacking. It has been reported that the use of oral tablets (200 mg five times daily) or topical ointment (5%), applied five times a day with the onset of symptoms may alleviate or abort secondary lesions in some cases. Primary HSV infections are usually treated with rest, fluids, antipyretics and gentle oral lavage. Acyclovir tablets (200 mg, five times per day) and intravenous acyclovir are approved for treating oral HSV infections in immunocompromised patients (Table of Medications). The intravenous dosing is 5 mg/kg administered over 1 hour, three times daily and resolution is generally rapid. Immunocompromised patients with severe infections may require hospitalization and intravenous acyclovir administration. The hospitalization can involve a few days of parenteral administration or placing the patient in observation for intravenous administration followed by oral outpatient dosing.

III. TRAUMATIC ULCERS

Traumatic ulcers may vary considerably in their clinical appearance based on the type, duration and magnitude of the initiating trauma. Low grade, chronic irritation commonly results in a focally ulcerated area of leukoplakia, whereas a more intense trauma may cause an ulcer of varying depth with peripheral erythema and considerable discomfort. Traumas such as chemical or thermal injuries often cause more diffuse ulcerations. Despite the spectrum of clinical manifestations, traumatic ulcers can usually be diagnosed from the patient's history. Occasionally the patient may not remember the event until questioned specifically about various forms of trauma, so specific questioning is required. Clinical examination may also identify the source of trauma, as with fractured teeth and restorations or malposed teeth. Once the diagnosis is made, the traumatic ulcer will heal without treatment after the source of irritation is removed. If necessary, symptomatic relief can be obtained by a variety of agents including topical anesthetics such as benzocaine or lidocaine in an adherent base (i.e., 2% viscous lidocaine mixed with Maalox or Milk of Magnesia in a 1:1 ratio (Table of Medications). Only in severe cases would an antibiotic rinse such as tetracycline be indicated to prevent secondary infection.

IV. CANDIDIASIS

Candidiasis is the most common oral fungal infection, occurs in both young and old patients and is prevalent in immunocompromised and cancer patients. Candida is an opportunistic fungus with many local and/or systemic factors involved in its conversion from a commensal to a pathogenic organism. In infants and the elderly, candidiasis may be related to immaturity or aging, respectively, of the immune system. Patients undergoing antibiotic therapy will sometimes manifest an overgrowth of candida as the populations of other microorganisms are reduced by the medication. Patients with endocrine imbalances including diabetes mellitus, pregnancy or those on systemic steroids are also prone to candidal infections as are malnourished individuals. Although *C. albicans* is the most common species involved, other potential species include *C. parapsilosis*, *C. tropocalis* and *C. glabrata*.

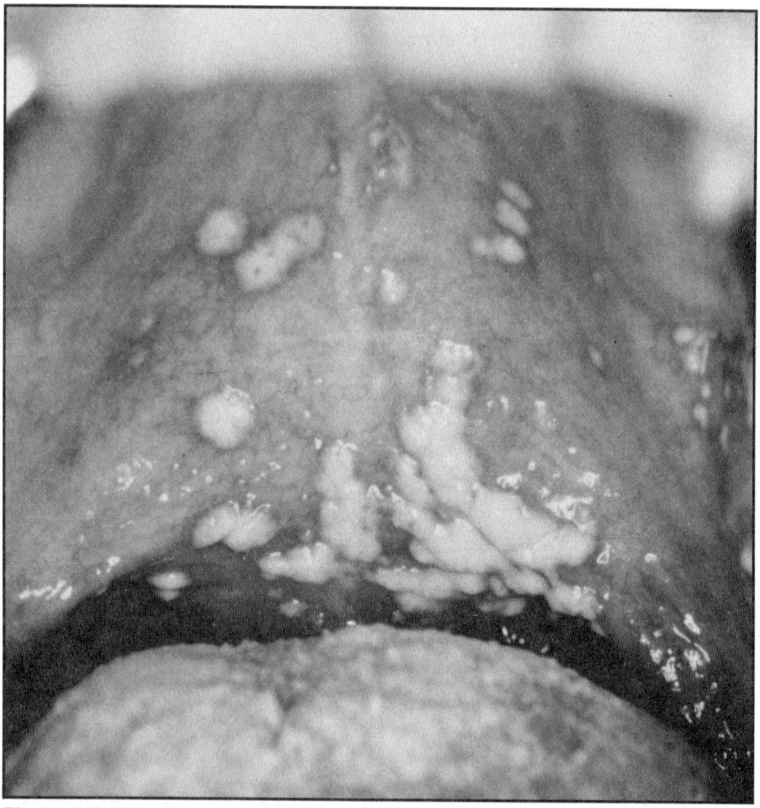

Figure 5-4: Pseudomembranous candidiasis - The typical curd-like lesions can be easily rubbed off leaving an erythematous bleeding base.

The classification of oral candidiasis infections is usually based on the differences in clinical presentation. Pseudomembranous candidiasis is the most common type with characteristic diffuse or multifocal white curd-like plaques that are loosely adherent to the mucosa. These plaques are easily wiped from the mucosal surface leaving an erythematous and sometimes bleeding base (Figure 5-4). Patients may complain of burning or tenderness, but in most cases symptoms are minimal. The erythematous form of candidiasis appears as red atrophic lesions, similar to what is seen after removing the white plaques in the pseudomembranous type. This form is frequently painful, and commonly associated with antibiotic or steroid use. A third form, hypertrophic candidiasis consists of asymptomatic, tenacious, large white plaques and is usually associated with chronic infections. Median rhomboid glossitis and inflammatory papillary hyperplasia of the palate may be the result of chronic hyperplastic candida infections. Angular cheilitis, an extraoral form of candidiasis is also relatively common and consists of painful fissured ulcers at the commissures of the mouth. Typically these lesions are seen in patients who have worn dentures for many years and have subsequently lost vertical dimension. Mucocutaneous forms of candidiasis may be localized or diffuse. The localized form consists of persistent pseudomembranous plaques involving the oral and vaginal mucosas accompanied by skin and cuticular lesions. A diffuse form of mucocutaneous candidiasis is apparently familial (autosomal dominant) with approximately half of the cases associated with an endocrinopathy such as hyperparathyroidism, Addison's disease, hypothyroidism or diabetes mellitus.

Candidiasis is an important opportunistic infection in patients infected with HIV and is the most common oral manifestation of this disease. While the pseudomembranous form is the most common in HIV-infected patients, angular cheilitis in a young patient or the erythematous form involving the gingiva or buccal mucosa multifocally are also associated with an underlying HIV infection. As with other infections, candidiasis in the immunocompromised patient is often atypical in its clinical presentation and course. In these patients, the infections are commonly refractory to the usual antifungal agents. Also, the immunocompromised patients are usually between 20 and 50 years of age rather than young or elderly. Although oral candidiasis does not define AIDS, it does appear to be a predictor of the development of AIDS in the HIV positive patient. In these patients oral candidiasis may also foretell the development of esophageal or pharyngeal candidiasis, Kaposi's sarcoma or other opportunistic infections within the following 3 to 12 month periods.

Candidiasis may be diagnosed on the basis of clinical appearance, culture, histologic examination, or cytologic examination using a 10% KOH preparation or gram stain. Cytologic smears demonstrate typical hyphae, whereas biopsy specimens reveal hyphae infiltrating the keratin or spinous cell layer of the epithelium accompanied by an inflammatory infiltrate and microabscess formation. Candida can be cultured on several media including blood agar or Saboraud's broth.

Candidiasis can be effectively treated topically with nystatin suspension or clotrimazole troches (Table of Medications). When dentures are present, they should be disinfected and the patient given instructions on proper care. Nystatin cream may be placed on the denture for topical application in cases of candida-induced denture stomatitis. Generally the topical medications are used for a period extending one week after the candidal lesions have disappeared clinically. In cases of severe candidiasis, chronic mucocutaneous candidiasis or infections in immunocompromised patients, it may be necessary to use systemic antifungal agents such as oral ketoconazole, oral fluconazole or intravenous amphotericin B (Table of Medications). Patients on these drugs should be monitored closely because of the potentially serious side effects. Ketoconazole can be hepatotoxic or may cause a hypersensitivity reaction, nausea or vomiting. Fluconazole may also be hepatotoxic or lead to exfoliative skin lesions. Amphotericin B should only be used by clinicians experienced in its use as nephrotoxicity, fever, hypotension, phlebitis and many other side effects are possible. Chlorhexidine gluconate mouthwash (Peridex™) 0.12% has also been advocated in HIV infected individuals as an effective adjunctive treatment for infections and as a deterrent for reinfection (Table of Medications).

V. ACUTE NECROTIZING ULCERATIVE GINGIVITIS

Acute necrotizing ulcerative gingivitis (ANUG) is an uncommon acute infection that primarily affects young and middle age adults, ages fifteen to thirty. The disorder is rare in children and the elderly. Commonly, the affected individual has a decreased resistance to infection and is experiencing emotional stress, which corresponds with its occurrence in students during examination periods. Fusiform bacilli and spirochetes are increased in number during the course of the infection, however, it has not been possible to induce the disease by inoculation. This finding supports the belief that the disease is not contagious and that multiple factors may be required for its occurrence. It is also interesting to note that smoking has also been implicated as a predisposing factor for the occurrence of ANUG.

The hallmark clinical manifestation of ANUG is necrosis of the interdental papilla, which usually involves the mandibular anterior teeth initially. These painful gray-white pseudomembranous lesions are hemorrhagic and spread to involve the marginal gingiva (Figure 5-5). Although generally limited to the gingiva, ANUG may also affect the soft palate and tonsils. Fetor oris is a prominent feature and patients may also manifest

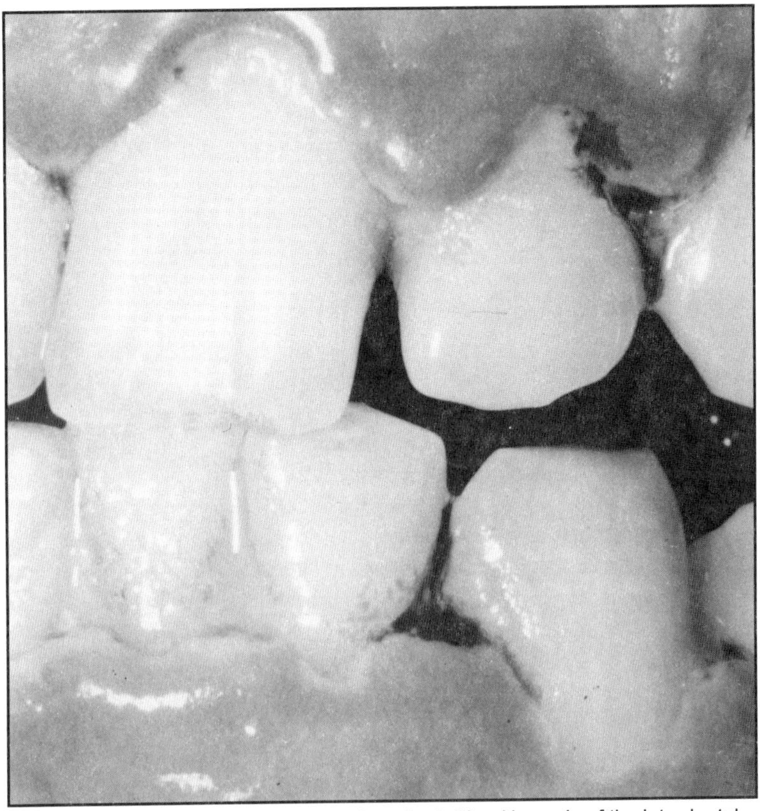

Figure 5-5: Acute necrotizing ulcerative gingivitis - Necrosis of the interdental papillae and marked erythema of the marginal gingiva accompany fever and malaise in this acute infection.

fever, malaise and lymphadenopathy. Oral hygiene is usually poor and, because of the pain, the individuals have difficulty maintaining adequate nutrition. Loss of alveolar bone can result if the condition becomes chronic, which is rare.

The diagnosis of ANUG is often obvious because of the characteristic clinical features. Differential diagnosis includes primary herpetic gingivostomatitis, erosive lichen planus and HIV-associated gingivitis/ periodontitis. Primary herpetic gingivostomatitis affects younger patients, involves more extensive areas of the oral mucosa, and the fever occurs prior to rather than concurrent with the oral lesions. Erosive lichen planus may also be confused with ANUG, but usually affects patients over thirty, involves areas other than the gingival margin and demonstrates the characteristic white, reticulated striae of Wickham. HIV-associated gingivitis and periodontitis may resemble ANUG.

The treatment of ANUG includes antibiotic therapy and local oral hygiene measures. Two hundred and fifty milligrams of penicillin every 6 hours is recommended for 7 to 10 days. Oral hygiene measures include debridement of the affected areas, a good home care program using a soft toothbrush, rinses with dilute hydrogen peroxide and close follow-up care. Interproximal cleaning may be difficult because of pain, but can be accomplished with toothpicks, irrigating devices or floss.

VI. NEOPLASMS

The appearance of both benign and malignant neoplasms, in the oral cavity, may simulate acute mucogingival conditions. Neoplastic lesions of mesenchymal or salivary gland origin may manifest as submucosal swellings of unknown duration, which are secondarily ulcerated and, thus, appear to be inflammatory. Neoplasms arising from the mucosal epithelium may also resemble inflammatory hyperplasia associated with chronic trauma. Other lesions associated with neoplasia such as leukoplakia and erythroplakia, may also be mistaken for mucogingival inflammatory lesions.

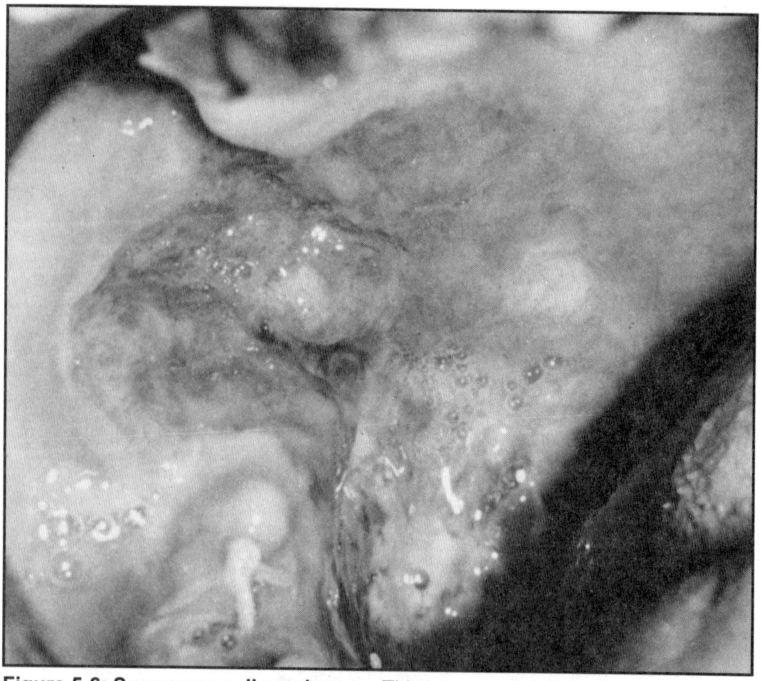

Figure 5-6: Squamous cell carcinoma - This large, crater-shaped ulcer with a rolled border is typical of intra-oral squamous cell carcinoma.

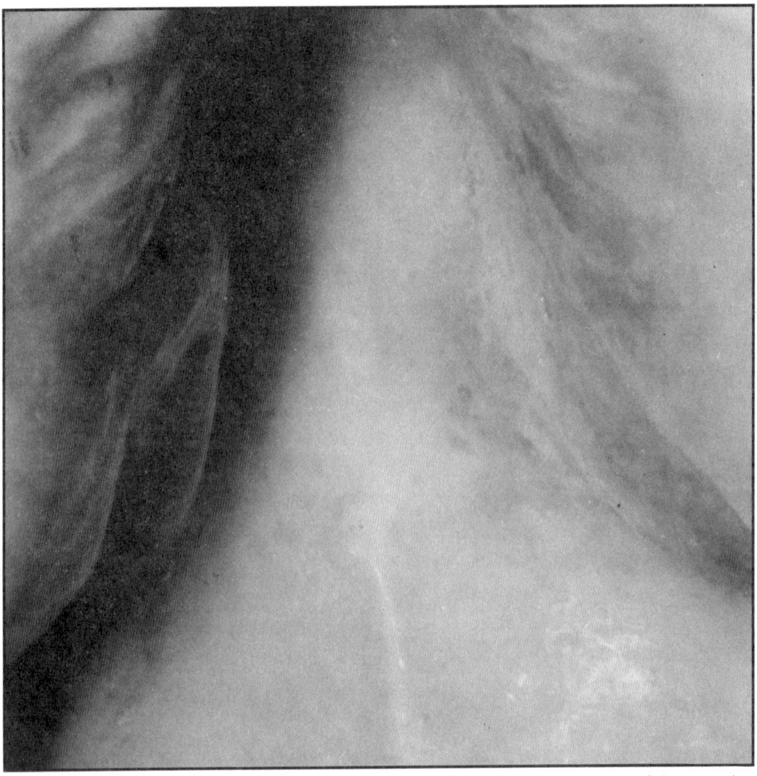

Figure 5-7: Kaposi's sarcoma - The palate is the most common site of the purple-red lesions of KS.

Squamous cell carcinoma is the most common oral malignancy and its clinical appearance often resembles traumatized or infected tissue. Commonly, the lesions are crater-shaped ulcers with rolled borders and peripheral vascularity (Figure 5-6). The most frequent sites for intraoral squamous cell carcinomas are on the ventral or lateral surfaces of the tongue, floor of the mouth, soft palate and tonsils. Unless secondarily infected or traumatized, squamous cell carcinomas are frequently asymptomatic, which is helpful in differentiating them from inflammatory lesions.

Kaposi's sarcoma associated with AIDS can also resemble an inflammatory lesion because of its vascular nature. As such, the diagnosis of this lesion in a patient whose HIV status is unknown can be difficult. The purple-red lesions may be flat, raised, or even nodular and involve the palate or the maxillary gingiva. Again, pain is an uncommon feature of this neoplastic proliferation, although rapid growth with the appearance of additional lesions occurs (Figure 5-7).

The definitive diagnosis of neoplastic lesions can only be accomplished by a biopsy. Excision is possible for smaller lesions though a border of normal tissue should always be included. For larger lesions, incisional biopsy with normal appearing peripheral tissue is recommended. The biopsy of ulcerated lesions must contain both the base of the ulcer and the periphery for an adequate sample. Additional clinical signs associated with head and neck neoplasms can include xerostomia, dysgeusia, dysphagia and dysphonia. The treatment of oral neoplasms varies widely depending on the nature of the tumor. Most benign neoplasms are treated by simple excision, whereas malignancies are treated by either surgery, chemotherapy, radiation therapy or a combination of these modalities. A detailed description of oral neoplastic therapy is beyond the scope of the text.

VII. MUCOSITIS

Mucositis is a frequent outcome of either local or systemic cancer therapy. The effects of therapeutic doses of radiation on the oral mucosa and salivary glands are well known to most dentists. Likewise, many drugs used systemically in the treatment of cancer and other diseases may cause inflammation and ulceration. In most cases, the primary etiology is obvious from the medical history, however, secondary infections make the diagnosis of these lesions challenging.

The oral lesions from radiation therapy appear to be dose related. Doses in the range of 4000 to 5000 cGys, as is given for lymphomas, generally produce fewer and/or less severe changes than the 6000-7000 cGys given for other carcinomas. The mucositis resulting from radiation can range from painful erythema to shallow ulcerated lesions (Figure 5-8). These lesions are secondary to impaired cell division in the basal cell layer. As such, this mucositis is traumatically induced but may represent a secondary infection such as candidiasis. When candidal infections are of the pseudomembranous or hypertrophic varieties, their diagnosis can generally be accurately based on clinical appearance alone. Atrophic forms cannot be distinguished from radiation induced mucositis by clinical appearance; therefore, cytology (e.g., gram stain or KOH wet prep) is recommended to determine the presence of secondary candidal infections. The skin surface in the radiation beam may also show erythema and temporary or permanent alopecia depending on the dose. These changes begin about 1 to 2 weeks after initiation of the therapy and persist for several weeks following completion. Unfortunately some radiation changes are permanent, including xerostomia caused by damage to the salivary glands and impaired alveolar vascularity that may lead to hypoxia and osteoradionecrosis. Oral ulcers and mucositis from radiation therapy are

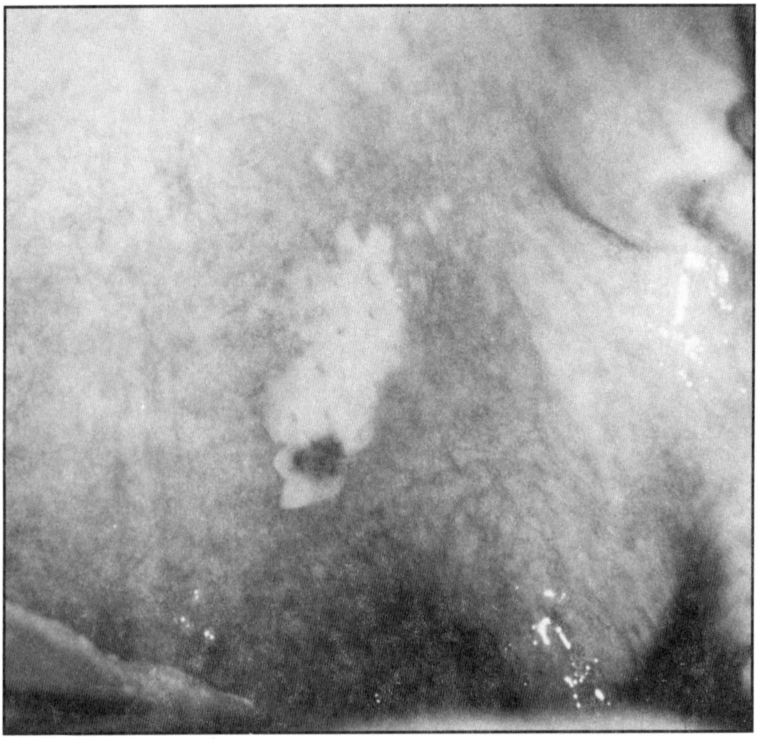

Figure 5-8: Radiation-induced mucositis - Hard palate lesion comprised of epithelial sloughing and an erythematous ulceration.

usually treated palliatively with topical solutions containing various combinations of diphenhydramine HCL (Benedryl), tetracycline, hydrocortisone, viscous lidocaine along with kaopectate, Maalox or Milk of Magnesia as a vehicle to prolong mucosal contact (Table of Medications). One tablespoon of the solution is swished in the mouth for one minute and then expectorated. If candidiasis is present, nystatin can be added to the solution or clotrimazole troches can be prescribed. Systemic anti-fungal medications such as ketoconazole or fluconazole may be used when oral pain prevents the use of topical medications. Frequent sips of water and less commonly, saliva substitutes are used to manage xerostomia. Among the saliva substitutes, Oral Balance™ appears to be more uniformly accepted (Table of Medications).

The oral mucositis secondary to chemotherapy manifests similar changes to those from radiation including erythema, ulcerations, candidiasis and xerostomia. In addition, during periods of leukopenia, patients may have recurrent herpetic infections and candidiasis that are atypical in their clinical appearance; therefore, viral cultures and candida cytology are needed to accurately diagnose lesions in these patients. Anti-fungal therapies previously described or acyclovir for HSV recurrence are indicated for positive cultures. When viral and candidal etiologies are ruled out, palliative topical solutions described for radiation patients may be used (Table of Medications). Oratect Gel™, an OTC oral adhesive preparation containing 15% benzocaine, has been shown to provide symptomatic relief for pain secondary to chemotherapy induced oral mucositis for up to three hours. The gel is applied topically to the affected mucosa with a cotton swab after the area is dried (Table of Medications). As with radiation induced mucositis, the mucositis resulting from chemotherapy is temporary and should resolve within two weeks of the cessation of therapy or with the improvement in leukocyte count.

VIII. REACTIVE MUCOSAL LESIONS

There are a number of reactive hyperplastic lesions involving the gingiva and mucosa that result from chronic, low grade irritation. Several of them may present as acute mucogingival lesions which may be mistaken by patient and clinician as a malignancy. The rapid growth potential of the lesion, relative lack of symptoms and the erythema secondary to increased vascularity and inflammation, is also characteristic of neoplastic growths. Because of the similarities in clinical presentation, these lesions must be differentiated on the basis of their histologic appearance.

The pyogenic granuloma is one of the more common reactive lesions which primarily involves the gingiva but may also affect other areas. Usually occurring as a pedunculated or sessile erythematous mass originating from the gingival crevice, the pyogenic granuloma may be secondarily ulcerated and tends to bleed easily (Figure 5-9). Often a sulcular foreign body such as calculus is the apparent cause of the lesion. Epulis granulomatosum is a less common lesion which, like the pyogenic granuloma, is composed of hyperplastic granulation tissue. In contrast, however, this lesion originates in an extraction site. Pregnant women have an increased incidence of gingival lesions composed of granulation tissue that are referred to as "pregnancy tumors". The elevated incidence probably results from hormonal changes in combination with some low grade irritant.

The peripheral giant cell granuloma (PGCG) is frequently indistinguishable on a clinical basis from the pyogenic granuloma. The PGCG is a highly vascular lesion found on the interdental and marginal gingiva which radiographically may show a cupping or "scooping out" of the bone at its base. Secondary ulceration of the surface is also common. The lesion is probably reactive, although a histologically identical lesion occurs centrally within bone associated with hyperparathyroidism.

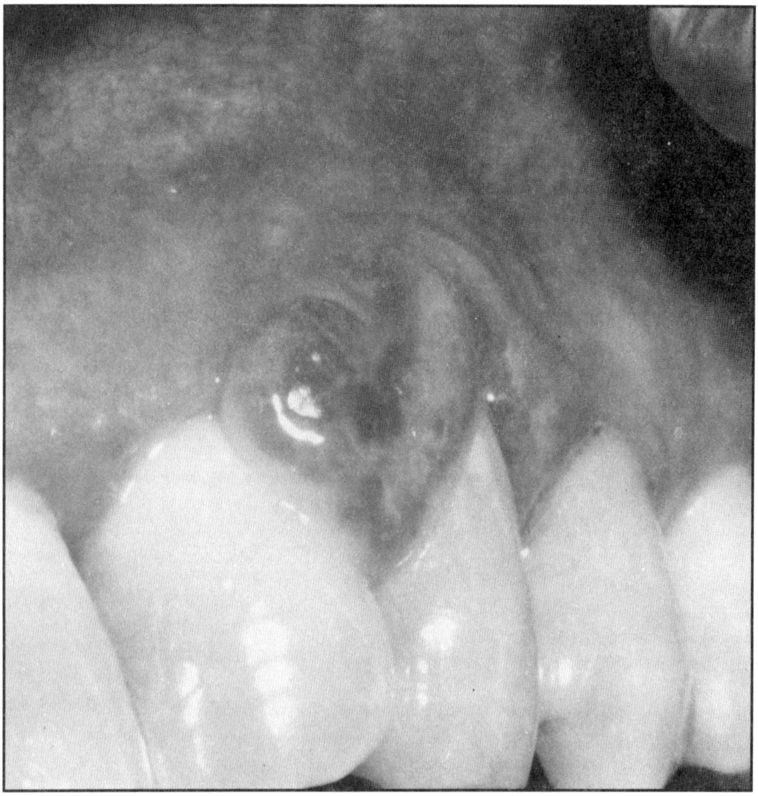

Figure 5-9: Pyogenic granuloma - Rapid growth and a tendency to bleed are characteristics of this reactive lesion.

Another reactive lesion occurring on the gingiva is the peripheral fibroma. The etiology of the lesion, whether neoplastic or reactive hyperplasia, is still debated. The clinical features mimic the lesions previously discussed except that fibromas tend to be the same color as the adjacent gingiva because they are less vascular and composed of more dense, mature connective tissue. Small amounts of mineralized substance resembling bone or odontogenic material may be found in these lesions, which has led to some confusion in the terminology used such as peripheral ossifying fibroma and peripheral odontogenic fibroma.

Regardless of the type, lesions in this group behave in a similar fashion and are treated in the same way. The recommended therapy is complete excision down to periosteum coupled with removal of any possible sources of irritation from the gingival sulcus (e.g., calculus).

A common reactive lesion that occurs on the buccal mucosa, labial mucosa and lateral tongue is the irritation fibroma. These sessile, domeshaped lesions are composed of dense, collagenized fibrous connective tissue. Sparse vascularity and minimal inflammation account for their relatively pale appearance. The lesions usually result from chronic trauma, especially biting, and some patients develop a habit of "chewing" or sucking on the lesion. As such, the surface of the lesion may be hyperkeratotic or ulcerated due to the continuing irritation. Diagnosis of an irritation fibroma is based on appearance and the identification of the initiating trauma (e.g., fractured teeth, impingement by removable prosthesis). Excision and histologic examination is the recommended treatment to rule out other entities such as neoplasms of minor salivary gland, mesenchymal or neural origin.

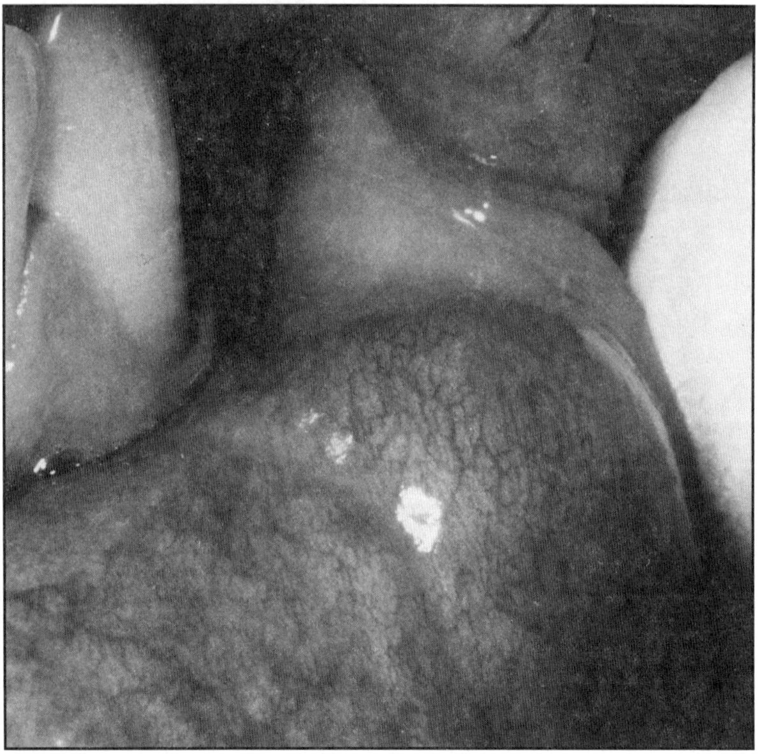

Figure 5-10: Mucocele - A bluish, raised swelling with an intact mucosal surface typifies a mucocele of the lip.

A final reactive lesion well known to practitioners is the mucocele or mucous escape reaction. These common lesions arise rapidly after trauma disrupts the duct from a minor salivary gland and mucin spills into the adjacent soft tissue causing what is essentially a foreign body reaction. Clinically, the lesions appear as raised, painless swellings, with a smooth intact mucosal surface and a bluish or translucent coloring (Figure 5-10). Lesions can occur throughout the mucosa but are most common on the lower lip. Patients frequently give a history of biting their lower lip followed by the appearance of a blister-like lesion which may spontaneously rupture then reappear. Some lesions resolve without treatment while others require excision, including the removal of the involved minor salivary gland. With excision, it is important to tell the patient that the lesions may recur because the surgery itself traumatizes additional salivary gland ducts.

IX. VESICULOBULLOUS AND EROSIVE DISEASES

This group of diseases can present a diagnostic challenge to the practitioner because of similarities in their clinical presentation. Careful attention to minor differences in history and clinical appearance is required to make an accurate diagnosis and institute proper therapy. Histologically, it is often necessary to obtain two specimens by biopsy; one to be fixed in 10% formalin for routine histopathologic examination, and one placed in an appropriate medium provided by the laboratory for immunoflourescence studies. Diseases in this group include pemphigus vulgaris, cicatricial pemphigoid, erythema multiforme, erosive lichen planus and lupus erythematosus.

Pemphigus vulgaris is the most common mucocutaneous disease in which acantholysis within the epithelium leads to the formation of vesiculobullous lesions. The lesions are the result of circulating IgG autoantibodies which cause loss of cellular adhesion. Complement also appears to play a role in this pathophysiologic process. Dentists have a significant role in the diagnosis of pemphigus vulgaris because about 60% of patients have oral manifestations prior to the appearance of skin lesions. The disease is most commonly seen in patients 30 to 50 years of age with no apparent sex predilection. Oral lesions consist of small to large vesicles, bullae or shallow ulcers. A positive Nikolsky sign can be seen but this is not specific for pemphigus. A positive Nikolsky sign refers to stripping of the epithelium or bullae formation from traction placed on the unaffected mucosa. Differential diagnosis includes the lesions discussed in this section, which can be distinguished via biopsy and immunologic testing. Histologic examination of pemphigus shows suprabasilar or intraepithelial clefting and the presence of round, hyperchromatic, acantholytic squamous cells called Tzanck cells. The basal cell layer stays intact having what has been described as a "tombstone appearance". Direct immunofluorescence demonstrates IgG antibodies in the areas of the intercellular desmosomes particularly near the basal cell layer. The majority of patients will also show circulating antibodies by indirect immunofluorescence testing. Treatment of pemphigus vulgaris usually involves the use of systemic corticosteroids such as prednisone, sometimes in combination with other immunosuppressive drugs, such as azothioprine, methotrexate or cyclophosphamide. One to two mg/kg/day of prednisone in divided doses is recommended to achieve symptomatic control followed by gradual tapering. Due to the problems associated with long-term use of these drugs, management of these patients is best accomplished by a physician.

Cicatricial pemphigoid is also an autoimmune disease involving IgG, IgA and complement. Other terms commonly applied to this condition are benign mucous membrane pemphigoid, desquamative gingivitis and gingivosis. Women are more commonly affected than men and the disease occurs in adults and the elderly. As with pemphigus, the oral lesions consist of chronic vesicles, bullae, erosions or erythematous areas, however, with pemphigoid the lesions tend to involve the gingiva and may heal with scarring. The larger lesions can be painful and may lead to poor oral hygiene and diet modifications. Other mucous membranes and occasionally the skin may also be involved and a positive Nikolsky sign can be observed. In contrast to pemphigus, the microscopic changes in cicatricial pemphigoid include sub-basilar clefting without acantholysis and the presence of a mixed inflammatory infiltrate in the lamina propria. IgG and occasionally IgA are found along the basement membrane area by direct immunoflourescence, but indirect immunofluorescence studies are usually negative.

As with pemphigus, systemic corticosteroids are the treatment of choice; however, even with high doses, results can be variable. .75-1.25 mg/kg/day of prednisone in divided doses is recommended to be tapered off following symptomatic control. Topical steroids including fluocinonide or betamethasone can also be used in a carrier such as a soft mouthguard (Table of Medications). Systemic immunosupression agents are used in refractory cases or to avoid steroid complications, but these treatments are again in the purview of the physician.

Erythema multiforme (EM) is an acute disease of unknown etiology. Approximately half of the patients, primarily young adults, will have oral involvement in the form of painful ulcers. The ulcerations vary in size and number, and can involve any area of the oral mucosa (Figure 5-11). The skin manifestations can include vesicles, bullae, plaques, macules and papules, but the pathognomonic presentation is the target or iris lesion. This lesion consists of concentric alternating rings of erythema and normal skin color located on the extremities (Figure 5-12). Additional signs and symptoms can include fever, headache and lymphadenopathy. In many

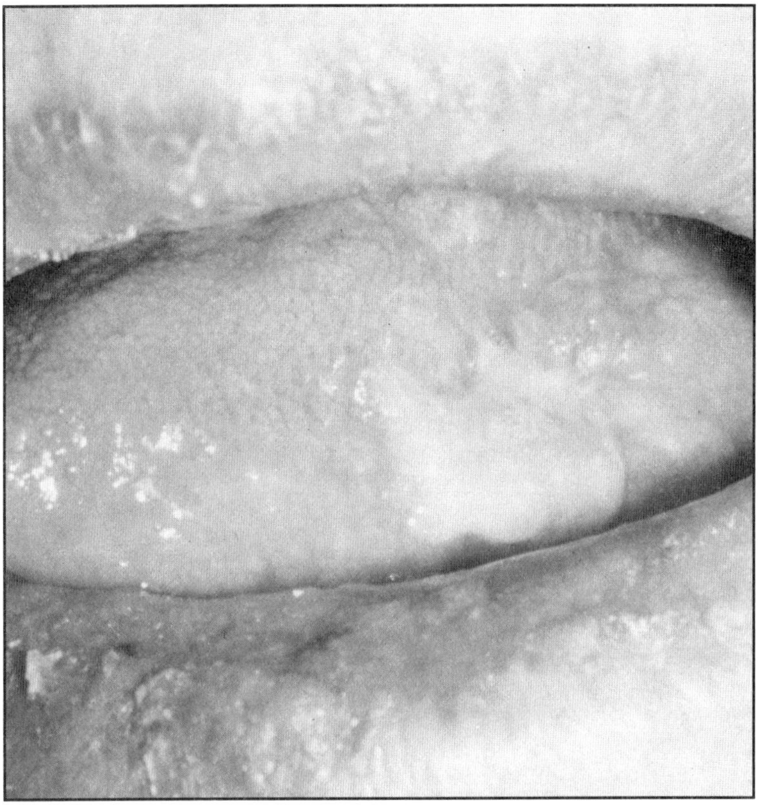

Figure 5-11: Erythema multiforme - The clinical and histologic appearance of the oral ulcers are non-specific and, in the absence of skin lesions, present a diagnostic challenge.

cases a precipitating factor, such as an infection (especially HSV), or the use of a particular drug can be identified, which has led to the suspicion that EM may represent a hypersensitivity reaction. Relapse is common and recurrent lesions may be similar to the first occurrence or be relatively mild with fewer, less painful ulcers.

When target lesions are present on the skin the diagnosis of EM can be made based on this finding. If only oral lesions are present or when the skin lesions are less specific, the diagnosis is more difficult and is complicated by the lack of unique histopathologic and immunopathologic changes. The differential diagnosis includes primary herpetic gingivostomatitis, aphthous stomatitis and the other lesions discussed in this section. Factors which favor the diagnosis of erythema multiforme over HSV infection include the presence of skin lesions, the relative lack of systemic symptoms, a negative viral culture, the absence of vesicles

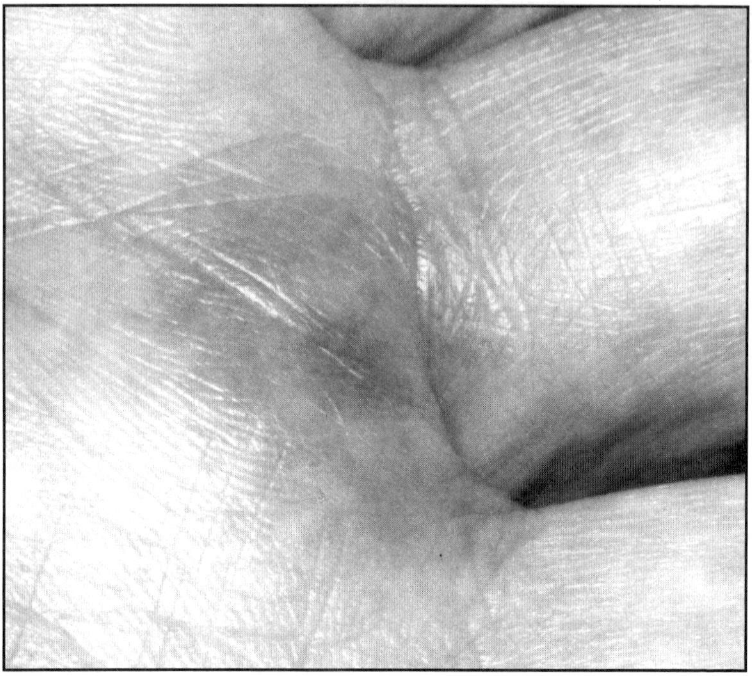

Figure 5-12: Erythema multiforme - the pathognomonic target lesion on the palms of the hands consists of concentric alternating rings of erythema and normal skin color.

preceding ulcers on the lips, tongue, buccal mucosa and palate, and the history of a precipitating factor. Aphthous ulcers can usually be excluded by history and from the limited number of ulcers. The acute onset, limited duration and non-specific histologic changes help differentiate EM from pemphigus vulgaris, cicatricial pemphigoid and lichen planus.

EM is a self-limiting disease which generally does not require treatment other than palliation, such as avoiding the ingestion of spicy foods and alcohol, taking analgesics as needed and using topical anesthetic rinses previously described. A severe form of EM known as the Stevens-Johnson syndrome is distinguished by extensive involvement of the mouth, skin, genitalia and eyes and more pronounced systemic manifestations. Systemic steroids are added to the aforementioned palliative therapies in patients with this condition.

Lichen planus (LP) is a mucocutaneous disease with many variations. The most common form involves white, reticulated mucosal lesions. Atrophic, bullous and erosive forms can present as acute lesions associated with pain and burning. The etiology is apparently a cell-mediated immune response involving the basal cell layer of the mucosa. With erosive LP, the oral lesions consist of erosions covered by a gray-white pseudomembrane with the typical white striae at the periphery (Figure 5-13). The lesions sometimes present initially as blisters and their pattern may change during the course of the disease. Skin lesions involve violaceous or scaly papules that occur on the flexor surfaces of the extremities, but skin lesions are not always present. Erosive LP involves males and females equally and mostly affects middle aged individuals.

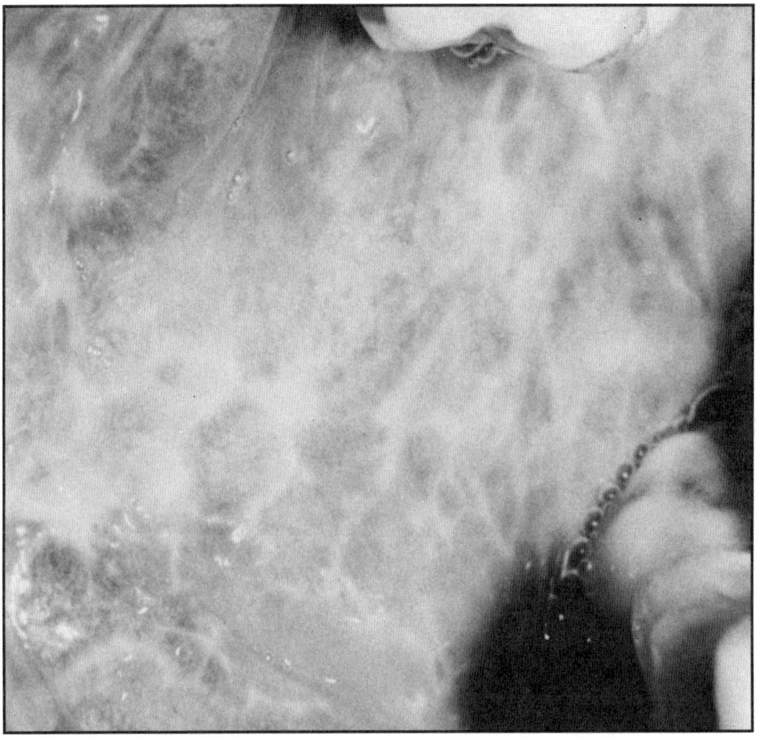

Figure 5-13: Lichen Planus - The erosive form of lichen planus in the buccal mucosa is characterized by erosions covered by a gray-white pseudomembrane.

The differential diagnosis of LP includes drug eruptions, cicatricial pemphigoid and erythematous candidiasis, which can be differentiated by biopsy with immunologic studies. Fortunately, lichen planus has a characteristic microscopic appearance that includes hyperkeratosis, irregular acanthosis with a "sawtooth" appearance of the rete pegs, liquefaction degeneration of the basal cell layer and a band-like infiltrate of lymphocytes in the lamina propria.

Palliative therapies are used to treat lichen planus as the lesions tend to wax and wane. For the erosive form, topical or systemic corticosteroids appear to be the most useful. Retinoids (systemic and topical) and dapsone (systemic) have also been used in severe cases (Table of Medications).

Another disease which must be considered when confronted with a patient suffering from erosive lesions of the oral mucosa is lupus erythematosus (LE). LE is an autoimmune disorder in which antibodies form to the epithelial cell's nucleus and cytoplasm. Apparently there is also a cell-mediated component to the disease because of the increased number of T lymphocytes and abnormal T cell function in patients with LE. There are three variations of LE: discoid (DLE), subacute cutaneous (SCLE) and systemic (SLE). The form that is least severe and most often affects the oral cavity is DLE, in which erosions and erythematous plaques may involve the gingiva, buccal mucosa or lips. Skin lesions consist of red plaques with hyperpigmented margins which heal with scarring and loss of pigment. DLE occurs most often in middle-aged females and may cause significant cosmetic problems because of its propensity for face and scalp lesions. SCLE has oral lesions similar to DLE, but the skin lesions last longer (weeks or months) and heal without scarring. Neither DLE nor SCLE are likely to progress to the more severe form of SLE in which systemic complications are more significant while skin and mucosal involvement are relatively mild. SLE is seen predominantly in females around age 30, and the initial symptoms may include malaise, fever and weight loss. An erythematous "butterfly" rash over the nose is the characteristic skin lesion, but the lesions of the heart, kidneys, lungs and joints are the primary concern for the clinician. Inflammatory glomerulopathy of the kidneys is often the cause of death in SLE patients, and heart lesions may require the use of prophylactic antibiotics to protect against the development of endocarditis from a bacteremia.

Microscopic changes in oral LE lesions include basal cell destruction with an inflammatory infiltrate of lymphocytes, often found around dilated blood vessels in the edematous submucosa. Also, the epithelial surface may be hyperkeratotic. Direct immunofluorescence demonstrates immunoglobulins (IgG, IgM, IgA) and complement deposited in a linear pattern along the basement membrane.

The differential diagnosis for patients with LE includes erosive lichen planus, pemphigus vulgaris, erythema multiforme and drug reactions. The clinical differences in the presentations of these lesions have been described, but the similarities in appearance require biopsy and often immunoflourescent studies to establish the diagnosis. The treatment consists of immunosuppressive agents, topical steroids, antimalarials or sulfones for DLE and systemic steroids for cases of SLE. Which drugs or combinations are used depends on the severity of the lesions.

X. SYSTEMIC INFECTIOUS DISEASES

The majority of known infectious diseases can manifest themselves either as a primary or secondary infection in the oral cavity. The lesions can range from localized dental infections involving the teeth or gingiva to systemic illnesses involving alveolar bone or soft tissue. Because these lesions can simulate many other conditions, the possibility of an infectious disease should be included in almost every differential diagnosis. In addition to the localized infectious processes previously discussed (herpes, HIV, Candida and ANUG), it is important to be familiar with the oral manifestations of systemic infections such as sexually transmitted diseases, deep fungal infections and tuberculosis.

Foremost among the sexually transmitted diseases is syphilis which, despite the present emphasis on "safe sex", is increasing in incidence. The primary lesion, the chancre, develops at the site of inoculation by the organism *Treponema pallidum* about 3 weeks after exposure. The lesion is usually a single ulcer with an indurated border, similar in appearance to squamous cell carcinoma in the oral cavity, and lasts about 4 to 6 weeks. Regional lymphadenopathy is present but resolves within the same time frame. Secondary syphilis presents 2 to 8 weeks following the chancre and consists of flu-like symptoms, lymphadenopathy and skin lesions. The nebulosity and commonness of the appearance are responsible for secondary syphilis being called the "great imitator". In a majority of cases, mucous membrane lesions are present and consist of non-painful ulcerations covered by a gray-white pseudomembrane. The lesions may be subtle and difficult to detect, are teaming with spirochetes and are potentially contagious. The secondary lesions also resolve in about 2 to 6 weeks even without treatment. The tertiary lesions of late syphilis consist of the gumma, a granulomatous lesion, which may involve the oral cavity, and virtually any other organ system. These lesions take years to develop and commonly affect the cardiovascular and central nervous systems. The diagnosis of syphilis is made by identification of T. pallidum, using darkfield microscopy; however, spirochetes indigenous to the oral cavity can complicate the diagnosis.

Numerous diagnostic serologic tests are available including the VDRL, RPR, ART, the fluorescent treponemal antibody absorption test (FTA-ABS) and the microhemagglutination test (MHA-TP). The recommended treatment for syphilis is with Penicillin G.

Gonococcal infections may involve the mouth through orogenital contact and consist of superficial ulcers with a gray-white pseudomembrane or a generalized erythema of the soft tissues. The lesions appear 1 to 14 days after contact. Penicillin is the treatment of choice after culture confirms the diagnosis.

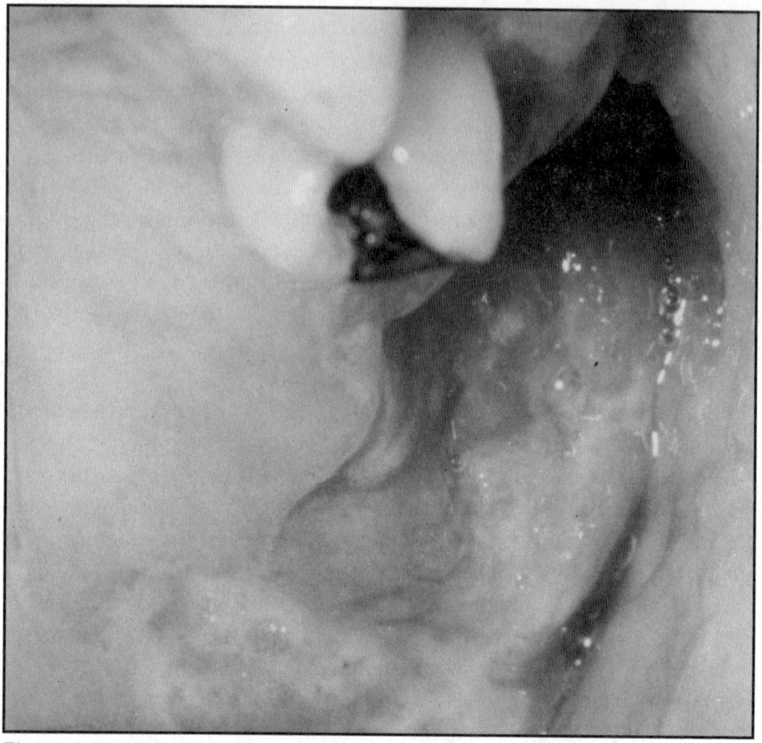

Figure 5-14: Histoplasmosis - Characterized by ulcerated lesions with rolled borders, typical of deep fungal infections and squamous cell carcinoma.

Tuberculosis and deep fungal infections usually present as secondary infections in the oral cavity with lungs being the primary site of involvement. The oral lesions consist of raised, granulomatous nodules or crater-shaped ulcers with rolled borders that resemble squamous cell carcinoma (Figure 5-14). Immunocompromised patients are at greater risk to acquire these infections; however, they are also found in otherwise healthy individuals. The diagnosis is made by microscopic identification of the organisms from either a biopsy or a culture. In the case of tuberculosis, a positive skin test using purified protein derivative (PPD) is also diagnostic. Treatment is accomplished by combinations of antimicrobial chemotherapeutic agents and is the responsibility of the physician.

XI. HIV - ASSOCIATED LESIONS

Several of the most important lesions found in HIV-infected patients were discussed earlier in this chapter. These are aphthous ulcers, herpes simplex infections and candidiasis, whose appearance in immunocompromised patients is characterized by their atypical presentation. Additional oral manifestations in AIDS patients are HIV-associated gingivitis and periodontitis (HIV-G and HIV-P respectively), oral hairy leukoplakia and Kaposi's sarcoma.

Periodontal lesions are common in HIV patients and range from mild gingivitis to rapidly progressive periodontitis. The lesions may be localized, diffuse or multifocal and tend to be unresponsive to standard periodontal therapy. HIV-G involves only the soft tissues (gingiva and alveolar mucosa) displaying a distinctive erythema of the marginal gingiva throughout the mouth. Pain, spontaneous hemorrhaging or bleeding with brushing may prompt patients to seek care. HIV-P is characterized by the same soft tissue necrosis coupled with rapid loss of periodontal attachment and bone loss without deep pocketing as is commonly seen in chronic inflammatory periodontal disease (Figure 5-15). Patients often complain

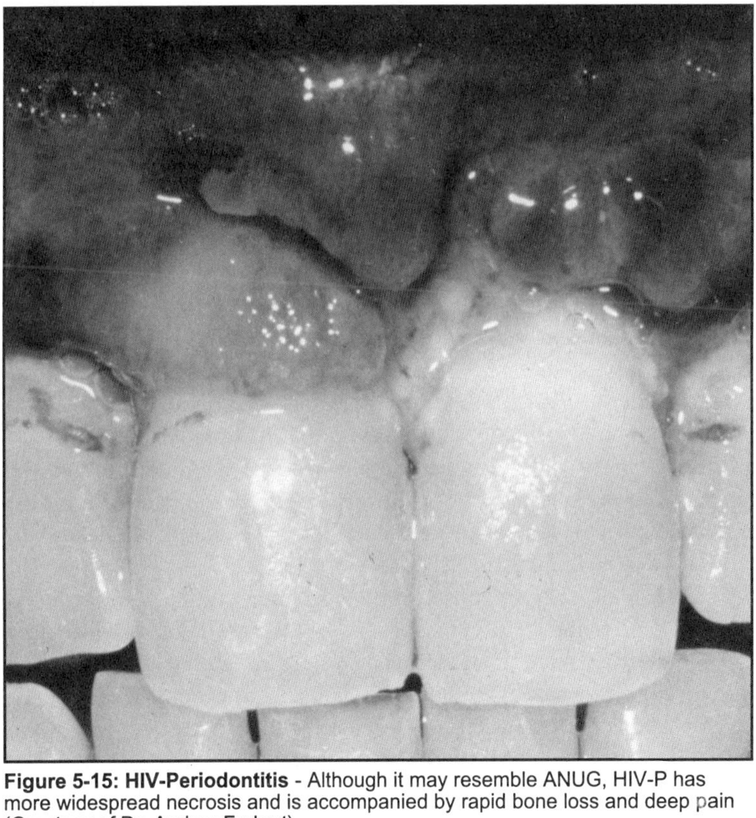

Figure 5-15: HIV-Periodontitis - Although it may resemble ANUG, HIV-P has more widespread necrosis and is accompanied by rapid bone loss and deep pain (Courtesy of Dr. Audrey Furkart).

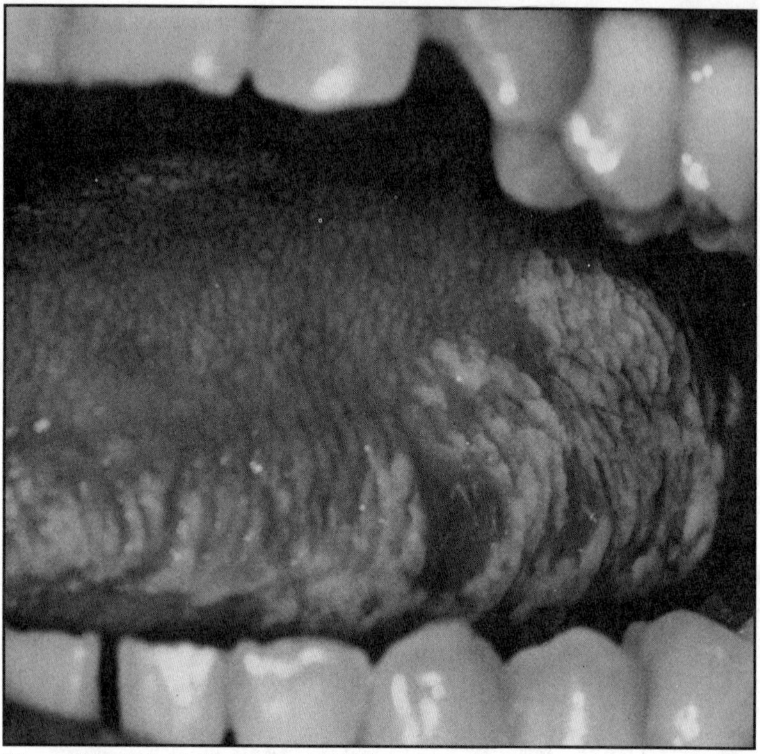

Figure 5-16: Hairy leukoplakia - The lateral tongue border is the most common site for this benign AIDS-related lesion characterized by corrugated areas of leukoplakia (Courtesy of Dr. Bobby Hassanzadeh).

of deep bone pain and the process may be multifocal with intervening areas of relatively healthy periodontium. The treatment for both conditions includes an intense patient home care program, scaling and root planing with povodine-iodine irrigation and the use of .12% chlorhexidine gluconate mouthrinse (Peridex™) three times daily. Due to the reported involvement of anaerobic organisms in HIV - G and HIV - P, metronidazole has also been advocated in treatment of these conditions (Table of Medications).

Oral hairy leukoplakia (HL), first described in 1984, has proven to be an indicator of a compromised immune system, primarily associated with an HIV infection. HL consists of asymptomatic, flat or corrugated areas of leukoplakia found predominantly on the lateral borders of the tongue, but occasionally involving other areas of the mucosa (Figure 5-16). The lesions of HL are usually bilateral and vary in size, though the extent of the lesions is unrelated to the progression of HIV disease. The presence of HL is significant because of its predictive value regarding the development of AIDS. It has been reported that the probability of AIDS developing in patients is 48% by 16 months and 83% by 31 months after the diagnosis of HL. It appears that Epstein-Barr Virus (EBV) is linked to the etiology of HL in HIV patients, and demonstration of the presence of EBV may be necessary to establish a definitive diagnosis. The microscopic features of HL include hyperkeratosis, which produces the "hairy" appearance, ballooning of mucosal squamous cells, typical viral-induced changes in the epithelium, a lack of submucosal inflammation and frequently the presence of Candida at the surface. The treatment of HL with antiviral drugs such as acyclovir is possible, but the lesions recur if the medication is discontinued. More importantly, it may not be necessary to treat HL since the lesion is benign and significance of the lesions relates to its prognostication in developing AIDS.

Kaposi's sarcoma (KS), the most common malignancy in AIDS patients, usually arises in the skin, but oral involvement occurs with the palate as the favored site. Oral KS may present as flat or nodular purple to red lesions which progress to lobulated, frequently ulcerated masses (Figure 6-17). Clinically KS could be mistaken for a pyogenic granuloma or hemangioma. Histologic features of KS consist of a proliferation of vascular spaces lined by atypical endothelial cells and a mononuclear inflammatory cell infiltrate. Smaller lesions can be surgically excised, while larger lesions may be excised, treated with chemotherapeutic agents or irradiated. Treatment is not curative but can be performed for cosmetic reasons or to eliminate pain or bleeding.

Health care providers should be aware of the broad spectrum of HIV oral manifestations and realize that an uncommon lesion occurring in the mouth (and sometimes resembling a common entity) or a common lesion with an unusual clinical presentation may be the harbinger of HIV infection.

Table of Medications

Rx.	Acyclovir capsules, 200 mg
Disp.	35 capsules
Sig.	Take 1 capsule by mouth five times daily for 7 days (Acyclovir Prophylaxis - All patients who are seropositive for HSV prior to bone marrow transplant begin acyclovir 200mg capsules t.i.d. before beginning conditioning chemotherapy and continue for 6 weeks. If oral mucositis develops and oral intake is compromised, then 5mg/kg of IV acyclovir every 8 hours is started. Oral acyclovir is reinstituted when oral intake is resumed)

Rx.	Acyclovir ointment - 5%
Disp.	15 gm tube
Sig.	Apply to affected area with cotton swab five times per day
Rx.	Acyclovir sterile powder
Disp.	5 mg/kg
Sig.	Infuse over 1 hour tid
Rx.	Benedryl elixir 12.5 mg/tsp (with equal parts of 2% viscous Lidocaine and/or tetracycline suspension) with equal part Kaopectate
Disp.	6 oz
Sig.	2 tsp as oral rinse for 1 minute three or four times each day
Rx.	Betamethasone diproprionate 0.05% ointment
Disp.	15 gm tube
Sig.	Apply to affected area in carrier provided once each day
Rx.	0.12% Chlorhexidine gluconate (Peridex Tm) rinse
Disp.	16 oz
Sig.	Rinse with 15 ml vigorously for 60 seconds and expectorate after breakfast and before bed (after meals if used t.i.d. for treatment of HIV-G or HIV-P)
Rx.	Clotrimazole - 10 mg troches
Disp.	70 troches
Sig.	Dissolve troche in mouth five times daily for 14 days
Rx.	Fluconazole - 100mg tablets
Disp.	15 tablets
Sig.	Take 2 tablets by mouth the first day then 1 tablet each day for 14 days (Patients with impaired renal function may require a reduced dosage)
Rx.	Fluocinonide - .05% gel
Disp.	15 gm tube
Sig.	Apply to affected area four times daily with cotton swab (or carrier provided)
Rx.	Ketoconazole - 200 mg tablets
Disp.	14 tablets
Sig.	Take 1 tablet daily by mouth for 14 days

Rx. Lidocaine viscous 2%
Disp. 450 ml bottle
Sig. Rinse with 1 tablespoon and expectorate every 2 hours for oral pain

Rx. Metronidazole tablets, 500mg
Disp. 28 tablets
Sig. Take one tablet 4 times a day for one week

Rx. Nystatin oral suspension - 100,000 U/ml
Disp. 60 ml
Sig. Rinse with 4 ml for 2 minutes and swallow four times daily

Rx. Oral Balance™
Disp. 42 gm tube
Sig. Apply to dry areas of mouth as needed

Rx. Oratect Gel™
Disp. 10.5 gm tube
Sig. Apply to dried areas of painful mucosa; allow dry for 30 - 60 seconds, apply up to 4 times daily

Rx. Tetracycline oral suspension 750 mg/tsp
Disp. 4 oz
Sig. 1 tsp four times daily, rinse in mouth for 5 minutes then swallow

References

CDC., "AIDS and human immunodeficiency virus infection in the United States: 1988 Update." *MMWR*. 38 (1989): 1.

Correll R.W., *Common oral soft tissue lesions*. Los Angeles: VA Western Dental Education Center, 1990.

Correll R.W., Wescott W.B., *Diagnosis, treatment and management of HIV-associated oral disease*. Los Angeles: VA Western Dental Education Center, 1990.

Ferretti G.A., et al., "Chlorhexidine for prophylaxis against oral infections and associated complications in patients receiving bone marrow transplants." *J Am Dent Assoc*. 114 (1987): 461.

Gold D., Corey L., "Acyclovir prophylaxis for herpes simplex virus infection." *Antimicrob Agents Chemother* 31 (1987): 361.

Greenspan D., *AIDS and the dental team*. Munksgaard, Copenhagen: Yearbook Medical Publishers, Inc., 1986.

Greenspan D., et al., "Oral "hairy" leukoplakia in male homosexuals: evidence of association with both papillomavirus and a herpes-group virus." *Lancet*. 2 (1984): 831.

Greenspan D., et al., "Relation of oral hairy leukoplakia to infection with the human immunodeficiency virus and the risk of developing AIDS." *J Infect Dis.* 155 (1987): 475.

Greenspan J.S., Greenspan D., "Oral hairy leukoplakia: diagnosis and management." *Oral Surg Oral Med Oral Pathol.* 67 (1989): 396.

Langlais R.P.; Bricker S.L.; Cottone J.A.; and Baker B.R., *Oral diagnosis, oral medicine and treatment planning.* Philadelphia: W.B. Saunders, 1984.

Miller C.S., Redding S.W., "Diagnosis and management of orofacial herpes simplex virus infections." *Dental Clinics of North America.* Philadelphia: W.B. Saunders, 1992.

Montgomery M.T., Redding S.W., Le Maistre C.F., "The incidence of oral herpes simplex virus infection in patients undergoing cancer chemotherapy." *Oral Surg Oral Med Oral Pathol.* 61 (1986): 238.

Redding S.W., Montgomery M.T., *Dentistry in Systemic Disease.* Portland: JBK Publishing, Inc., 1990.

Regezi J.A., Sciubba J., *Oral Pathology, clinical-pathologic correlations.* Philadelphia: W.B. Saunders, 1989.

Rose L.F., Kaye D., *Internal medicine for dentistry.* 2 ed., St. Louis: CV Mosby, 1990.

Shafer W.G., Hine M.K., Levy B.M., *A textbook of oral pathology.* 4 ed., Philadelphia: W.B. Saunders, 1983.

Silverman Jr. S., "AIDS update: Oral findings, diagnosis, and precautions." *J Am Dent Assoc.* 115 (1987): 559.

Winkler J.R., et al., "Diagnosis and management of HIV-associated periodontal lesions." *JADA.* Supplement, November, 1989.

Zysset M.K., et al., "Systemic Lupus Erythematosus: A consideration for antimicrobial prophylaxis." *Oral Surg Oral Med Oral Pathol.* 64 (1987): 30.

6 Lacerations

Brookie D. Armstrong, D.D.S.

Robert A. Dale, D.D.S.

Scott D. Schumann, D.D.S.

Lacerations are a common type of wound that may be treated by medical and dental health care professionals alike. This is especially true of perioral and intraoral wounds. This chapter will present the salient aspects of intraoral and extraoral wound evaluation and management.

I. ANATOMY OF THE SKIN

The treatment of lacerations requires an understanding of skin anatomy and wound healing. This knowledge improves decisions concerning selection of an appropriate suture material and closure technique.

The four principle layers of skin are the epidermis, dermis, superficial fascia and deep fascia (Figure 6-1). The superficial fascia is also referred to as the subcutaneous layer. The skin's many functions include: 1) bodily protection against mechanical trauma, heat injury and bacterial invasion, 2) assisting in the regulation of body temperature via vascular plexi and sweat glands, and registering environmental stimulation via sensory organs. Each layer of skin and fascia is present throughout the body's exterior; however, the thickness of the layers varies with anatomical location. This variability is one factor to be considered in choosing the appropriate suture needle. For example, a small, delicate needle is suitable in the thin skin of the eyelid, whereas a larger, stronger needle is indicated for the thicker skin in the palm of the hand.

The ***epidermis*** is the outermost layer of skin and contains no organs, nerve endings or vessels. This layer is vital in providing protection against bacterial or chemical invasion. The epidermis is composed of four microscopic layers of which the stratum germinativum (basal layer) and the stratum corneum (keratinized, or horny layer) are the most important. The former provides cells for new epidermis formation following injury and the latter gives the skin its final cosmetic appearance.

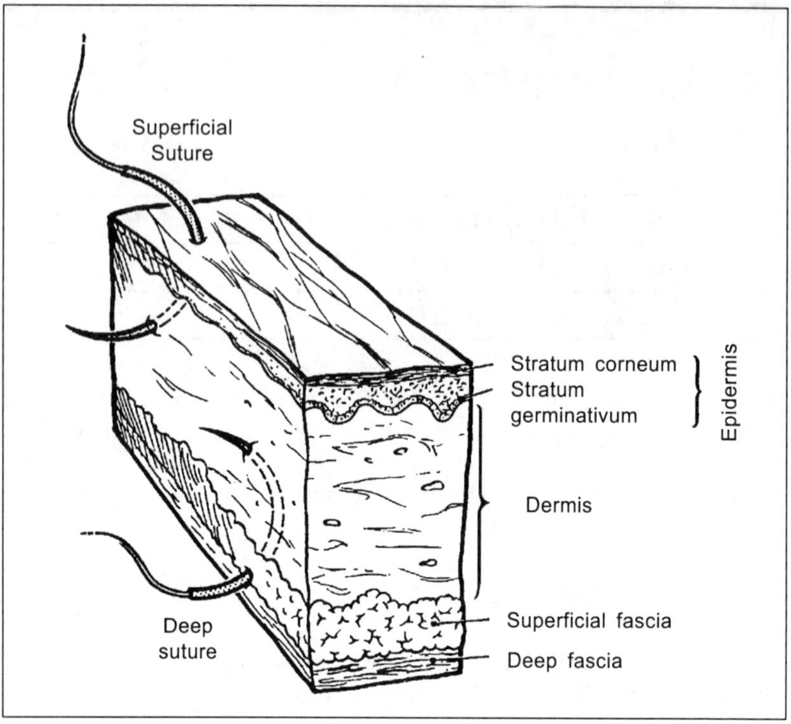

Figure 6-1: Principal Layers of the Skin for Suture Location.

The ***dermis*** resides immediately beneath the epidermis and is comprised primarily of connective tissue. The prominent cell type within this layer is the fibroblast. However, the dermis also contains macrophages, mast cells and lymphocytes, all of which are important in wound healing. Other dermal structures include nerve fibers, vascular plexi, hair follicles and the accompanying sebaceous glands, as well as the apocrine and exocrine sweat glands. The dermis is the most important skin layer in the wound repair process because collagen, the basic structural component of the skin, is formed by fibroblasts in the dermis. The dermis is much thicker than the epidermis and, as such, is the anchoring site for both superficial and deep sutures.

The ***superficial fascia*** lies under the dermis and consists of loose connective tissue, fat and sensory nerves. The primary functions of this layer are to provide insulation against heat loss and some measure of protection against trauma. There are several consequences of injury to this layer, one of which is infection because devitalized fat can promote bacterial growth. Also, injuries to this layer have the potential for creating dead space which, if not adequately evacuated or closed, can lead to hematoma formation and further increases the risk of infection.

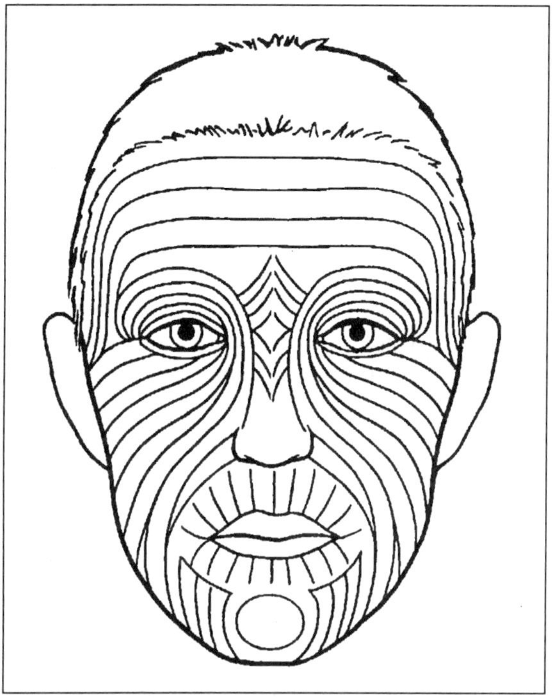

Figure 6-2: Natural Skin Tension Lines of the face.

Beneath the superficial fascia is the ***deep fascia***, which is a dense and discrete fibrous tissue layer. The main function of this layer is to support and protect muscles and other soft tissue structures. A secondary function is to provide a barrier against the spread of infection from the skin and superficial fascia. Lacerations reaching this layer require closure in order to re-establish its protective and supportive functions.

In addition to the anatomical layers, the skin is influenced by static and dynamic forces. The skin is under natural static tensile forces over the entire body. It is this ***static tension*** that must be considered in wound edge debridement and revision because it will affect the final morphology of a scar. While it is tempting to excise jagged edges in a wound, an irregular, but well adapted laceration will likely heal with a less noticeable scar than would a revised wound in which the revision creates a tissue deficit requiring increased tension for primary closure. ***Dynamic forces*** are different from static forces but, like static forces, are important in wound healing. These forces are created by underlying muscle contraction, which compresses the skin and results in wrinkle lines. Dynamic forces are most visible in the face during facial expressions (Figure 6-2). Lacerations perpendicular to these dynamic tension lines heal with wider scars than do those that are parallel to them. It is important to consider these forces when suturing lacerations, when elective excision of a foreign body is planned and when incising for drainage of facial abscesses.

II. WOUND HEALING

While the anatomy of the skin is important in wound healing, there are a myriad of other factors that ultimately affect the outcome. Normal wound healing is thought to occur in three phases, although the process is actually a collection of ongoing and intertwined events.

The ***initial phase***, or substrate phase, of wound healing is the immediate vascular response to an injury. Included in this phase are both vasospasm and the coagulation cascade, which are critical to hemostasis. An inflammatory response begins immediately following the vascular reaction to injury. Polymorphonuclear leukocytes and smaller numbers of lymphocytes may be found in a wound within the first three hours following injury. These cells continue to increase in number during the first forty-eight hours. Macrophages begin to appear in the wound within twenty-four hours and become actively involved in phagocytosis. Macrophages also play a role in the stimulation of fibroblast reproduction and neovascularization. All of these cell types are important in the control of bacterial invasion and the suppression of infection. New blood vessels and fibroblasts begin to form at the edge of the wound during this phase. Within twelve hours, intact cells at the wound edge begin to form pseudopod structures which facilitate cell migration and replication. Once cell replication begins, the new cells move over the wound surface connected by desmosomal attachments. This new cell layer is formed over the damaged dermis, but beneath the hemostatic coagulum. The new epithelial cell covering acts to protect the wound while healing proceeds. Continued epithelial cell replication reforms a normal epidermis. This re-epithelialization process occurs in all wounds, even the small puncture wounds caused by suturing. Epithelial "plugs" that form in suture punctures may be trapped in the wound during healing if the sutures remain in place too long. These plugs, or "tracks," contribute to a less desirable cosmetic result.

Phase two or the proliferative phase of wound repair is established by the fourth or fifth day following injury. Macrophages are the predominant cell type initially, however, fibroblasts increase in number as the phase continues. Vascular granulation tissue containing new capillaries, fibroblasts, macrophages and mast cells fill the wound when the second phase is fully established. The first fibrils of collagen within the wound have no cross links with the collagen fibrils on the edge of the wound until the fifth or sixth day. The intrinsic mechanical strength of the wound is developed as the collagen fibrils become cross-linked and mature.

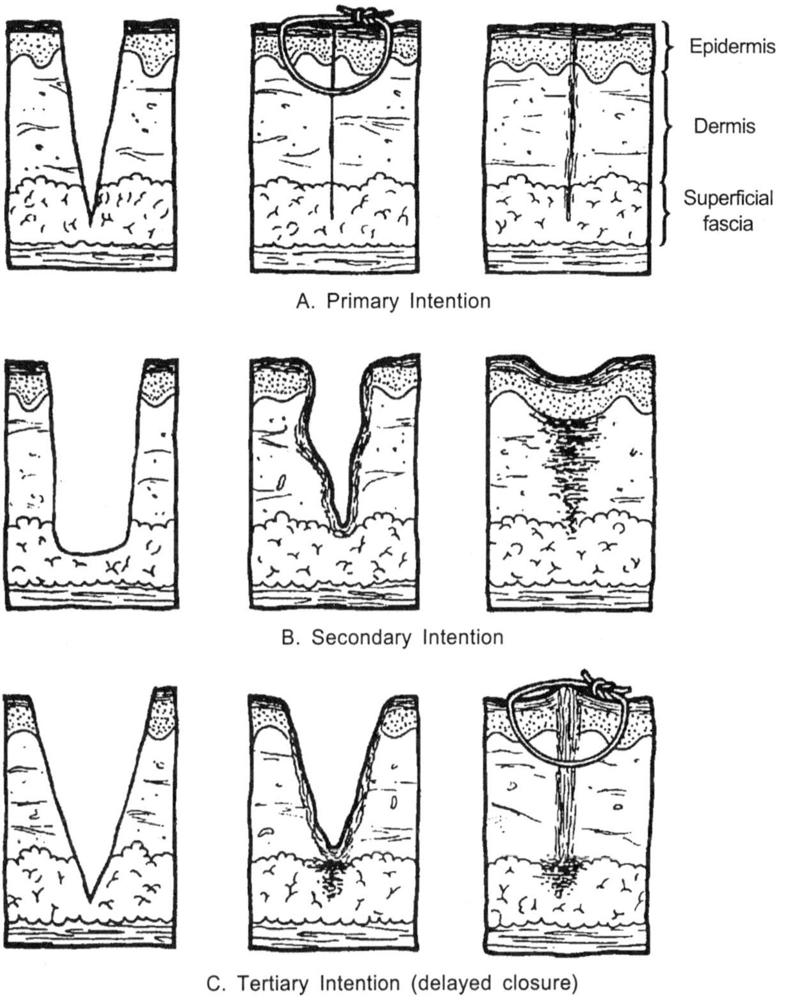

Figure 6-3: Types of Wound Healing.

Phase three, or the remodeling phase, is a gradual transition from the second phase and does not end until healing is complete. At the beginning of this phase, fibroblasts and macrophages decrease in number and wound vascularity diminishes. During this phase, many of the existing collagen fibrils are broken down by collagenases and new fibers are laid down. Generally, the fibers that remain in the scar are those that are parallel to the lines of tension, thereby imparting mechanical strength to the wound tissue. Even though collagen undergoes numerous changes in the remodeling phase, abnormal tissue architecture may remain for years following the injury.

Clinically, wound healing is generally classified into one of three types of union (Figure 6-3). This classification provides guidelines for the management of a wound based on the time from injury, the level of contamination and the amount of tissue damage. Relatively clean wounds with minimal tissue damage, such as those created from shearing forces, usually heal best by ***primary intention***. In this type of healing, the wound is closed by some type of mechanical intervention such as sutures, skin tape or staples. Wound closure by primary intention must take place within the "golden period" of three to six hours post injury, except in highly vascularized areas such as the head and neck when this time period may be extended to eight to twelve hours following the injury. This type of healing generally produces the least amount of scar formation.

A wound that involves significant tissue damage, such as an avulsion, ulceration or infarction, may heal by ***secondary intention***. In this process, wound edges either cannot or should not be sutured, and healing proceeds via granulation tissue formation followed by re-epithelialization. The inflammatory processes in this type of healing are more pronounced than with primary repair. In addition, significant secondary intention requires the formation of more granulation tissue with more pronounced wound contraction. Within granulation tissue are modified fibroblasts and myofibroblasts that contain the contractile proteins responsible for wound contraction. Contraction is a process common to all wounds and is essential in reducing the size of an open wound. This reduction in wound area is accomplished through centripetal movement of the surrounding skin. Healing by primary intention involves a combined process of contraction and epithelial migration, whereas healing by secondary intention occurs essentially by contraction alone. Because there is more granulation tissue formed in this type of wound and thus more contraction, fibrous tissue formation is more pronounced, resulting in a larger scar.

A third type of healing is that of ***tertiary intention***, or delayed closure. Wounds that are too contaminated to close primarily and have not suffered significant tissue loss or devitalization are candidates for this process. This description usually applies to wounds that are over twelve hours old, to wounds caused by human or animal bites, or to wounds caused by high velocity missiles such as bullets. Healing by tertiary intention involves thorough debridement and irrigation, followed by three to four days of observation and mechanical closure.

Complications in wound healing may arise as a result of technical errors, anatomical variability, systemic drugs and diseases (Table 6-1). With advanced aging, the skin undergoes changes which can complicate healing. Thinning of the dermis is caused by changes in cell morphology and decreased vascularity that result in a significant loss of tensile strength. These changes render the tissue less resistant to injury and impede the

Table 6-1: Factors Associated with Wound Healing Complications

Technical Factors	Anatomical Factors	Drugs	Systemic Conditions
Inadequate wound preparation Excessive suture tension Reactive suture material Local anesthetics	Static or dynamic skin tension Oily skin Pigmented skin	Corticosteroids Penicillamine Colchicine anticoagulants antineoplastics NSAIDs	Advanced age Alcoholism Diabetes Uremia Severe anemia Malnutrition Ehlers Danlos' syndrome Osteogenesis imperfecta Marfan's syndrome Ionizing Radiation Immunosuppression

ability of the dermis to support sutures. In elderly individuals, therefore, sutures are prone to tear the skin, thus making tapes a more common choice for closing wounds. Advanced age is also associated with slower wound healing, which is presumably a manifestation of the decreased vascularity.

Chronic corticosteroid use, such as in post-organ transplant patients and severe asthmatics, is another factor which causes an alteration of skin anatomy. Corticosteroids exert an inhibitory effect on collagen fiber synthesis and an enhancing effect on collagen degradation, both of which delay the rate that a wound gains tensile strength. Thinning of the epidermis and an increased fragility of small vessels are additional corticosteroid-induced effects which retard healing. Ecchymosis is commonly manifested with insignificant trauma because these changes result in tissue that is easily traumatized and prone to bleed.

Another healing problem created by corticosteroid therapy is the drug's anti-inflammatory action. Inflammation is essential during the initial phase of wound healing. To combat the negative effects of corticosteroids, supplementation with vitamin C, vitamin A, zinc sulfate and anabolic steroids can be helpful. Vitamin A and C can be administered systemically and may reverse some of the skin changes seen with corticosteroid use. The dose is 500 mg of ascorbic acid per day and 50,000 International Units of vitamin A per day. While vitamin C is safe in these patients, vitamin A acts as an antagonist to the corticosteroids and may interfere with the therapeutic effects of the corticosteroid on the underlying systemic disease. Vitamin A can be applied topically to the wound in the form of a water soluble cream and will not interfere systemically with the corticosteroid therapy. The possibility of adrenal suppression must also be considered when treating patients on chronic corticosteroid therapy. Such patients could suffer an acute adrenal crisis when stressed. To avoid this life-threatening problem, the administration of supplemental corticosteroids at the time of injury should be considered. The recommended dosage is 200 to 400 mg of IV hydrocortisone or its equivalent.

Other drugs which can alter wound healing are nonsteroidal anti-inflammatory drugs (NSAIDs), anticoagulants and antineoplastic agents. Like corticosteroids, NSAIDs can decrease the extent of inflammation and thereby be detrimental to wound healing. This effect is dose-dependent; however, no adverse effects have been reported with present therapeutic doses. Anticoagulants can delay healing by increasing the potential for hematoma formation. Antineoplastic drugs are purported to interfere with healing by disrupting cell proliferation which is essential to the healing process. However, the metabolic suppression by antineoplastic drugs is apparently too weak to interfere with the rate of tensile strength gain in wound healing. Most of the concerns about antineoplastic drug effects on wound healing, therefore, have not been substantiated by either clinical or experimental evaluation. The blunting of cell-mediated immunity by cytotoxic drugs, however, remains a valid concern and as such, wound infection rather than disrupted wound healing, is the primary concern with these agents.

There are several diseases and conditions which can affect wound healing. Chief among them are diabetes mellitus, uremia, Ehler Danlos Syndrome and malnutrition. The mechanism of poor healing in the diabetic appears to result from both a reduction in collagen accumulation and local tissue hypoxia secondary to diabetic atherosclerosis. Diabetics are also more susceptible to infection, especially in the extremities, because of a deficiency in polymorphonuclear leukocyte chemotaxis. Diabetics undergoing surgery experience infections approximately 10% of the time. In wounds of a traumatic nature, some studies have reported that the risk of infection is five times greater in diabetic patients than in non-diabetic patients. In addition to the poor healing and susceptibility to infection, the loss of vibratory and pain sensation secondary to neuropathies in diabetics decrease their awareness of an infection or ulceration. The most important factors in wound management of diabetic patients are the control of blood sugar and the use of adjunctive antibacterial therapy.

In uremics fibroblast growth is inhibited and, thus, so is collagen formation, resulting in a decrease in wound tensile strength. In patients who are malnourished, a decrease in the amount of ingested protein causes a deficiency in the amino acids needed for fibroblast mitosis and collagen synthesis. Most of the previously mentioned factors alter wound healing by affecting collagen formation. However, in Ehler-Danlos syndrome, poor wound healing appears to result from an increase in skin elasticity. This abnormality is secondary to an increased number of elastin fibers and an abnormal arrangement of collagen fibers in these patients.

Irradiation produces an obliterative endarteritis with subsequent chronic ischemia which predisposes any injury to infection and poor wound healing. In such situations, it is critical that all devitalized tissue be meticulously removed and the wound surgically closed primarily for wound healing to occur normally.

In all of the aforementioned systemic diseases, adjunctive hyperbaric oxygen therapy may be required to achieve complete wound healing.

Other potential complications of wound healing involve anatomical factors and abnormal scar formation. The region of the body in which the injury occurs and the skin tension lines in the area can significantly affect scar size. For example, wounds involving the extremities or the anterior thorax heal with the most noticeable scars, while lacerations of the eyelid typically heal with the least evident scars. Likewise, injuries perpendicular to dynamic skin tension lines heal with wider scars than do wounds that are parallel to the tension lines. Furthermore, patients with pigmented and oily skin tend to heal with more noticeable scar formation. Proliferative scarring is a major concern to both the health care professional and the patient. Two types of proliferative scarring are the hypertrophic scar and the keloid. Hypertrophic scars remain within the boundary of the original injury and usually form in areas of stress such as in the skin overlying joints. Although the cause is unknown, this type of scar can be minimized by decreasing wound contraction time and by reducing the inflammatory response. It has been reported that scar hypertrophy is related to the length of time a wound is in the inflammatory or substrate phase before moving into the proliferative phase of healing. Hypertrophic scarring can also occur in tissue deficient wounds that are closed primarily under excessive tension. In contrast to the hypertrophic scar, a keloid extends beyond the boundaries of the original wound and is not iatrogenic. Keloid formation is most common in the butterfly area of the sternum, mandible, ear, abdomen and deltoid. The cause is unknown but may be related to the production of excess melanocyte stimulating hormone. Because keloid formation does not occur in all wounds within the same patient, it appears that this complication is not a systemic healing defect. The treatment of keloid formation can involve local injections of corticosteroids, compressive dressings and surgical revision.

In view of all the potential complications of wound healing, one can see the importance of an accurate patient history, good surgical technique and careful follow-up of mechanically repaired wounds. Patient's concerns about wound healing are justified, in many instances, and should not be overlooked in post-operative instructions. Taking the time to advise patients about what to expect during the healing process can alleviate much unnecessary anxiety.

III. PATIENT HISTORY

Like patients, all wounds are unique, each requiring individualized treatment. A thorough history must be obtained for each patient to include a past medical history, past surgical history, current review of systems, medications and allergies. Of critical importance are questions concerning diseases such as diabetes or liver and kidney disorders, which can significantly influence wound healing and infection. Awareness of medications that can alter the normal healing process such as corticosteroids, immunosuppressants, anticoagulants and inhibitors of platelet aggregation is also critical. Questions should also be asked to assess the patient's potential to develop keloids. A history of the present injury must include information about when and where the injury occurred, as well as how it happened. It is also important to identify possible underlying medical causes for the injury such as hypotension, syncope or seizures. Information regarding the patient's tetanus immunizations must also be obtained (Appendix D).

While all traumatic wounds are considered contaminated, the concentration of the bacterial inoculum and the time elapsed since the injury determine the likelihood of subsequent wound infection. Research does not support the use of prophylactic systemic antibiotic coverage for uncomplicated minor wounds and lacerations. Systemic antibiotics have no practical effect unless therapeutic blood levels or, more importantly, therapeutic tissue levels are attained within four hours from the time of injury. However, with visibly soiled and contaminated wounds, and in

Table 6-2: Indications for Antibiotic Therapy

- Wounds Greater than 4-6 Hours Old
- Crushing Wounds
- Lower Extremity Wounds
- Human Bites
- Cat Bites
- Severely Contaminated Wounds
- Complicated Hand Wounds
- Infection Prone Host (Immunocompromised, Diabetes, etc.)

patients with diseases that lower host resistance, antibiotics are recommended for injuries less than four hours old (Table 6-2). Topical antibacterials can be effective in re-establishing the bacterial balance when patients present after the four hour time period with wounds associated with a large bacterial inoculum. The most common infecting organism in traumatic wounds is gram positive *Staphylococcus aureus*, although gram negative organisms also occur frequently. *Pasteurella multocida* is the most common infecting organism from animal bites and is responsible for 80% of all cat bite infections. Antibiotic therapy should include a cephalosporin for *S. aureus* and gram negative infections, and oxacillin or dicloxacillin for animal bites. Studies are inconclusive regarding the efficacy of antibiotics with dog bites, though research overwhelmingly supports the use of antibiotics in cat bites and scratches. A dog bite can usually be treated like any other minor wound and closed by primary approximation following thorough cleaning and irrigation. However, primary closure of either a human bite or a cat bite will almost always develop a clinical infection. This undesirable outcome is secondary to the virulence of the oral organisms in cats and to the high concentration of oral bacteria in humans.

There are two anatomic areas in which the wound management of bites should be modified. Bites on the face are more resistant to infection and are usually sutured in both cat and dog bites to prevent gross disfigurement. Such wounds still require careful follow-up. In contrast, cat or dog bites of the extremities, especially the hands, are best left to heal by secondary intention. This approach is warranted because of the decreased blood supply in the hands, which increases the incidence and dissemination of infection. Rabies exposure must also be explored in all animal bites and treatment rendered if indicated.

The term "Golden Period" refers to the amount of time required for an inoculum to reach the critical level of 100,000 bacteria per gram of tissue. Studies have demonstrated that wound infection is likely when bacterial contamination attains this concentration. This period is important because it defines when and how a wound can be closed. The length of the golden period is variable and depends on such factors as the anatomic location of the wound, the type of wound and the degree of contamination. In general, most wounds should be closed within three to six hours following the injury. Head and neck wounds have an extended time period during which closure by primary union is considered safe. The abundant blood supply in the head and neck extends the closure time to eight to twelve hours in a clean wound. If a wound cannot be closed within the Golden Period, careful consideration should be given to allowing the wound to close by secondary or tertiary intention.

IV. PHYSICAL EXAMINATION

A limited physical examination should be conducted for all patients who have sustained a laceration injury. When examining the wound itself, the practitioner must thoroughly debride and irrigate each laceration and achieve hemostasis. It is important to remember during these maneuvers that soft tissue wounds generally involve some level of pain and discomfort. One of the initial steps in wound management is to screen for the presence of foreign bodies and the loss of local function and sensation. Sensory and motor examinations should be performed to rule out the presence of peripheral nerve damage before local anesthetics are used.

The presence of a foreign body in the wound of a conscious patient may sometimes be signaled by the patient's sense that something is present in the wound. Visual explorations should be conducted carefully because objects are oftentimes small and hard to detect. Manual palpation and radiographic assessment can be useful adjuncts to help confirm or deny the presence of foreign bodies in the wound. Metal, teeth and many types of glass can be visualized radiographically.

All lacerations must be thoroughly evaluated by digital and visual inspection to the depths of the wound once contributing factors have been ruled out and all personal injuries have been identified. The use of local anesthetic agents may be necessary for patient comfort prior to the final cleansing and debridement to allow exploration of deep wounds and underlying structures.

V. ANESTHESIA

Of all the local anesthetic solutions commonly used in the management of skin lacerations, lidocaine with epinephrine is the most popular (Table 6-3). A 1% solution of lidocaine can block nociceptive stimuli, but often leaves the sensations of touch and pressure intact. A 2% solution is recommended to obtund all sensation. The elimination of all stimuli is important for adequate pain control since it is common for anxious patients to confuse the sensations of pain and pressure. The use of epinephrine in local anesthetic is recommended to extend the period of effective anesthesia and to aid with temporary hemostasis. The fear of epinephrine induced ischemia in the extremities, such as fingertips, nasal tip and ears, has been thought for years to be a contraindication to its use in local anesthetic. However, the remote chance of this adverse effect is outweighed by the aforementioned benefits.

Topical anesthetics have been recently utilized to anesthetize very simple wounds, especially in children. The most often discussed topical anesthetic is a mixture of tetracaine, epinephrine and cocaine which is referred to by the acronym TAC. When compared to lidocaine, TAC has been shown to provide equivalent anesthesia for the repair of dermal

Table 6-3: Properties of Local Anesthetics

Agent	Concentration	Onset of Action: Infiltration	Onset of Action: Block	Duration of Action
Lidocaine with epinephrine	1% or 2%	Immediate	4-10 min	60-120 min for a block
Mepivicain	1%	Immediate	6-10 min	90-180 min for a block
Bupivicaine	0.25%	Slower	8-12 min	240-480 min for a block
TAC*		5-10 min	-	20 min

*Equal parts of 0.5% tetracaine + 1:2,000 epinephrine + 11.8% cocaine

lacerations. Unlike injected lidocaine, the administration of TAC is painless and there is no distortion of the tissue margins. TAC may be applied directly to the wound or indirectly on a saturated gauze. After waiting five to ten minutes, the wound may be repaired. Studies have shown a 95% success rate in placing sutures without eliciting pain in wounds that were 5 centimeters or less in length and five millimeters deep. TAC was found to be most efficacious for facial and lip injuries. However, a greater potential for infections and for toxic or fatal reactions was reported if the drug was used in amounts higher than the maximum recommended dose.

VI. ANESTHESIA TECHNIQUES

The administration of local anesthesia into the wound should be accomplished after the wound has been cleaned, provided the patient can tolerate the discomfort associated with cleaning. Needles should not be inserted into dirty wounds because deeper tissues may become inoculated with surface contaminants. When it is necessary to obtain anesthesia before the wound is cleaned, a block is recommended at a site distant from the wound itself. The two methods most often suggested for administrating local anesthetics are direct wound infiltration and the parallel margin infiltration. In the ***direct infiltration*** method, the anesthetic is injected directly into the wound. The proper depth is just beneath the dermis at the junction of the superficial fascia. Tissue resistance in this area is less, and sensory nerves are more easily contacted by the spreading solution. A small bolus of anesthetic agent is injected into the wound, the needle is withdrawn and then reinserted into an unanesthetized area and another bolus injected.

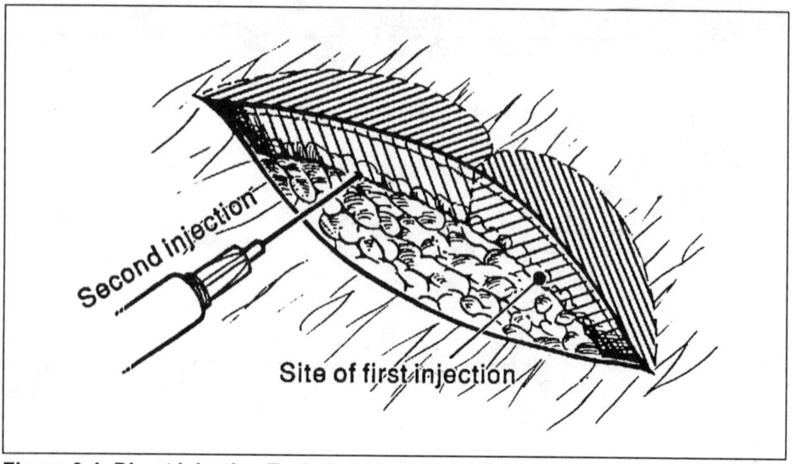

Figure 6-4: Direct Injection Technique for Wound Anesthesia.

This process should be repeated until all edges of the wound are anesthetized (Figure 6-4). The direct technique is less painful than some other methods because the needle does not pass through intact, sensory competent skin with each injection. However, the direct technique is principally indicated for small lacerations without visible contamination. A second method, the ***parallel margin*** technique is preferred for dirty wounds to minimize the spread of infection. The needle is inserted through the intact skin to

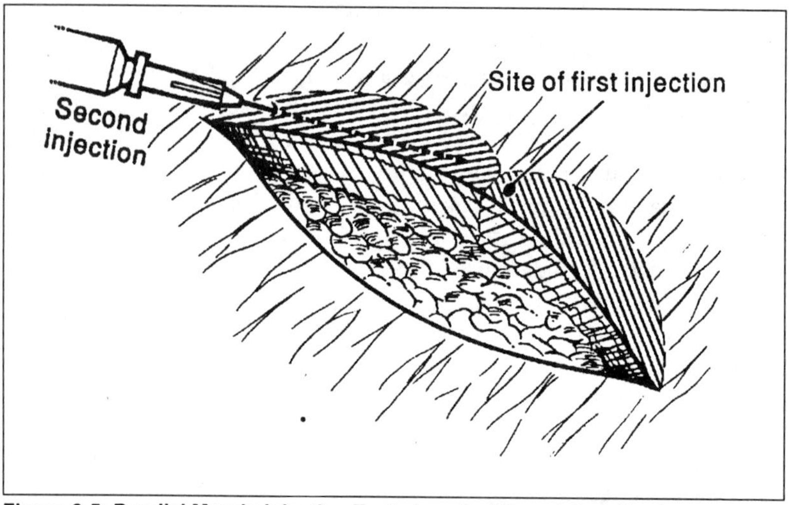

Figure 6-5: Parallel Margin Injection Technique for Wound Anesthesia.

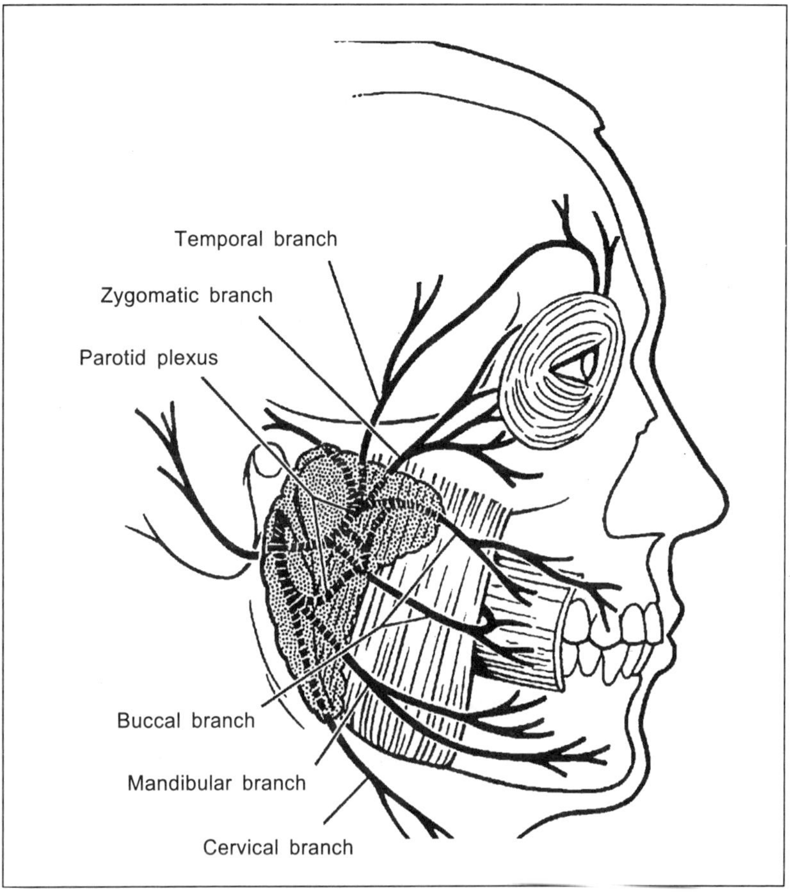

Figure 6-6: Facial Nerve Anatomy.

the dermis-superficial fascia plane, rather than through the wound itself, starting at one end of the laceration. The needle is advanced in a direction parallel to the edge of the wound to the opposite end of the laceration or until the full length of the needle is reached. A track of anesthetic agent is injected as the needle is withdrawn. In a wound that is longer than the needle, the procedure is repeated by starting at the end of the first track until the full length of the wound has been anesthetized. This process is repeated on all sides of the wound until complete anesthesia is obtained (Figure 6-5).

The techniques for intraoral blocks and infiltrations are discussed in Appendix A. Peripheral nerve blocks are beyond the scope of this chapter.

VII. DAMAGE TO UNDERLYING STRUCTURES

After local anesthesia is obtained, a thorough and accurate examination of the wound's extent must be conducted. Even a small laceration sometimes overlies serious structural damage, as in the case of a small scalp laceration associated with a depressed skull fracture. The eye and periorbital tissues are also susceptible to serious injury from relatively minor trauma. The parotid gland and the facial nerve are two important vital structures lying just anterior to the ear which can be injured by penetrating cheek lacerations. Saliva leaking from a cheek wound or bloody fluid from Stensen's duct intraorally are indicators of underlying parotid gland injury. All five branches of the facial nerve should be tested (Figure 6-6). The temporal branch competency can be assessed by asking the patient to contract the forehead and elevate the eyebrows. Zygomatic branch function is tested by noting whether the patient can open and close their eyes in a symmetrical manner. Competency of both the buccal and mandibular branches can be evaluated by assuring symmetrical muscle contraction during smiling and frowning. Finally, the cervical branch function may be evaluated by noting symmetrical contraction of the platysma muscle.

Imaging can be an invaluable adjunct in wound examination to detect underlying fractures and the presence of foreign bodies. Beneficial imaging techniques include plane films, computed axial tomography (CAT scan) and magnetic resonance imaging (MRI). These techniques are especially helpful in cases of head trauma to detect subdural hematoma formation which can result in significant post-trauma morbidity and mortality.

Table 6-4: Types of Skin Injuries

Type of Injury	Cause of Injury	Character of Injury	Incidence of Infection	Scarring Potential
Shearing	Sharp objects	Minimal cell destruction		
Avulsion	Object strikes skin at an angle. Caused by tension force on tissue	Blood supply is often interrupted causing tissue to be devitalized with possible necrosis	++	++
Crushing	Blunt object striking skin at right angle. Caused by a compression force on the tissue	Often have ragged edges with increased incidence of tissue devitalization	+++	+++

VIII. TYPES OF SOFT TISSUE INJURIES

In the management of traumatic wounds the goals are to restore function and to achieve acceptable esthetics. The mechanism of injury is a key factor in determining the required technique of repair and the potential for subsequent wound infection. The types of traumatic injury are classified as, shearing, avulsion and crushing (Table 6-4). ***Shearing injuries*** are commonly caused by sharp objects, like glass and knives. The prognosis for shearing injuries is usually favorable because tissue damage is confined to the area of insult. These lacerations are generally managed by primary closure, have a low incidence of wound infection, and the resulting scars are usually more esthetically acceptable than avulsion or crushing injuries. ***Avulsion*** injuries occur when an object strikes the skin at an angle resulting in a triangular laceration and creating a flap of skin as a consequence of tensile forces. Because the blood supply to the flap is interrupted on two sides, ischemia can result in devitalization and necrosis. As such, avulsion injuries are associated with greater cell destruction, potential ischemia, a higher incidence of infection, and more scarring than shearing injuries. When blunt objects strike the skin in a perpendicular direction a ***crushing or compression*** type of injury is likely. The wound edges are typically ragged and are accompanied by more widespread devitalization of skin and superficial fascia. Crushing injuries generally require extensive cleaning, irrigation and debridement. Prophylactic antibiotics are usually recommended and the resulting scars more commonly require surgical revision.

IX. WOUND PREPARATION

The purpose of wound preparation is to disinfect the wound and to remove the non-vital tissue, debris and foreign objects from the site of injury. There are four phases in wound preparation which include hair removal, cleaning, irrigation debridement, wound trimming and hemostasis. To prevent further contamination of the wound and to protect the practitioner from contracting disease, routine infection control measures should be followed. These measures include hand washing, the use of sterile gloves, a mask and head covering. Prior to wound cleaning it must be decided if hair adjacent to the wound should be removed. Today, hair removal is a controversial issue because recent research suggests that removal is associated with higher infection rates. Two studies have demonstrated an increase in wound infection rates in shaved versus non-shaved patients, while a third study found that shaved patients have a greater incidence of wound infection than either patients who received a depilatory agent or were unshaven. However, these studies examined surgical wounds and presently there is no data

Table 6-5: Wound Cleaning Agents

Agent	Antibacterial Activity	Tissue Toxicity	Systemic Toxicity
Povidine-iodine surgical scrub	Bacteriocidal against gram negative and gram positive bacteria	Can be toxic & painful to tissue in the wound	Rare
Povidine-iodine solution	Same as povidone-iodine scrub	Not toxic to tissue in the wound	Rare
Chlorhexidine	Bacteriocidal against gram positive bacteria weakly against gram negative bacteria	Can be toxic to tissue in the wound	Rare
Hexachlorophene	Bacteriostatic against gram positive bacteria and poorly active against gram negative bacteria	Can be toxic to tissue in the wound	Rare, teratogenic with chronic use
Hydrogen peroxide	Weakly antibacterial	Toxic to red blood cells	Rare

concerning hair removal in traumatic wounds. There are case reports of infections resulting from hair becoming inadvertently buried in wounds. Hair shafts can harbor bacteria, while sebaceous glands and hair follicles do not appear to contain bacteria under normal conditions. However, the hair shafts can be successfully cleansed using standard antiseptic solutions and techniques. Therefore, when planning hair removal, careful consideration should be given to whether hair removal would facilitate wound management. In sparse hair bearing areas, the practice of shaving the patient is generally unnecessary, whereas, in heavy hair-bearing regions such as the scalp or a bearded face, shaving facilitates laceration closure. When hair removal is indicated, the hair around the wound can be clipped with scissors, then shaved with a razor that has a recessed blade. Such a protocol will decrease the chance of epidermal or dermal injuries which can promote bacterial invasion and result in a post surgical infection. The only location where hair removal is contraindicated is the eyebrow, because the unpredictable nature of hair regrowth in this area can lead to cosmetically unacceptable results. In addition, eyebrow hair is an excellent landmark and can aid in proper alignment during wound closure.

To ***cleanse a wound*** the patient should be in a supine position to improve access to the wound and to prevent a vasovagal reaction. Sterile materials needed for cleansing include several 4x4 sponges, an appropriate wound cleaning solution, saline for irrigation, two all purpose bowls and a 35 cc syringe with an attached large, blunted needle (or the plastic catheter

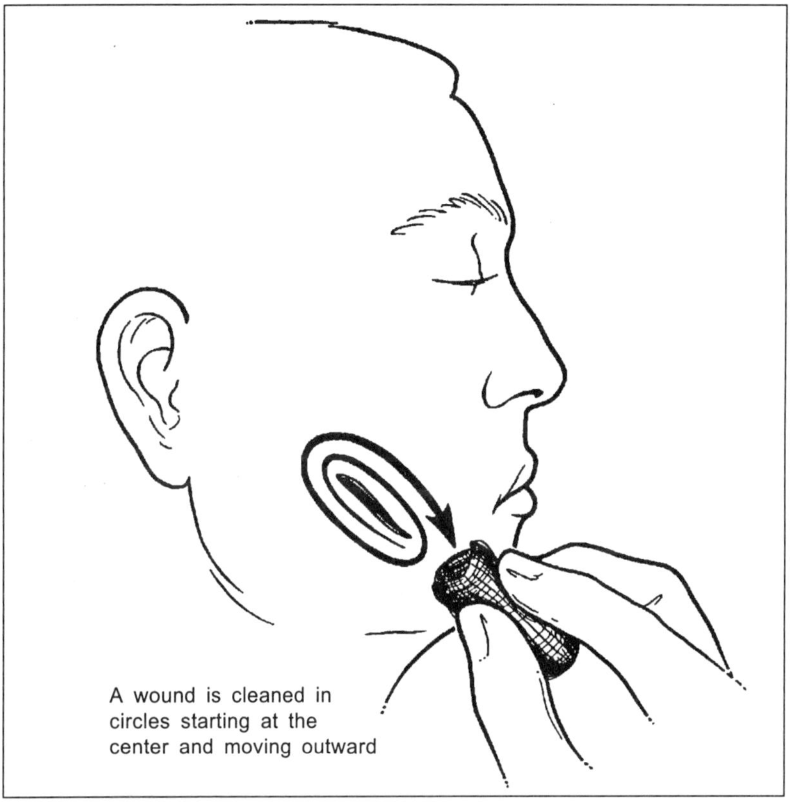

Figure 6-7: Wound Cleansing Technique.

from an angiocath). The cleaning solution is placed in one bowl and the saline in the other. There is little research information concerning the use of skin cleaning agents in traumatic wounds. Most of the information about the effects of cleaning solutions was derived from studies that compared the efficacy of these agents in elective surgery patients or lab animals. The ideal cleaning agent should have a broad spectrum of antimicrobial activity, be minimally toxic and act rapidly in addition to preparing and disinfecting skin. The most commonly used skin preparation compounds are the iodophors (Table 6-5). The goal of scrubbing with the cleanser is to clean the skin surrounding the wound, rather than to scrub the wound itself, since the detergent can be toxic to wound tissue. The technique for scrubbing the wound involves circular motions beginning at the wound margins and gradually projecting outward (Figure 6-7). Scrubbing is performed with a sponge that should be discarded, rather than reused, as reuse would introduce organisms into the cleansed wound. If considerable amounts of dirt, grease or tar are present, vigorous scrubbing with a soft nail brush is appropriate. This procedure is important because it will help to minimize or eliminate cosmetically unacceptable tattooing. Wound cleaning should be repeated with new sponges impregnated with cleaner for two to three minutes or until the skin is visibly free from contaminants and dried blood.

Irrigation is the most effective way to reduce bacterial counts on the wound surface and remove clotted blood, non-vital tissue, foreign bodies, dirt and other debris. Irrigation also removes fibrin coagulum, which can encase bacteria and small particulate contaminants isolating them from the effect of antibiotics. Sterile saline is the most commonly used solution for wound irrigation. High pressure irrigation is superior to the low pressure streams achieved with bulb type syringes. A 19-gauge needle attached to a 35 cc syringe and held 1 to 2 inches from the wound can deliver 8l pounds per square inch (psi) of pressure which is quite effective in cleaning a contaminated wound. Irrigation pressures higher than 70 psi may cause local tissue damage and should be avoided. The amount of irrigation fluid should range from a minimum of 100 cc to whatever volume is needed to eliminate contaminants. Following irrigation, it is important to visually reassess the presence or absence of foreign bodies in the wound. Useful instruments in foreign body removal are the Adison tissue forceps and a #11 blade.

Tissue debridement is another important part of wound preparation. Debridement involves the removal of non-vital tissue and tissues heavily contaminated by particulate matter. Devitalized soft tissue, either fat, muscle or skin is an ideal culture medium for bacterial growth. The devitalized tissue inhibits leukocyte phagocytosis, and the anaerobic environment further limits leukocyte function. Debridement of non-vital tissue is oftentimes difficult because the exact limits of debridement are unclear. Thus, surgical judgment and repeated examination of the wound is required. The skin edges should be gently debrided to remove any badly contused portions of tissue. With jagged edges, trimming can convert an irregularity into a straight line to improve wound closure and cosmetic outcome. As a rule, a ragged wound with viable tissue edges is repaired by putting the "puzzle pieces" back together and preserving as much tissue as possible. This is especially true in the face, where it is better to preserve skin which may die, rather than removing tissue with survival potential. If the laceration is vertical or diagonal and results in an overhang, the overhanging dermis and epidermis should be trimmed to develop a laceration that is perpendicular to the skin. This provides a better chance for adaptation of the wound edges.

The viability of crushed or avulsed tissue may be difficult to clinically determine during the acute phase of injury. The main indicator of necrosis is the failure to bleed when cut. Bright red bleeding from wound edges is usually a dependable confirmation of skin viability. However, in acute trauma, hypovolemic shock and arteriovenous shunting of the dermal plexus may obscure the diagnosis. To overcome this problem, intravenous fluorescein has been recommended to more accurately predict skin flap viability. The usual dose is 15 mg/kg in Caucasians to 20 mg/kg in blacks. Because the drug rapidly diffuses from the intravascular fluid space to the extra cellular fluid space, fluorescein can be used to predict tissue perfusion. Fifteen minutes after administration, the skin or flap is examined in a dark room with a Wood's lamp. A yellow fluorescence indicates tissue viability, whereas a purple coloration suggests an area of impending necrosis. This technique does not provide a quantitative assessment, however, and is not completely reliable. A variation of this technique is dermofluormetry, which has been shown to be a reliable predictor of digital replantation perfusion. The test requires only 1.5 to 2.0 mg/kg of fluorescein and can be repeated several times over a 24 hour period. A fluorescein perfusion ratio of less than 20% indicates soft tissue necrosis, whereas a value of greater than 50% is associated with flap survival.

X. INFECTION

According to the American College of Surgeons Committee on Control of Surgical Infections, traumatic wounds can be classified as either contaminated or infected. One study demonstrated that 62% of civilian wounds contained less than 10^2 organisms per gram of tissue prior to treatment. Eighteen percent of the wounds contained 10^2 to 10^5, organisms per gram and 20% contain greater than 10^5 organisms per gram. It is now generally accepted that all wounds with greater than 10^5 organisms per gram will become infected. When the infecting organism is B-hemolytic streptococcus, or when massive tissue damage exists, fewer organisms can lead to wound infection. It appears that wound infection is principally determined by the time between the initial injury and the treatment of the wound and the quantity of bacteria in the wound. Other factors, such as the condition of the local area and systemic host resistance, may also influence the risk of wound infection. Severely injured patients demonstrate diminished and delayed hypersensitivity responses and poor neutrophil chemotaxis. Other systemic factors which may potentiate wound infection are shock, malnutrition, diabetes mellitus, arteriosclerosis, cancer chemotherapy, corticosteroid medications, extremes of age and obesity. Local factors that contribute to the proliferation of bacteria are dead space, hematomas, irradiated tissue, heavy contamination with dirt and necrotic, devitalized or crushed tissue. Soil has organic infection-potentiating factors that can severely compromise wound resistance. When considering the use of antibiotics, it is important to remember that the length of time a wound is open is indirectly correlated with the effectiveness of systemic or topical antibiotics. This is primarily because the fibrin coagulum which contains bacteria effectively protects the organisms from the antibiotic effects. Also, the degree of contamination within the wound can diminish the outcome of antibiotic therapy. Finally, environmental conditions, such as cooling and desiccation of the wound, may further reduce antibiotic effectiveness.

XI. HEMOSTASIS

Although hemorrhage from cutaneous wounds can appear overwhelming, it is seldom life-threatening, except when major underlying vascular structures are injured. There are multiple methods of hemorrhage control available to the practitioner. The standard treatment is applied ***sustained pressure***. Direct pressure is frequently all that is needed to stop the bleeding in most soft tissue wounds involving small vessels and capillaries.

Electrocautery is also an effective and rapid method to achieve hemostasis of small blood vessels. A high frequency electrical current ranging from 2 to 18 million cycles/second, with relatively high amperage and low voltage will produce coagulation from the heat of the current. Although a small amount of tissue may be charred, there is no evidence that wound healing is impaired by this technique. The tissue trauma can be minimized and coagulation made more effective by placing the active electrode of the electrosurgical unit in contact with a small hemostat that accurately grips the site of hemorrhage. A relatively dry field and a ground electrode are required for effective electric current to pass through the tissues. As such, frequent suctioning or sponging is necessary.

Additional methods of hemostasis for small vessels include the injection of a ***vasoconstrictor*** into the wound or the topical application of ***hemostatic agents*** such as aluminum chloride, ferric sulfate, silver nitrate and topical thrombin. Bleeding from larger blood vessels may require ***ligation*** with a suture to stop the hemorrhaging. Indiscriminate clamping of bleeding vessels in an open wound should be avoided because of the potential to damage underlying vital structures, especially in the maxillofacial region and upper extremities. After clamping the hemorrhaging vessel with a fine pointed hemostat, a resorbable suture can be tied around the vessel; or for a more secure ligation, the suture may be passed through the adjacent tissue before being tied. In the past, clamping or crushing small blood vessels was used as the sole method of achieving hemostasis. Although this avoids placing sutures (which act as foreign bodies), this method is not a reliable form of hemostasis. Whatever method is used, proper suction, lighting and assistance should be available for exploration and precise control of bleeding vessels.

XII. SUTURING ARMAMENTARIUM

Surgical needles are designed to carry suture material through tissues with minimal trauma. The needles are comprised of heat treated stainless steel to maximize strength and ductility. All surgical needles have three basic components: the eye, the body and the point. The needle eye can either be closed, French (split or spring), or swaged (eyeless). The ***closed eye*** is the traditional loop with either a round, oblong or square shape. ***French eye*** needles are a series of interconnected loops that act as ridges to catch and hold the suture in place at various positions. These two types of eyed needles must be threaded and require that a double strand of suture material be pulled through the tissue. A ***swaged suture*** has the needle and suture joined together into a continuous unit. A hole or channel in the end of the needle is closed around the suture in a swaging process, resulting in a design that is convenient to use and causes less tissue trauma than either the closed or French eye needles (Figure 6-8).

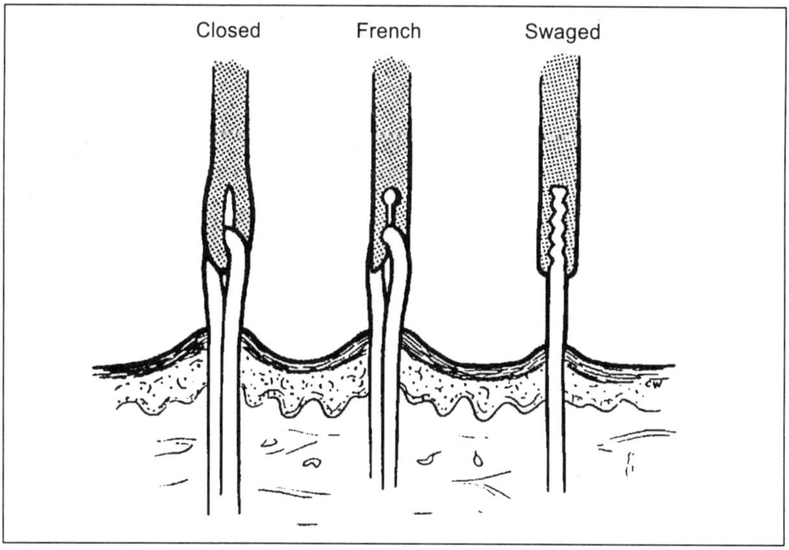

Figure 6-8: Tissue Displacement Caused by Different Needle Eyes.

The body of a needle may be round, oval, rectangular, triangular or trapezoidal in cross section. Some needles employ longitudinal ribs on the concave or convex surface to reduce rotational movement in the needle holder during suturing. The longitudinal shape of the body may be straight, half curved, curved or compound curved (Figure 6-9). When suturing, it is the body of the needle which is grasped with the suture forceps.

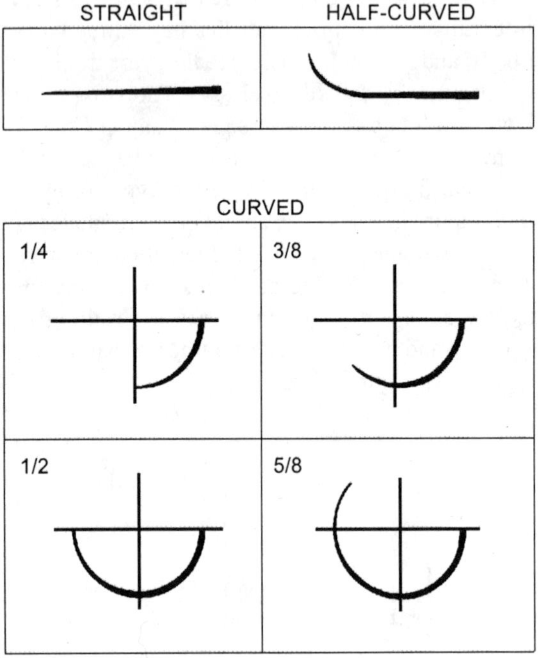

Figure 6-9: Types of Suture Needles.

Selection of the appropriate needle length, width and curvature depends on the size, depth and type of tissue to be sutured. ***Straight needles*** are usually used in tissue that is easily accessible allowing direct digital manipulation. ***Half curved needles*** are rarely employed because while the curved portion of the needle passes easily through the tissue, the remaining straight portion of the body cannot follow the curved path without bending or enlarging the path. ***Curved needles*** are the most frequently used shape because they allow the greatest maneuverability in a confined space. The compound curved needle was originally developed for anterior segment ophthalmic surgery to permit precise, uniform bites of tissue. The initial curvature of the needle affords reproducible short, deep bites into

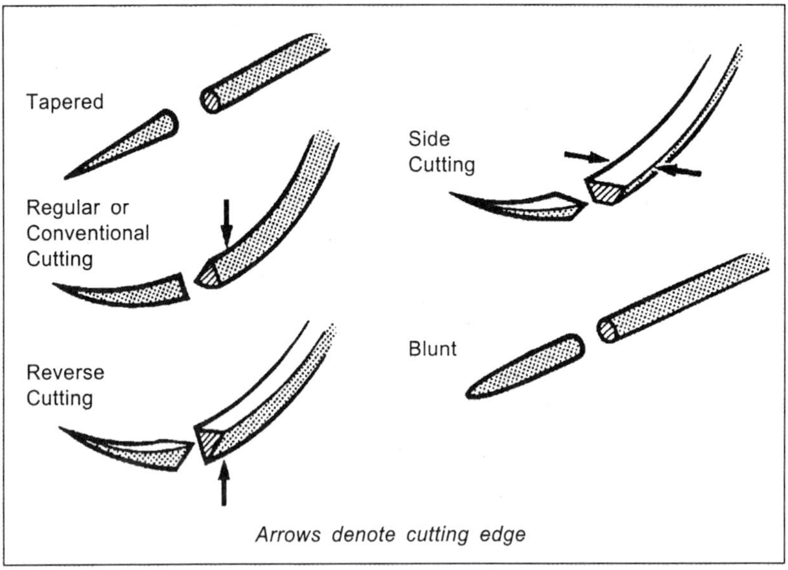

Figure 6-10: Types of Suture Needles.

the tissue, and the curvature of the remaining portion forces the needle out of the tissue, everting the wound edges. The design also aids in the equidistant placement of the suture on both sides of the laceration.

The point of the needle begins at the extreme tip and extends to the maximum cross section of the body. Each specific point is designed to the required sharpness to smoothly penetrate the type of tissue to be sutured. The basic designs include; cutting, reverse cutting, side cutting, taper and blunt points (Figure 6-10). A ***conventional cutting needle*** has two opposing cutting edges with a third inside cutting edge forming the apex of a triangular configuration. The inside edge is located on the concave portion of the needle and cuts toward the margins of the incision or wound. The ***reverse cutting needle*** differs in that the third cutting edge is located on the outer or convex curvature of the needle. Thus the flat surface is closest to the edges of the incision or wound which decreases the risk of tissue tear. Also, the hole left by the needle leaves a wide wall of tissue for the suture to be tied against. ***Side cutting or spatula needles*** are flat on top and bottom, and were intended for use in ophthalmic surgery. The design enables the needle to separate or split through the thin layers of scleral or corneal tissue and then to travel within these tissue planes. The ***taper point needles*** consist of a tapered body with a round blunt tip. The needle will not cut through tissue but rather is intended for blunt dissection in the suturing of friable parenchymal tissues such as liver and kidney resulting in the smallest possible hole.

There is no universal needle labeling or coding, as each manufacturer has its own nomenclature. Needle size and shape can be determined by examining the package on which the needle is drawn to scale.

Characteristics of an ideal ***suture material*** include strength, ease of handling, irritation potential and resorption characteristics. The suture should be as strong as the tissue being sutured and the strength should be maintained until the tissue is sufficiently healed to withstand tensile forces. Ease of handling includes such concerns as facilitation of knot tying, knot security and the passage of the suture through tissue. The suture should not irritate the tissue, and the potential for suture induced infection should be negligible. All suture materials act as a foreign body to human tissues regardless of the type.

Sutures can be classified by their absorbability, by their configuration (such as monofilament or multifilament) and by size or diameter. A ***monofilament suture*** is made of a single strand which makes it less likely to harbor microorganisms and easy to tie down; however, knot security is a problem. A ***multifilament suture*** consists of several filaments twisted or braided together. This design, which affords good handling and tying qualities, also increases tissue drag and provides areas for bacteria adherence. The sizes and tensile strengths for all suture materials are standardized by specific regulations. Stated numerically, the more zeroes (0's) in the number, the smaller the diameter of the strand thus, a 5-0 suture is smaller than 2-0 suture. The tensile strength is directly proportional to the diameter of the suture.

Sutures which are dissolved or digested by enzymes or hydrolyzed by tissue fluids are called absorbable (Table 6-6). Absorbable sutures should absorb completely, rapidly, predictably and with minimal inflammation once the suture has served its purpose. If the material is not significantly affected by enzymatic reaction or hydrolysis, then it is classified as nonabsorbable and the body will encapsulate or wall off the suture. Of the absorbable sutures, plain gut has the poorest tensile strength and the most rapid

Table 6-6: Properties of Absorbable Sutures

Type of Suture	Strength Retention	Absorption Rate	Tissue Reactivity
Plain gut	1 week	2.5 months	++++++
Chromic gut	3 weeks	3.0 months	+++++-
Vicryl	2-3 weeks	2-3 months	+++++
Polydioxanone	2-6 weeks	7 months	++++

resorption, while polydioxanone is the most resistant to resorption maintaining tensile strength over the longest time period. Chromic gut and polyglactin sutures behave similarly with intermediate absorption rates.

Cat gut suture is the prototypical absorbable suture and the name is derived from the former use of violin (kit) strings for surgical sutures. Today, surgical gut is derived from the submucosa of sheep intestines and the serosa of beef intestines. Purification of the tissue yields collagen-rich ribbons that are twisted together and dried under tension. When dry, the strands are polished, cut, packaged, and sterilized using CO^{60} irradiation. These procedures produce a suture that, while not a true monofilament, looks and behaves like one. To remain pliable, gut must be kept moist and thus is packaged in alcohol. As the suture material dries out, friction increases, making it is more formidable to tie. Because the material is not braided knot tying is less cumbersome. Many of the shortcomings of gut sutures are a reflection of its complex and non-uniform composition, which results in variability of strength and duration. Generally, gut has a 10-day life span in healthy tissue, however, the suture may lose significant strength much sooner in an acidic, infected tissue or in a fluid environment. In addition, gut can be difficult to tie and knots difficult to secure. Also, because of the sutures configuration, gut can promote bacterial growth and has been associated with increased infections relative to other sutures. Sugarman's research found gut to have 100 times the bacterial adhesion of nylon and the most of any suture examined by the study.

Chromic gut is plain gut tanned with chromium salts. This process produces a suture with improved strength and delayed dissolution characteristics. The average reported duration of chromic gut is about 3 weeks. Knot security of chromic gut is superior to plain gut, however, the handling properties are equally problematic. Despite the additional processing step, the cost of the suture is the same as untanned or plane gut. The tissue's inflammatory response to chromic gut is only slightly less than the tissue response to plane gut. Chromic gut sutures would appear superior to plain gut when a resorbable suture is indicated.

Collagen sutures are prepared from the long flexor tendons of cattle. Following a series of treatments, the tendons are converted into a collagen-rich viscous gel that can be extruded into monofilament-like strands. Because both gut and collagen sutures are comprised of collagen, most of their properties are the same. A minor difference between the two is that collagen sutures are a more pure collagen product. Like gut, the suture is available in either plain or chromic forms.

Dexon (polyglycolic acid or PGA), is a polymer of hydroacetic acid, a naturally occurring metabolic by-product. The material is processed and extruded into a fine monofilament, which is braided to make the suture more flexible. The suture is available in uncoated and coated forms (Dexon S, Dexon Plus), and the coating facilitates knot tying and passage through tissue. The tensile strength of Dexon is superior to that of natural absorbable sutures, and this strength is more stable in a fluid environment. Research studies support the claim that these sutures are stronger than silk, cotton polyester and gut sutures of comparable size. Although Dexon is more durable than gut sutures, little tensile strength remains after 14 to 21 days. Since Dexon is a synthetic material, it is harsher and stiffer than natural products. To overcome this drawback the strands are weaved into a braid to increase the handling characteristics, however, this also increases tissue drag. Also, Polyoxamer 188 is applied to the suture to produce an absorbable coating, and this process reduces knot security. Because of this, an extra throw is recommended when tying knots with Dexon. Resorption occurs differently with Dexon in that the process involves the hydrolysis of ester bonds within 15 to 30 days. As such, the tissue response is milder than with gut or silk, which may speed wound healing, reduce scar formation and minimize the potential for infection. The improved incidence of infection with PGA may also be related to the bactericidal nature of the suture's degradation products.

Vicryl is a copolymer of glycolic and lactic acid in a 9:1 ratio, hence the name polyglactin 910. The material is very similar to Dexon in handling and mechanical properties. Vicryl is braided and coated with calcium sterate and a copolymer of lactide and glycolide. Both Vicryl and Dexon can be used in infected tissue, as there is no accelerated decline in strength or increased rate of resorption.

Polydioxanone (PDS) is made from polymerized paradioxone, which produces a flexible suture that can be made into monofilaments of all sizes. This advantage alleviates the need to braid the suture and, thus, avoids the undesirable features of increased bacterial adherence, tissue drag and size. However, special care is required when tying because of the inherent elasticity of the material. The tensile strength of PDS is superior to that of other monofilaments, and the duration of this strength exceeds that of Vicryl. Bacterial adherence is less than with PGA, gut or Vicryl, and absorption occurs by hydrolysis.

Unlike the absorbable sutures, ***nonabsorbable*** sutures are not hydrolyzed by the body and must be removed by the practitioner at a later date (Table 6-7).

Silk sutures are fabricated from the filaments of natural silk obtained from silk worm larvae. The sutures are composed of 70% natural silk and 30% extraneous material. Silk has a lower tensile strength than most nonabsorbable materials, however, in contrast to absorbable materials, the short-term strength is sufficient to provide acceptable tissue healing before the suture's binding ability is lost. The main advantage of silk is its favorable handling characteristics. The material is easy to tie, forms soft, nonirritating knots and has good knot security. A second advantage is cost, as silk is the cheapest of all the commonly used suture materials.

Table 6-7: Properties of Nonabsorbable Sutures

Type of Suture	Strength Retention	Tissue Reactiviy
Cotton	Decreases with time. All strength lost within 2 years.	+
Mersilene (Dacron)	Indefinite	+
Polypropylene (Prolene)	Indefinite	+
Silk*	All strength lost	++++++
Nylon†	Decreases with time. All strength lost within 5 years.	+

* Classified here as nonabsorbable even though it usually cannot be found after 2 years
† Classified here as nonabsorbable even though it will be completely degraded in 5-6 years

The tissue response to silk may be the most severe of all suture materials and is a definite disadvantage of the material. This reaction is cellular, with generalized inflammation in the area of the suture. Because of this response and the braided configuration of the material, the potential for infection is great. To minimize these problems silk is usually coated with either wax or silicone oil. An alternative suture material is recommended in a wound that is infected or contaminated.

Cotton sutures are comprised of a naturally occurring fiber that is braided and performs in a manner similar to silk. As such, the tissue response to the suture is severe and it is contraindicated in contaminated or infected tissue. The material is more often used as a ligature than to mend lacerations.

Nylon (polyamide) sutures are probably the most widely used skin suture. The material is a synthetic polyamide polymer that is available in monofilament and multifilament braided forms. Several studies have shown nylon to be among the best suture materials for minimizing infection, thus making the material suitable for use in contaminated and infected tissues.

Polypropylene (Prolene) sutures are derived from the polymerization of propylene. The product is melted and extruded into monofilament strands. The resulting elasticity is a major benefit, allowing a healing wound to expand without marking the skin from increased suture tension.

Polypropylene and steel are among the least reactive suture materials available, and the reaction that does occur is largely acellular. Because of this minimal tissue response and the monofilament construction, prolene is suitable for infected and contaminated tissues.

Dacron (Mersiline) is one of the strongest synthetic materials and it is comprised of braided polyester. The suture is usually coated with Teflon to improve handling properties and to minimize the capillary or wicking action common to braided sutures. Teflon pieces, however, may flake off and become a source of inflammation. ***Stainless steel*** sutures are derived from drawn, low carbon, iron-alloy strands that are available in monofilament and multifilament forms. The tissue reaction is mild and may be the least severe of any of the nonabsorbable sutures. Although corrosion products can cause a tissue response, stainless steel has also been shown to be the least infective suture material. Handling properties are a drawback; however, knot security is good if the sutures are tied correctly.

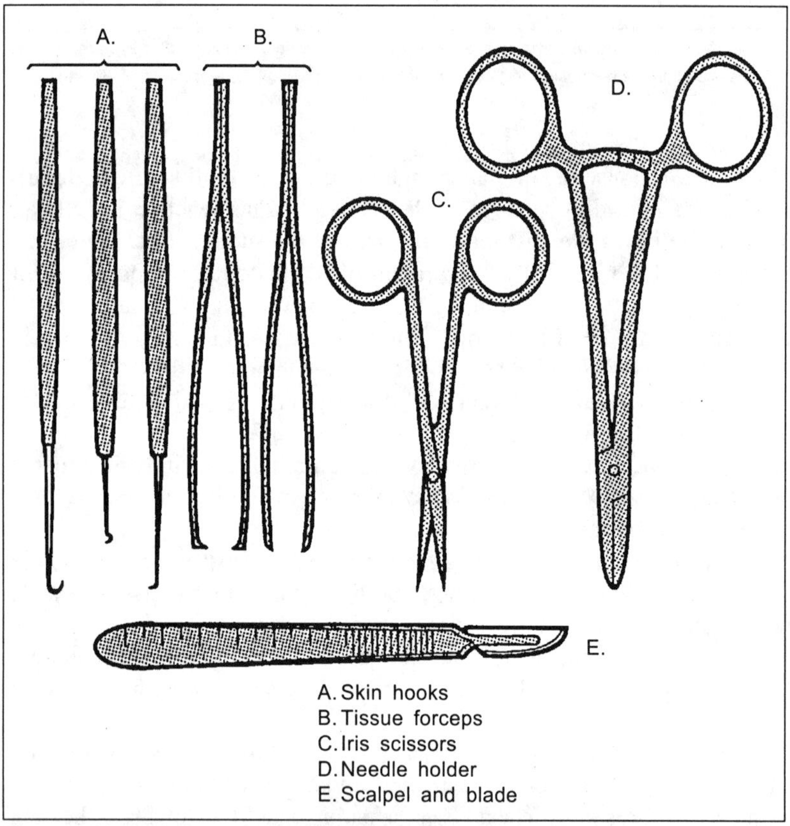

Figure 6-11: Basic Instrument Setup for Repairing Lacerations.

XIII. SUTURING INSTRUMENTS

The basic instrument setup used to repair soft tissue lacerations includes fine Adison forceps with and without teeth, a scalpel handle with a #15 blade, skin hooks, a needleholder and small scissors for doing wound debridement (Figure 6-11).

The ***needle holder*** of choice has a locking handle and is held with the thumb and ring finger through the rings. The index finger is placed along the length of the needle holder to provide stability and control (Figure 6-12).

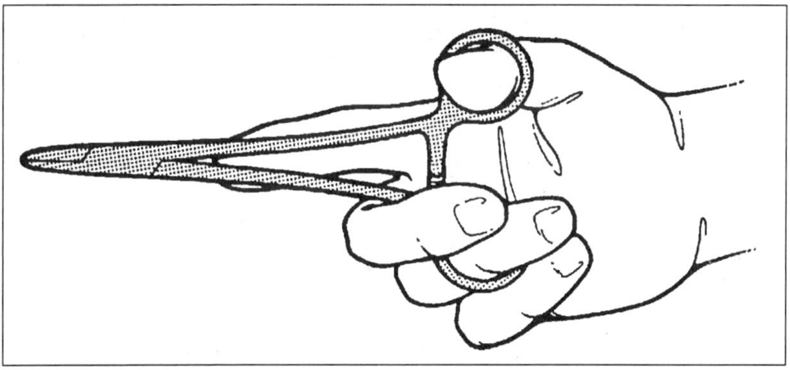

Figure 6-12: Correct Hand Position for Grasping the Suture Holder.

Needle holders are made of noncorrosive, high strength, quality steel alloy with jaws designed to secure needles. The jaws of some needleholders have diamond-cut surfaces, while others have a tungsten carbide insert to increase jaw hardness. The jaws may be short or long, broad or narrow, slotted or flat, concave or convex, and smooth or serrated. In choosing a needle holder, one should be selected that matches the size of the needle. To avoid breakage the needle should be grasped away from the swaged or eye region, approximately ¼ to ½ of the distance from the swaged area to the point (Figure 6-13).

Likewise, the suture needle should not be crushed or crimped with needle holders in the swaged area where the suture joins the needle. The tips of the needle holder should meet before the rest of the jaws come together to assure the most positive grasp of the needle. The needle should not rock, twist or turn, but should feel stable. The needle holder should not be closed beyond the first or second ratchet to avoid fracture of the needle precipitated by excess force. The tissue pickups facilitate suturing by securing the tissue as the needle is being passed. The needle should enter the tissue at right angles and the needle holder rotated so the needle

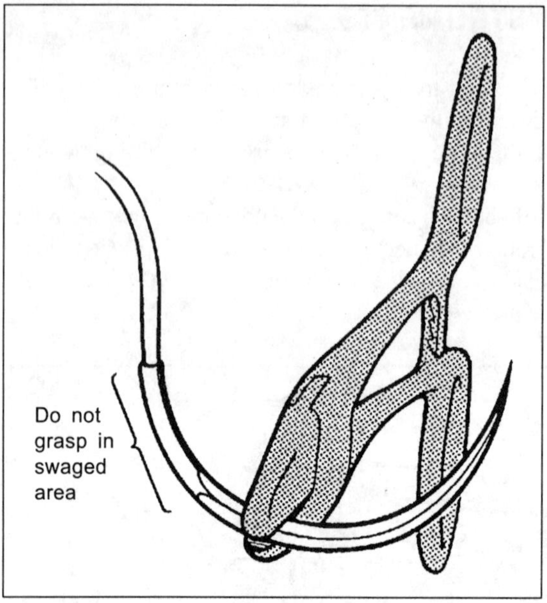

Figure 6-13: Correct Placement of Suture Needle in the Needle Holder.

continues to pass through the tissue at right angles (Figure 6-14). Tearing of the tissue may occur if the needle is directed into the tissue at an angle less than 90 degrees. Sutures should be evenly spaced about 1 to 3 mm from the wound edge.

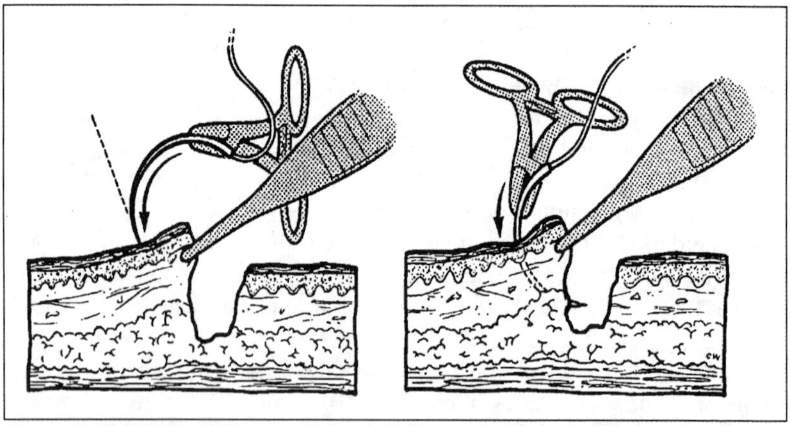

Figure 6-14: Needle is Directed Perpendicular to the Soft Tissue.

XIV. COMMONLY USED SUTURE TECHNIQUES

Following wound debridement, irrigation and the repair of other injuries such as bony fractures, decisions must be made regarding wound closure. Surgical principles dictate that the choice of wound closure begins with the simplest and progresses to the more complex. Such choices include primary closure, skin grafts, local or regional rotation flaps, and distal free-tissue transfers. This chapter will focus on primary closure, leaving the more complex techniques for those with greater expertise.

The wound must first be isolated with sterile drapes prior to suturing and a sterile field maintained throughout the procedure. ***Primary closure*** is preferred whenever possible. Healthy, non-edematous tissues, without heavy bacterial contamination are good candidates for primary closure. In experimentally contaminated wounds, primary closure has prevented infection associated with prolonged exposure of repaired vascular injuries. Closing the wounds minimized bacterial inoculation and desiccation of the wound. Clinically, however, primary closure in the face of heavy contamination results in wound infection nearly 100% of the time. In preparing the wound, tissue margins should be sharply debrided and should bleed easily in the process. In the face, however, every attempt should be made to save tissue for cosmetic reasons. Suturing should begin by aligning landmarks (such as the vermillion border, birthmarks) and should extend bidirectionally to the ends of the wound. If no landmarks are present, suturing should begin in the middle of the laceration and close bidirectionally toward each end. This type of closure is accomplished by "halfing" the remaining portion of the laceration and halfing again, and so on, until the wound is closed (Figure 6-15).

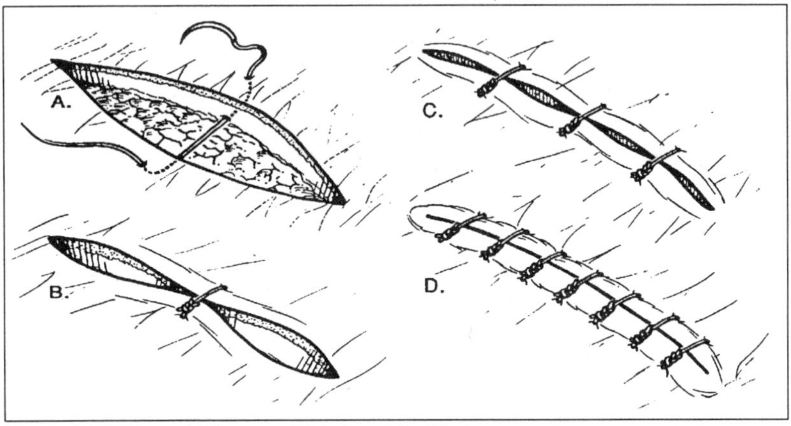

Figure6-15: Wound Closure with Interrupted Sutures.

When the esthetics of a resulting scar are important, it is critical to use the finest needle and suture that will oppose the tissue properly, and to have the majority of the appositional tension in the dermal layer. The epidermal sutures should be placed with minimal tension. These objectives can be accomplished by using any of the interrupted or continuous subcuticular stitches. A vertical or horizontal mattress suture can also be used in an interrupted fashion (Figure 6-16). Eversion of the opposing flaps is esthetically desirable to compensate for wound contracture and, thereby, minimize the scar width. A horizontal mattress is preferred when eversion is desired.

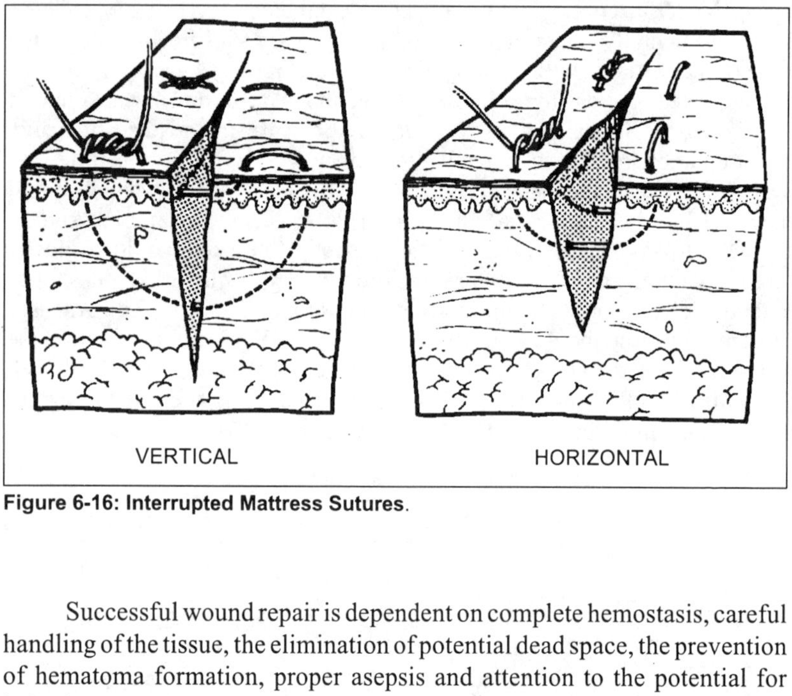

Figure 6-16: Interrupted Mattress Sutures.

Successful wound repair is dependent on complete hemostasis, careful handling of the tissue, the elimination of potential dead space, the prevention of hematoma formation, proper asepsis and attention to the potential for infection. As with non-viable tissue, a hematoma provides a fertile medium for bacterial replication and, thereby, greatly increases the risk of infection following wound repair. In deep wounds, multiple layers of sutures are needed to close the wound and prevent dead space formation (Figure 6-17) while more superficial wounds generally need a single layer for acceptable apposition. Subepithelial sutures should be resorbable, and are passed in an inverted manner. Burying the knot will help prevent the "spitting" of the knot during healing. When placing deep sutures, remember that fat has no tensile strength. Also, sutures placed tightly in fat often cause ischemia and necrosis, thus increasing the chances for infection. Like fat, muscle fibers do not support sutures well. As such, the overlying fascia, which has a high collagen content, should be included when suturing muscle. Because most wounds achieve only 60% of their final tensile strength, in two weeks, resorbable subepithelial sutures should consist of a synthetic material that requires enzymatic dissolution rather than hydrolysis for absorption. Enzymatic absorption is slower and will extend the sutures effective duration. A synthetic absorbable material can also be used in a continuous subcuticular stitch that pierces the skin on both ends of the wound. This allows the subcuticular suture to be removed by pulling on the extruded suture. An interrupted suture technique is preferred subcutaneously to a continuous one, to avoid the total loss of dermal retention should the suture break. Proper alignment of the subcutaneous layers allows eversion of the margins, which prevents formation of a depressed scar as the wound contracts during healing. The closer the coadaptation of the dermal edges, the narrower the resulting scar will be.

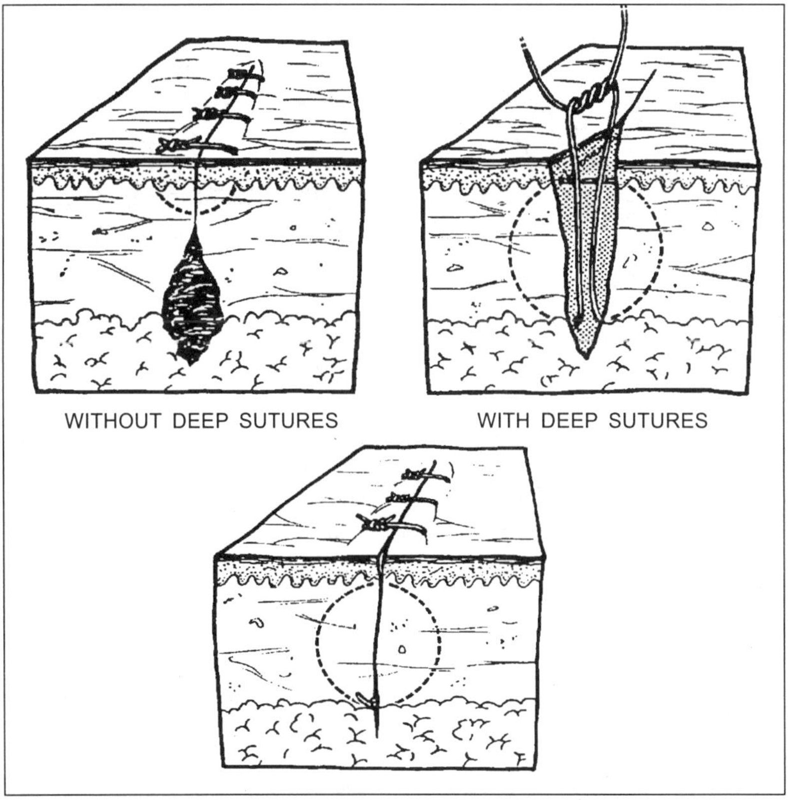

Figure 6-17: Placement of Deep Sutures to Prevent Dead Space and Improve Edge Adaptation.

When tissue debridement yields a wound that gaps, undermining the dermal tissue with blunt dissection may afford a tension free closure (Figure 6-18). When this technique is employed, the tissue should be undermined along the entire length of the wound. Sutures are placed with minimal tension to avoid enlarging the suture needle tracks. The needle is passed so that the points of entrance and exit closely approximate the wounds edges. When a running epidermal stitch is used, the suture is placed very near the edge of the wound, and the bites spaced to avoid overlap. Larger bites of the subcutaneous tissue are needed with superficial, interrupted sutures to avoid inversion of the skin edges.

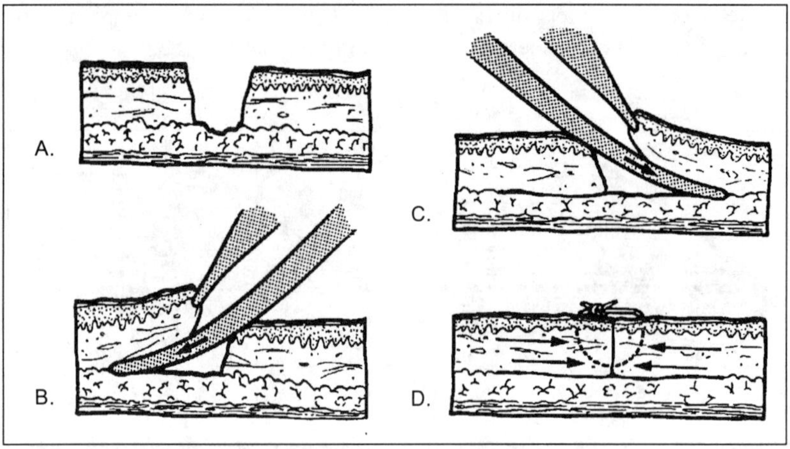

Figure 6-18: Blunt Dissection to Allow Tension-Free Closure.

The ***knot*** used to secure the suture will vary according to the material used, the location, depth and purpose of the stitch. Generally, the suture only needs to be tied tight enough to oppose the tissue without slipping. Strangulation of the tissue should be avoided and postoperative edema should be anticipated in deciding on a suture tension. When tying a knot it is recommended to throw two times in one direction so the suture will lie down flat, then a reverse throw to secure the knot. After the first loop is tied, traction should be maintained on one end of the strand to avoid loosening. When the two ends of the suture are pulled in opposite directions with a uniform rate and tension, the knot may be secured with less possibility of breakage. The suture line can be of greater cosmetic acceptance during the healing phase if the knots are all tied on the same side of the incision. Extra throws add bulk but not strength to the knot.

However, when using synthetic monofilaments several extra throws are needed because of the smooth surface and elasticity of the material. The knot should be small and the loose ends cut as short as possible to minimize the opportunity for bacterial adhesion and foreign body tissue reaction. Excessive tension should be avoided to prevent suture breakage and the creation of large track marks created by the suture material. Clamps and hemostats should not be used to grasp any portion of the suture which will remain *in situ*.

XV. SPECIAL PROBLEMS IN SUTURING

Puckering occurs when the lengths of the wound margins are unequal. It is common for a pucker to appear at the end of the suture line just prior to complete approximation of the skin. To remedy this problem, the wound should be extended by removing an elliptical section of tissue (Figure 6-19).

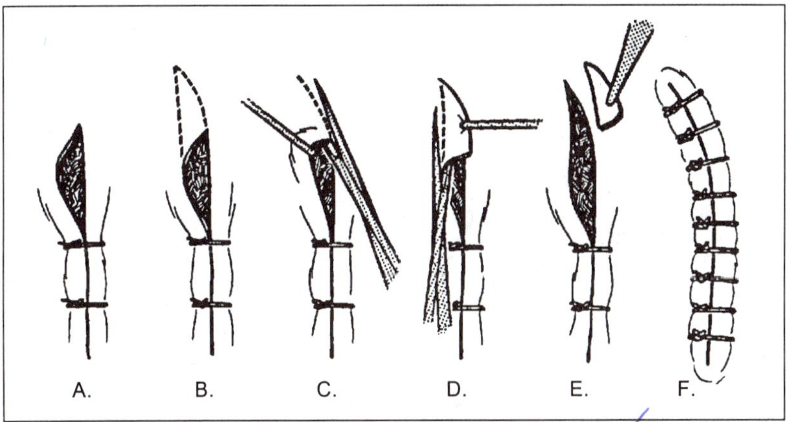

Figure 6-19: Correction of Puckering by Removal of Tissue.

Unequal flap thickness is also commonly encountered in injuries. This problem can be managed by advancing the fat from under the thicker flap into the dead space of the thinner flap (Figure 6-20).

Tissue avulsion occurs when a minimal to moderate amount of skin has been lost. Undermining the skin should allow for primary closure without undue tension (Figure 6-20). When primary closure is not possible, either a full thickness graft, or a split thickness graft can be used for primary wound healing. However, in most cases, scar revision will still

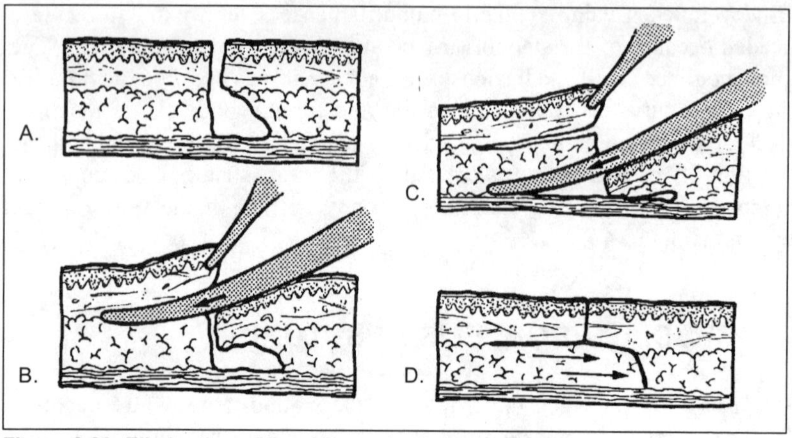

Figure 6-20: Elimination of Dead Space by Fat Advancement.

be needed at a latter date to achieve cosmetically acceptable results. Occasionally, a portion of tissue, such as the tip of the nose is either dangling by a small pedicle or is completely detached. In such a case the severed portion should be washed thoroughly in saline solution, the fat removed and the detached tissue sutured into place.

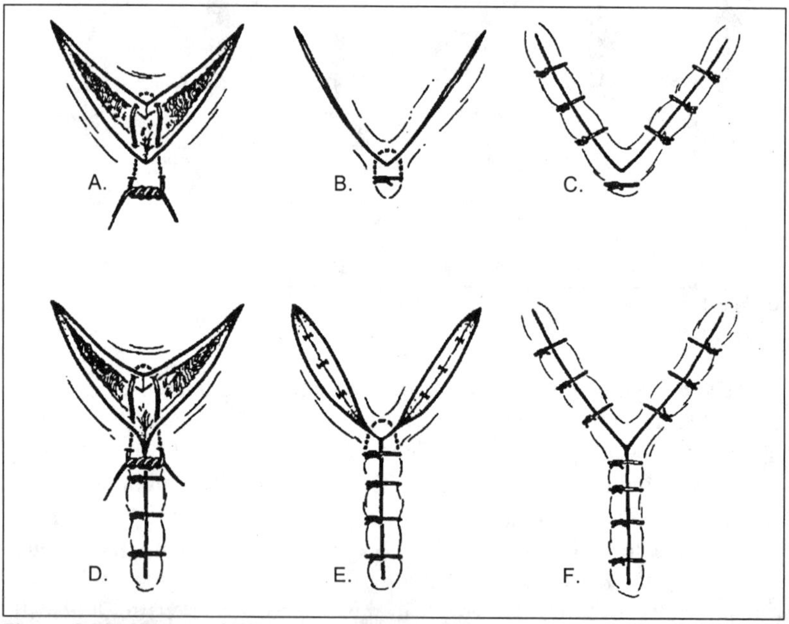

Figure 6-21: Closure of "V" and "Y"-Shaped Flaps.

V and Y shaped flaps or triangular injuries present special problems because necrosis of the skin triangle is almost certain to occur if tissue approximation is accomplished by skin sutures alone. Treatment options include placing a transverse dermal stitch between the tip of the triangle and opposing apex, followed by loosely tying the skin sutures to ensure that the blood supply to the triangle is not endangered. A second option is to close the V shaped incision as a Y by not extending the apex of the triangular flap. Suturing is performed on both sides of the flap simultaneously beginning at the base (Figure 6-21).

Stellate lacerations with contused edges often appear as if there has been tissue avulsion. However, when the tissue is pieced together, the wound is, in reality, a complex of short linear lacerations (Figure 6-22). Also, these lacerations tempt one to excise the jagged flaps to achieve a more cosmetic result. This temptation should be resisted to avoid creating an avulsion injury. These wounds underscore the importance of closely examining an injury and repositioning the flaps prior to suturing.

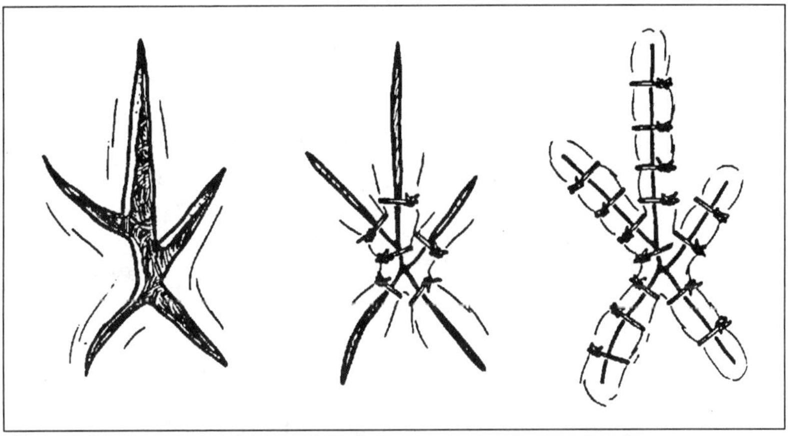

Figure 6-22: Closure of Stellate Lacerations.

Lip lacerations require special attention because of the inherent difficulties in achieving a cosmetic apposition of the mucocutaneous border. In full thickness lip lacerations this problem is compounded by the nearly inevitable contraction of the scar which can produce shortening of the lip, notching of the lip margin and eversion of the mucocutaneous border. These undesirable outcomes can be avoided by the careful approximation of the vermilion skin junction as an initial step in flap alignment. When a full-thickness flap is involved, the first suture should take a firm bite through the mucocutaneous junction of the vermilion border (Figure 6-23).

The placement of traction on this suture will then facilitate the accuracy of the remaining sutures. The closure of deep or full-thickness lacerations must be made in layers, with careful attention to the approximation of the obicularis oris muscle. Inattention to this detail can result in a depressed scar. All sutures are placed from an extraoral approach, closing the mucous membrane and the muscular layer first with fine silk or monofilament mattress sutures through both layers. The vermilion border is then brought together with close attention to anatomical alignment. The skin sutures should be removed on the fourth day and the mucous membrane-muscle sutures are removed on the eighth day.

Through and through lacerations create a communication between the skin and the intraoral environment. It is recommended to suture the

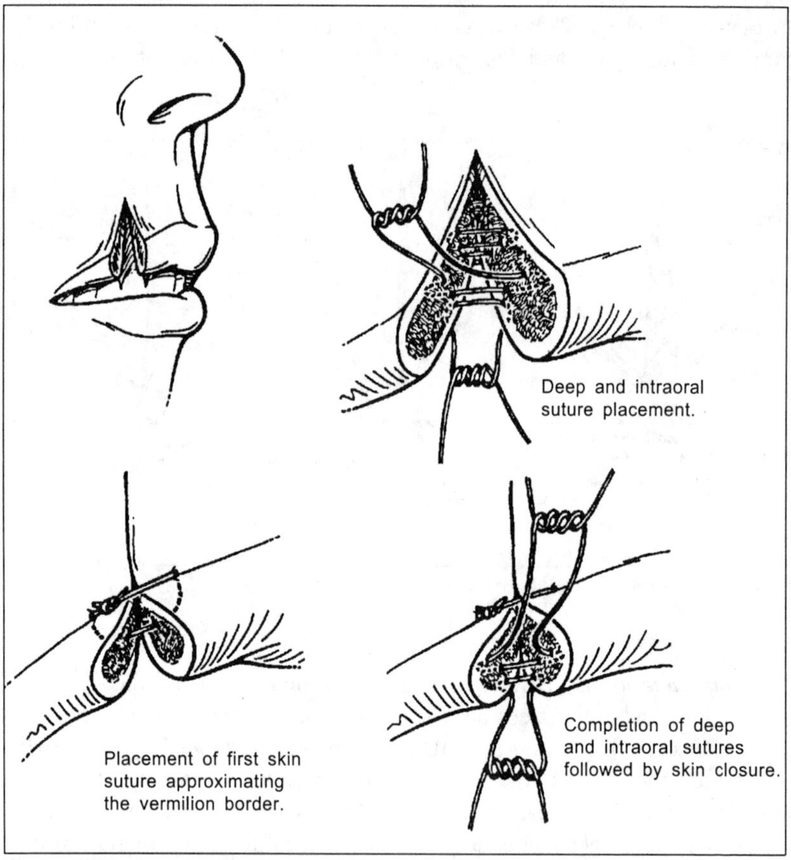

Figure 6-23: Closure of a Lip Laceration.

oral mucosa first to minimize further contamination of the wound from saliva and the oral flora. In such cases, tight mucosal closure should be achieved with nonresorbable sutures, followed by irrigation and cleansing of the remaining extraoral wound prior to skin closure. Through and through lacerations are sometimes difficult to diagnose, especially in vestibular lacerations that can travel along the alveolus before exiting. Exploration of all intraoral lacerations with a blunt instrument is recommended to rule out this possibility. Puncture wounds from teeth rarely require much more than a thorough cleaning. Through and through lacerations usually occur following a fall or blow on the chin and, as such, the wounds are frequently contaminated. When through and through wounds are contaminated it is recommended that the patient be placed on a week of antibiotics and be given a tetanus shot.

Tongue lacerations are frequently self-inflicted following a fall or a blow to the chin. The bleeding from such an injury can be intimidating, however, hemostasis usually occurs within minutes with direct pressure from a cotton gauze. Sutures should be used to approximate the edges of a deep tongue wound even though healing of the tongue is generally extremely rapid without them. Features about the tongue that should be remembered during suturing are the uncontrollable continuous muscle actions and profuse blood and lymph supply. Either tying a suture through the tip of the tongue or grasping the tongue with a towel clamp can aid in controlling the movement. Sutures should be placed wide and deep, and should be tied very loosely. Sutures placed deep in the muscle should be aligned in an anterior/posterior direction. A large stout needle and fairly heavy suture (silk or chromic gut) should be inserted and tied loosely. It is helpful to place an instrument such as a closed hemostat or the scalpel handle between the suture and the tongue while the knot is being tied. Edema is quite severe during the first 48 hours and tight sutures will either cut through tissue too quickly or produce deep necrosis and excess scar tissue. Swelling of the tongue may be so severe that a tracheotomy is required to maintain airway patency; however, this is uncommon for wounds in the anterior two-thirds.

Gingival degloving results from stripping the gingival tissue away from the alveolus. The dangling flap oftentimes appears too small to cover the area of exposed bone giving the illusion of an avulsion injury. The tissue should be examined for gross contamination and blood clots on the connective tissue side, and rinsed with saline. The tissue can then be stretched with finger pressure and cotton gauze to it's original size. If stretching is unsuccessful, then blunt dissection is recommended to free up the flap. Once extended, the tissue should be sutured with either silk or chromic gut through the interdental papilla and the superior edge of the adjacent gingiva

(Figure 6-24). Direct pressure with cold, wet cotton gauze will help with adaptation of the tissue to the underlying bone. The patient should be instructed to keep the area clean with frequent rinsing and not to pull the lip out to look at the injury until the sutures are removed in one week.

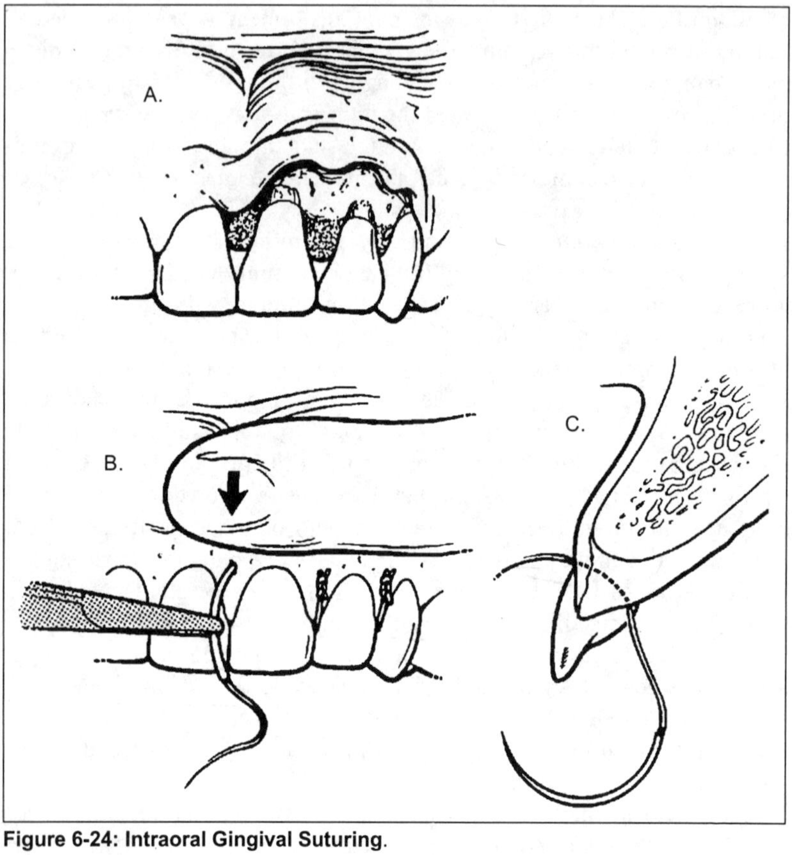

Figure 6-24: Intraoral Gingival Suturing.

Cheek lacerations can result in injuries to the seventh cranial nerve and/or the parotid gland. Seventh nerve function should be evaluated as previously described. When glandular parotid tissue is involved in a wound, a discharge of clear fluid is likely within a few hours following the insult. This seeping of salivary fluid usually ceases without incident. To treat this injury, the parotid capsule should be closed and the wound drained prior to suturing the skin over the wound. When Stensen's duct is severed, a polyethylene tube of suitable size should be inserted into the proximal end of the duct and retained there by a resorbable suture.

The mucous membrane of the cheek is then punctured with a fine scalpel and the distal end of the tube is passed into the mouth. The hole in the mucous membrane can be closed with a stitch that stabilizes the tube, thus converting an external salivary fistula into an internal one. The tube can be removed in 7 to 10 days.

Ear and ***nose*** lacerations are complex and require additional expertise to manage well. For example, if these wounds are sutured in a straight forward manner, notching usually results from contraction of the scar tissue. To avoid this unacceptable outcome, the technique of halving and stepping is recommended (Figure 6-25). A triangular wedge of skin down to the cartilage is removed from the upper portion of the wound and an identical area of cartilage is removed from the lower portion. Suturing is then carried out by imbrication. Because the viability of the auricular cartilage is poor, efforts to suture large, avulsed segments are not commonly successful. Reattachment is more successful, however, when the detached fragment is small. It is imperative that retained ear wound segments have an adequate blood supply.

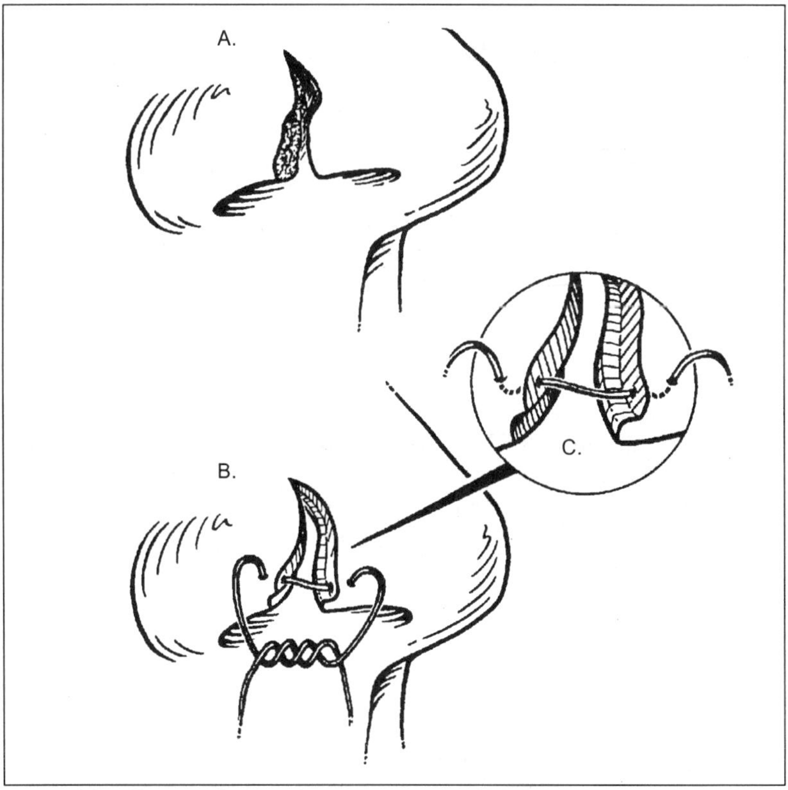

Figure 6-25: Closure of a Nasal Laceration Using Halving and Stepping.

Eyelid lacerations as with lacerations of the ear and nose, require expertise that is beyond the scope of this book. Such wounds should be referred to persons skilled in their management.

Bite wounds may be human or animal in origin. The bacterial content of animal saliva is species-specific, thus it is imperative to know the type of animal responsible prior to making a decision on wound closure. For example, because of the bacterial concentration and virulence associated with human, cat and pig bites, such wounds are very prone to infection and are not recommended for closure. Instead, such wounds are best treated with intravenous antibiotics, debridement and topical antimicrobials. In contrast, dog bites can usually be closed safely. However, caution is advised in wounds from older dogs where there is a higher incidence of periodontitis, resulting in higher salivary bacterial counts. Studies suggest that dog bites can be closed primarily, the patient placed on antibiotics and followed closely. Should infection develop, the wound may be reopened and allowed to heal by tertiary intention. Deep puncture wounds from canine teeth should not be closed primarily.

XVI. ALTERNATIVE WOUND CLOSURE METHODS

Although suturing is the standard method of wound repair, tissue adhesives, tissue staples and adhesive tapes represent other options. The use of ***cyanoacrylate tissue adhesive*** to close facial lacerations has shown promising results. The cyanoacrylate (Histoacryl) is applied to the skin edges which are held together for 30 seconds until polymerizations occur (i.e., the glue becomes opaque). Most studies, however, have not included lacerations longer than 3 cm, eyelid lacerations or lacerations involving the mucocutaneous junction of the mouth. Also, deep hemorrhagic wounds and those with ragged edges have not been studied. Some authors feel that the polymer forms a barrier between the wound edges that prevents wound apposition and, thereby, delays healing. In addition, the incidence of wound infection with tissue adhesives has been significantly higher than with sutures according to some experimental studies.

The use of ***metal staples*** offers the advantage of greatly decreasing the time required to approximate wound edges. However, studies have shown that stapled wounds have less elasticity and less ability to absorb energy without disrupting the wound compared to closure with a monofilament nylon suture. In addition, the resulting scar is rarely cosmetically acceptable. Staples are not recommended in the facial region or when the distance from the stapled skin to underlying bones, vessels or internal organs is less than 5 mm. With traumatic wounds, in general, the decision to use staples rather than sutures should be based on whether the time saved would offset the potentially undesirable effects. In using staples, the wound edges are forced together with tissue forceps until the margins evert. Tension is applied to one end of the incision, and the staples are gently placed across the wound to uniformly span the incision line. The rectangular design of the staples minimizes both tissue trauma and staple rotation following placement. The approximation of the wound edges prior to stapling minimizes tissue compression and the space between the staple crown (top) and the skin surface minimizes crosshatching marks (Figure 6-26).

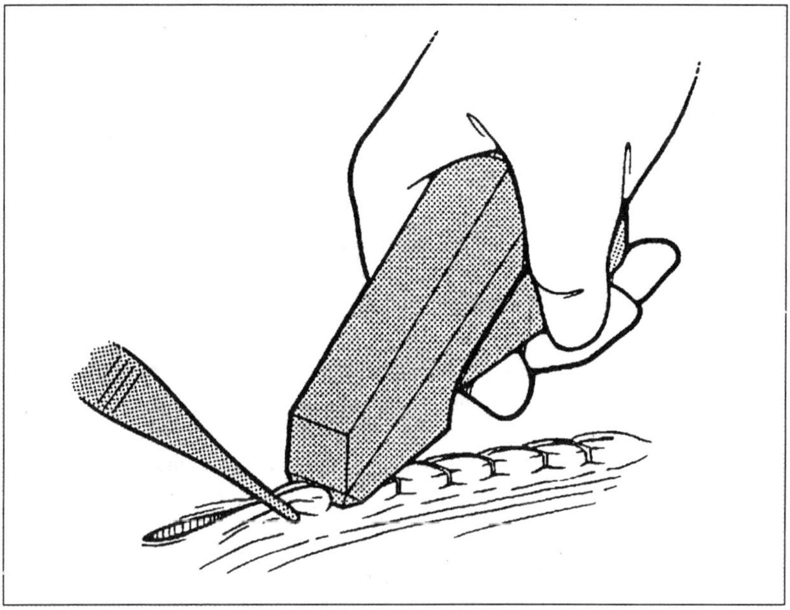

Figure 6-26: The Use of a Stapler for Wound Closure.

Steristrips are sterile adhesive strips which can be used for initial wound closure or for wound retention following early suture removal. There is some clinical evidence that wounds closed with these tapes develop tensile strength faster than sutured wounds. It is proposed that adhesive strips allow stress to be more uniformly applied to collagen fibers. The initial fibers to cross the wound aid in rapid fiber orientation and, thereby, increase tensile strength. Adhesive strips, however, cannot bring deeper tissues together and the strips do not promote hemostasis at the wound edges. In addition, eversion and fine approximation of wound margins is difficult if not impossible with tapes, and mildly depressed scars frequently result.

Nonetheless, skin closure tapes can be an effective alternative to sutures or staples if tensile strength, cosmetics and resistance to infection are not critical factors (i.e., with shallow clean wounds where esthetics is a minor concern). Retention of the tapes can be increased by using a liquid skin adhesive, such as tincture of benzoin. The benzoin-prepped skin can keep tape in place through daily showers for approximately two weeks.

XVII. WOUND DRESSING AND CARE

Small, repaired wounds, especially in the head and neck region, usually need no post-repair dressing, however, a simple Band-Aid may be used if a covering is desired. A topical antibiotic ointment such as Neosporin may be applied over the sutures. Although the value of such topical antibiotics is questionable in reducing subsequent infections, it does serve to keep the wound moist.

A dressing material should not adhere to the wound surface and it must also allow exudate to drain from the wound. In addition, a dressing should allow the wound to remain moist throughout the healing period as desiccation of the wound will deter the healing process. Most dressings have a non-adherent base which contacts the wound and a gauze covering over the base to absorb exudate. A dressing should also be resistant to bacterial contamination. Finally, the dressing should protect the wound by immobilizing it, because most wounds are initially very susceptible to disruption by even minor forces. A dressing is probably not needed following the first 24 to 48 hours in head and neck wounds. However, once the dressing is removed, it is important that the wound is kept clean.

After the wound has been repaired and any necessary medication and dressing applied, the patient should be instructed in caring for the wound. Wound cleanliness is the foremost factor in preventing secondary infection and delayed healing. Because wounds of the face and scalp are often closed primarily and left uncovered, cleanliness is even more important. With undressed wounds, patients should be instructed to shower daily and clean the wound with soap and water or hydrogen peroxide. The cleaning should be performed with the fingers avoiding material that can snag on the sutures such as a washcloth. Following cleaning, the wound should be gently patted dry with a soft towel. In contrast, wounds that are dressed or bandaged should be kept dry and clean. The skin surrounding the wound should be well cleaned before the patient is released to alleviate the need for post-dressing cleaning by the patient. A follow-up appointment should be made for the patient in 2 to 3 days to change the dressing and evaluate the healing process.

In addition to desired wound care, the patient should be instructed to watch for signs of infection (Table 6-8). Upon detection of any of these signs the patient should return for an evaluation and necessary treatment. When an infection develops during the healing process, early suture removal, irrigation, drainage and antibiotic coverage should be considered. In choosing an antibiotic, a single agent with low toxicity is preferred. Multiple antibiotics should be used only when the first choice is not effective or with serious infections. A culture and sensitivity test is recommended before therapy begins in case the patient fails to respond to initial antimicrobials. A semisynthetic penicillin such as oxacillin or a broad spectrum cephalosporin is usually effective in the prevention or treatment of traumatic wound infections.

Table 6-8: Signs of Wound Infection

- Wound tenderness
- Erythema over 1 cm from the wound edge
- Induration over 0.5 cm from the wound edge
- Purulence
- Dehiscence
- Regional lymphadenopathy

It is also prudent to discuss the possibilities of scar formation with patients because there are many factors that affect the outcome of wound healing. In addition, the physical appearance of a wound varies considerably during healing which can concern patients. It may take a year or more for a scar to obtain its final appearance and what may initially be intolerable to the patient, in most cases, will become acceptable as healing and remodeling continue. Patients should also be advised that the traumatized area may be temporarily temperature and touch sensitive for several weeks.

Finally, the need for tetanus prophylaxis must be assessed for each patient. Contaminated wounds with extensive devitalized tissue are considered more tetanus-prone, although tetanus has developed in seemingly insignificant wounds. The risk of tetanus is determined by a combination of factors to include: the type of wound, the age of the wound and the environment in which the wound occurred (Table 6-9). The tetanus immunization status of the patient is based on whether or not the initial series of shots was administered and the length of time elapsed since the last booster (Appendix D).

Table 6-9: Considerations for Tetanus Prophylaxis

Tetanus Prone	Age of Wound	Tissue Condition	Source of Contamination	Bacterial Level
+	< 24 hrs old	No devitalzed tissue	any wound that does not fit in the 2 categories below	Clean
++	< 24 hrs old	Crush injuries, puncture wounds & wounds extending into muscle	Pavement, wood, industrial sources & human bites	Moderate
+++	> 24 hrs old	Devitalized tissue that cannot be completely debrided	Sewers & Barnyards	High

XVIII. SUTURE REMOVAL

Sutures that include both the epidermis and dermis allow an ingrowth of fibroblasts and collagen along the sutures resulting, in suture tracks. Permanent suture tracks will appear if sutures are left in placed for more than a week in skin that contains a high concentration of sebaceous glands. In general, sutures should be removed from traumatic head and neck wounds in 3 to 5 days. When esthetics are of concern, epidermal sutures should be removed in 3 to 4 days and replaced by adhesive strips placed for a one week period. In areas where sebaceous glands are not present, such as the plantar and palmar surfaces, full-thickness sutures can be left in place for two or more weeks without the risk of suture track formation. Intraoral sutures are normally left in place for one week. Sutures are removed using an aseptic technique following cleaning of the wound with an antiseptic. Hydrogen peroxide can also be applied to remove dried blood encrusted around the sutures. The sutures are picked up with cotton forceps and cut on one side of the knot as close to the skin as possible. The knot is grabbed and the suture is gently pulled through the wound. The wound edges should be taped to prevent widening of the scar following suture removal when esthetics are essential. It is also important for patients to understand that removal of the sutures does not mean the wound is completely healed. The wound will have a low tensile strength for some time after the sutures are removed and, as such, reopening or dehiscence can occur if the wound is exposed to excessive trauma.

References

Bonadio W.A., "Efficacy of TAC topical anesthetic for repair of pediatric lacerations." *Am J Diseases of Child.* 142 (1988): 203-5.

Bucknell T.E., Ellis H., *Wound Healing for Surgeons.* London: Bailliere Tindall, 1984.

Chung H., Weinburg S., "Suture materials in oral surgery: A review." *Oral Health* 68 (1978): (10) 31-4.

Cocke W.M.; White R.R.; Lynch, D.J.; Verheyden C.N., *Wound care.* New York: Churchill Livingstone, 1986.

Cruse P.F., "A five year prospective study of 23,649 surgical wounds." *Surg* 107 (1973): 206-9.

Dagher F.J., *Cutaneous Wound.* New York: Futura Publishing Co, 1985.

Finley J.M., McConnell R.Y., *Emergency wound repair.* Baltimore: University Park Press, 1984.

Graham B.H., Gordon L., et al., "Serial quantitative skin fluoresceine: a new method for post-operative monitoring of vascular perfusion in revascularized digits." *J Hand Surg.* 10 (1985): (2) 226-30.

Gravett A.; Sterner S.; Clinton J.; Ruiz E., "A trial of povidone-iodine in the prevention of infection in sutured lacerations." *Ann Emerg Med.* 16 (1987): 167-71.

Hotter A.N., "Physiologic aspects and clinical implications of wound healing." *Heart & Lung.* 11 (1982): 522-30.

Hunt T.K., "Disorders of wound healing." *World J. Surg.* 4 (1980): 271-77.

Malamed S.F., *Handbook of local anesthesia.* St. Louis: C.V. Mosby Co., 1986.

McGraw J.B., "The value of fluorescein in predicting the viability of arterialized flaps." *Plastic Reconstr Surg.* 60 (1977): 710.

Pollack S.V., "Wound healing: A review." *J. Dermatol Surg & Oncol.* 5 (1979): 389-93.

Robsin M.C., "Disturbances of wound healing." *Ann Emerg Med.* 17 (1988): 1274-78.

Seropian R., Reynolds B., "Wound infections after preoperative depilatory versus razor preparation." *Am J. Surg.* 121 (1971): 251-54.

Sharp W.V., et al., "Suture resistance to infection." *Surgery.* 91 (1982): (1) 61-3.

Steele M.t.; Sainsbury C.R.; Robinson W.A.; Salomone J.A.; Elenbaas R.M., "Prophylactic penicillin for intraoral wounds." *Ann Emerg Med.* 18 (1989): 847-52.

Sugarman B., Musher D., "Adherence of bacteria to suture material." *Proced Soc Exp Biol Med.* 167 (1981): (2) 156-60.

Trott A., *Minor wound care.* New York: Medical Examination Publishing Co. Inc., 1985.

Varma S.; Ferguson H.L.; Breen H.; Lamb W.V., "Comparison of 7 suture materials in infected wounds: An experimental study." *J. Surg Res.* 17 (1974): (3) 165-70.

Wound closure manual. Ethicon, Inc. 1985.

7 Dentoalveolar Trauma

Robert A. Dale, D.D.S.

Dentoalveolar injuries are those involving the teeth, soft tissue and the adjacent alveolar bone. Examples of these injuries include tooth avulsions and subluxation, with or without alveolar bone fractures, and fractures of the tooth structure itself (crown or root). These injuries are associated with various types of external trauma such as motor vehicle accidents (MVAs), fisticuffs, etc., and are most common in children and young adults. The purpose of this chapter is to focus on the types of dentoalveolar injuries, their diagnosis, management and prognosis.

I. PATIENT EVALUATION

When evaluating a patient with dentoalveolar trauma it is useful to have a standardized questionnaire to guide the examiner in gathering data (Table 7-1). It has been shown that when such a form is not used, approximately fifty percent of the needed information is not solicited. While entering this data, it is important that the practitioner be cognizant of and investigate the systemic extent of the patient's traumatic injuries paying particular attention to the patients physical status. Even in an emergency room where the dental professional may not be the first to examine the patient, the dentist cannot defer this responsibility. Like any other member of the medical team, the dentist has unique expertise that can assist the primary physician in treating the patient. However, as a member of this team, if the dentist is ignorant of the patient's systemic injuries and the implication of these injuries, then the dentist is at risk to harm the patient.

A. History of the Traumatic Event

In any examination it is vitally important to listen to what the trauma patient is telling you. Oftentimes, patient complaints about seemingly vague problems will guide the astute listener to an area requiring treatment.

Historically, the examiner should ascertain when the accident happened, where it occurred, how it happened, and what treatment may have

Table 7-1: Essential Examination Information

1. Patient Information	**2. Accident Information**	**3. Findings from Previous Medical & Dental Examinations**
Address	Type	Date
Phone	Location	Time
Age	Time	Findings
Sex		Treatment
		Medications
4. Historical Information	**5. Systemic Examination**	**6. Head & Neck Examination***
Chief Complaint	Blood Pressure	Lacerations
Past Medical History	Pulse	Hematomas
Past Surgical History	Respirations	Swellings
Medications	Head & Neck Injuries	Abrasions
Allergies	Other Body Injuries	Ecchymosis
Past Dental History	Neurologic Assessment	Bony steps
Loss of Consciousness	Vomiting	Facial Bone Fractures
Headaches	Headache	Hemoptysis
Nausea & Vomiting		Cerebrospinal Fluid (ears or nose)
		TMJ Range of Motion
		TMJ Pain on Movement
		TMJ Pain on Palpation
7. Intraoral Examination*	**8. Avulsion Information**	**9. Radiographic Examination**
Tooth Fractures	Storage Media	Type Taken
Electric Vitality Readings	Condition of Tooth	Angulation
Percussion Response	Time out of mouth	Method of Holding Film
Mobility	Tetanus Immunizations	
Color (shade)		
Alveolar Fractures		
Mandibular Fractures		
Maxilla Fractures		
Tooth Displacement	**10. Diagnosis**	**11. Treatment**
Occlusion		
Periodontal Health		
Laceration		
Hematomas		
Swellings		
Abrasions		
Gingival Health	**12. Medications**	**13. Recall**

*The size, location and type of injuries should be noted

already been rendered. In addition, it is very important to know when the injury occurred, especially when tooth avulsion or alveolar fracture is involved. In these cases the prognosis worsens as the time from injury increases. Knowing where the injury occurred can be important in determining the possibility of foreign body contamination and the need for tetanus prophylaxis. Understanding how the injury occurred can assist the examiner in looking for other injuries and foreign bodies. For example, patients injured when impacting the windshield in an MVA may have glass particles buried in the wounds. Likewise, the direction of the force may guide the examiner to specific types of injuries (i.e., trauma to the symphysis is associated with subcondylar fractures of the mandible and cervical cord injuries). Finally, an awareness of prior treatments for the dentoalveolar injury may influence what needs to be done, as well as the prognosis. In such cases, a consultation with the person who originally treated the patient may be helpful. For example, in cases where teeth were replanted, or need to be replanted, the prognosis will be effected by how the tooth was handled and how it was stored prior to replantation.

B. Past Medical History

Systemic disorders may affect the type of treatment rendered and the prognosis, as well as how and where the treatment is delivered. For instance, patients with insulin dependent diabetes mellitus (IDDM) who have significant peripheral disease, patients who are immunosuppressed and patients who have had mandibular radiotherapy are prone to infection and may heal poorly. Supportive measures such as attempts to improve systemic health, antibiotic therapy or hyperbaric oxygen treatment (HBO) may be necessary. Likewise, patients taking oral anticoagulants or suffering from significant hepatic disease may require systemic or local measures to achieve hemostasis.

C. Past Surgical History

Of additional importance is knowledge concerning the types of surgical procedures the patient has undergone, including dental surgery, and any untoward sequela. The surgical history will oftentimes disclose medical problems which the patient neglected to mention in the medical history. For example, the patient who denies bleeding problems in the medical history may acknowledge having to be hospitalized following a tooth extraction because of heavy, prolonged hemorrhaging.

D. Physical Examination

Vital signs should be recorded for every patient to include the blood pressure, heart rate, respiratory rate and temperature. The entire head and neck should be carefully examined for lacerations, abrasions and contusions. The presence of facial asymmetry should be noted and facial bones palpated for evidence of fractures. Epistaxis is a frequent finding following head injuries and can indicate either a nasal fracture or the intrusion of a tooth into the floor of the nasal passage. When facial fractures are discovered or suspected the patient should be referred to the Oral and Maxillofacial Surgery or ENT services for evaluation and treatment. The presence of a basilar skull fracture may be signaled by periorbital ecchymosis (Raccoon Eyes), ecchymosis behind the ear (Battle's sign) or the drainage of cerebrospinal fluid through the ears or nose. All positive findings should be charted as to location and size and the reader is referred to Chapter 8 for a more detailed discussion regarding facial fracture management.

A gross neurological assessment should be preformed on patients suffering a dentoalveolar injury. Loss of consciousness, vomiting, dizziness, visual disturbances and severe headaches suggest an underlying neurologic injury. The neurological status of the patient may, in part, be determined by observing the patient's responses to questions, the character of their speech, their orientation to time, place and person, and by noting the presence of lethargy and gait disturbances. The motor component of Cranial nerves II to XII can generally be assessed by observing and conversing with the patient. In contrast, sensorial competency requires a brief clinical examination. Severe head injuries may also be assessed by the Glasgow Coma Scale which determines the patient's ability to perform three neurologic functions; eye opening, motor response and verbal response. Injury to the cervical spine (C-spine) must also be ruled out for all head injury cases, prior to manipulating the head or neck. Hence, any patient assessments requiring such movement must await this decision. The presence of skull fractures, neurologic deficit or cervical spine injury require the attention of a neurologist.

Sedative agents or narcotics should be avoided in victims of trauma until it is certain that no intracranial damage exists. Narcotics can increase intracranial pressure, and thereby worsen a closed head injury and the sedative effects from either agent can hamper patient assessment. Other bodily injuries to the extremities and the trunk should be identified and recorded, and referred to a surgeon for treatment.

E. Examination of Oral Soft Tissue

Both extraoral and intraoral blood and debris should be removed before the oral examination is preformed so that the full extent of the injuries can be determined. The location, shape, depth and size of intraoral lacerations and abrasions should be recorded. Lacerations should be cleaned and explored manually and radiographically looking for foreign bodies and assessing whether the lacerations extend completely through the lip, cheek or tongue. The proximity of the laceration to important anatomic structures such as salivary ducts and nerves should also be noted. Areas of bleeding from the gingival crevice may indicate occult trauma and should be charted. Swellings or hematomas in the floor of the mouth or buccal vestibule may signify a fractured mandible, hence, when noted, this potential relationship should be explored.

F. Examination of Oral Hard Tissue

The range of mandibular opening, lateral and protrusive movements should be determined, noting deviations on opening and closing. The presence of temporomandibular joint (TMJ) sounds and pain must be determined and evaluated. This information is essential for diagnosing traumatically induced TMJ capsulitis or disk displacements.

The border of the mandible and maxilla should be palpated to detect bony ledges (stepping) or segmental mobility indicative of a fracture. The alveolus should also be palpated for fractures which often approximate gingival lacerations. Alveolar fractures are commonly discovered at the time tooth mobility is checked and an entire alveolar segment moves.

The occlusion should be examined to insure that the teeth interdigitate with maximal closing. Abrupt changes in the occlusal plane or the presence of open bites, anterior or posterior, may also signify a fracture. All teeth should be carefully examined remembering that the presence of one injury does not preclude the existence of others. For example, fractured teeth may have also sustained a luxation injury on closer evaluation.

Teeth should be examined for fractures and the extent of the fractures (enamel, dentin or pulp) noted. The mobility of the teeth should be checked in the horizontal and vertical planes. Increased mobility may indicate injury to the periodontal ligament (PDL), alveolus or possibly a root fracture. Teeth which have been displaced from their normal position should also be noted. Occlusal discrepancies may indicate displacement of teeth, root fractures or fractures of the mandible or maxilla. Permanent teeth, which are injured or are suspected of being injured, should be checked for vitality using thermal, electrical and percussion tests. The color of injured teeth should also be recorded because changes in tooth shade are frequently the first manifestation of pulpal injury.

Immediately following a traumatic tooth injury, the response to vitality tests is equivocal and, hence, should never be the sole basis for a decision to institute prompt endodontic therapy. The criteria used to diagnose pulp necrosis are: 1) Unresponsive to vitality testing, although this must be interpreted carefully since some nonvital teeth give false readings, 2) Radiographic changes, usually seen as a periapical radiolucency, 3) Change in tooth color, usually becoming more gray in color, 4) Sensitivity to percussion, and 5) Fistula formation. Great care must be exercised in reaching the diagnosis of pulp necrosis, especially in luxation injuries where abnormal signs and symptoms may resolve with time.

Controversy exists between some authors concerning the value of vitality testing on recently traumatized teeth. However, many studies support the use of this diagnostic modality. In a study by Zadik involving children between the ages of 6 to 14 years old with uncomplicated dentinal crown fracture, the author concluded that a positive response to vitality testing at the time of injury is an acceptable prognostic indicator. The study suggested that pulpal response to electric vitality tests was a more accurate diagnostic aid than was pulpal response to thermal testing. In another study of almost 4,000 teeth, Ravn found that 97% gave a positive response to vitality testing immediately after injury. Rock, in a study involving 500 human teeth, found that the best predictor of continued tooth vitality was a vital response at the time of injury. As Andreasen points out, the results of vitality tests at the time of the injury may also serve as a valuable baseline for diagnostic comparisons at follow-up appointments. A tooth which gave a vital response at the time of injury and was unresponsive at subsequent appointments would carry a different prognosis than one that was initially negative and later elicites a vital response.

G. Radiographic Examination

Radiographs of the hard tissues provide information about root development, crown and root fractures, alveolar fractures, tooth displacement, maxillary and mandibular fractures, dental caries and bone loss. Radiographs of soft tissue lacerations involving the lips, cheeks or tongue may be needed to detect the presence of impacted foreign bodies such as tooth fragments. Chest and abdominal radiographs are indicated when teeth have been traumatically avulsed and aspiration is suspected.

In cases of dentoalveolar trauma, there is no standard series of radiographs recommended however, Andreasen found in a study that a combination of occlusal and selected periapical radiographs (taken at different angles) disclosed most tooth displacements. A panoramic radiograph can provide similar information when such capability is available. A lateral radiograph of the anterior teeth can depict facial alveolar fractures and facially displaced roots.

Radiographic technique is important in reaching a proper diagnosis following dentoalveolar trauma. The use of film holders is preferred to methods such as hand holding the film because the seriologic film variation is improved and allows for a more accurate comparison over time. Also, root fractures are best detected when the central beam of the x-ray is directed parallel to the long axis of the fracture. Deviations from this objective may incorrectly show a single fracture as multiple fractures or may fail to reveal a fracture at all.

H. Prognosis

The prognosis for retaining traumatized teeth is determined by the development of pulpal necrosis, root resorption, internal resorption and, in the case of root fractures, the type of hard tissue union. All of these sequela are generally radiographic determinations. The most favorable prognosis would be one in which none of these sequela developed. A favorable outcome may still be realized in the presence of pulp necrosis, provided that successful endodontic treatment is initiated. Following root canal therapy, the prognosis is favorable in the absence of progressive inflammatory resorption. Root resorption occurs in approximately 74 to 96% of replanted teeth.

In children there are many considerations that influence the treatment approach. Foremost among them is the child's ability to cooperate or, in the absence of cooperation, the skill of the practitioner to render the child cooperative via pharmacologic or nonpharmacologic methods. Suggested modalities of pharmacologic management are listed in Appendix 1.

A second important consideration in the treatment of deciduous teeth is the length of time until exfoliation. Average tooth development and eruption times are listed in Appendix 2 for both primary and permanent teeth. The amount of root formation in the succedaneous permanent tooth, the amount of natural primary tooth resorption and the relationship of the primary tooth root to the forming permanent tooth crown are important factors to consider when choosing a treatment approach in the pediatric patient. Generally, permanent teeth begin to erupt when one-half of the root is formed and enter the oral cavity with three-fourths of the root development complete.

Parents of children suffering dentoalveolar trauma of the primary dentition must be informed that damage to the permanent teeth may have occurred at the time of injury. Evidence of this injury may be immediately present or may not be manifested until several years later.

II. TYPES OF TRAUMATIC DENTOALVEOLAR INJURIES

There are many ways to classify dentoalveolar injuries. Some methods are based on an Arabic numbering classification while others are based on a Roman numeral system. Perhaps the system most easily understood is one that is based on a description of the injury. There are several such systems that define the injuries similarly, but they differ on how the injuries are grouped under major headings. One such classification was provided by the World Health Organization in 1978 and later modified by Andreasen. This type of system is presented here (Table 7-2). Regardless of the system used, it is important to recognize that dentoalveolar injuries have two major components: pulpal injury and periodontal injury.

Table 7-2: Types of Dentoalveolar Injuries

Crown Fractures	**Displaced Luxations**
uncomplicated	Extrusive
complicated	Lateral
	Intrusive
Crown/Root Fractures	Avulsion
uncomplicated	**Alveolar Fractures**
complicated	
	Soft Tissue
Root Fractures	
Nondisplaced Luxations	
Concussion	
Subluxation	

A. Tooth Fractures

Crown fractures may be divided into uncomplicated and complicated categories (Figure 7-1). ***Uncomplicated crown fractures*** are those injuries which result in fractures of the enamel alone or in a combination of enamel and dentin. If the fracture is incomplete causing no loss of tooth structure it is referred to as either a ***craze, a crack or an infraction***. Such injuries do not cross the dentoenamel junction. In contrast, ***complicated crown fractures*** involve the enamel, dentin and pulpal tissues. Both complicated and uncomplicated crown fractures may extend into the root (Figure 7-2). ***Root fractures*** are classified by the location of the fracture on the root. Usually the fractures are segregated into coronal or incisal third fractures, midroot fractures and apical third fractures (Figure 7-3). Root fractures typically involve all three tooth tissues (cementum, dentin and pulp) and most are oriented horizontally or obliquely. Vertical root fractures are rare and occur most commonly in the posterior teeth.

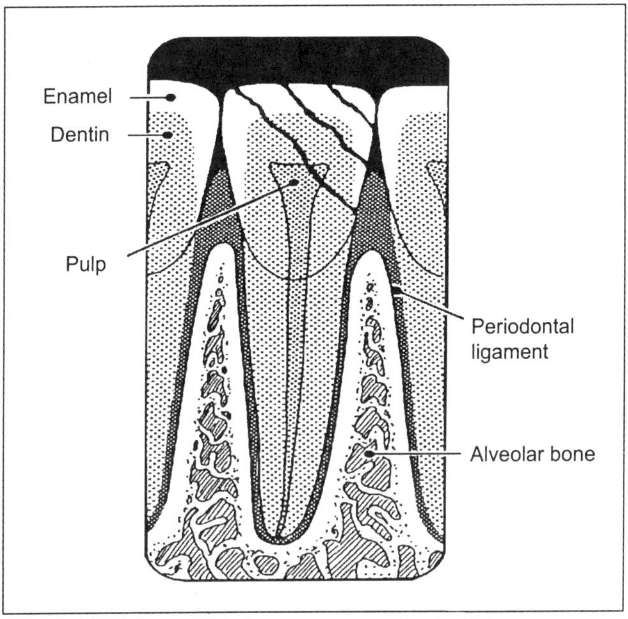

Figure 7-1: *Uncomplicated* crown fractures involve (1) the enamel only, and (2) the enamel and dentin. *Complicated* crown fractures involve (3) the enamel, dentin and pulp.

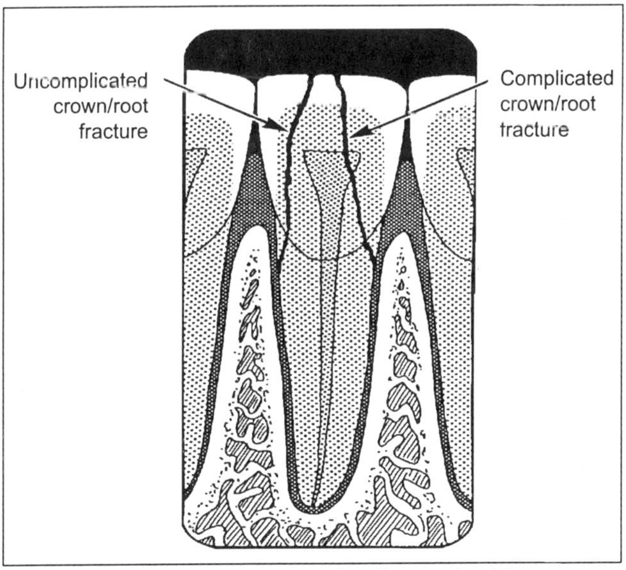

Figure 7-2: An uncomplicated crown/root fracture involving the enamel, dentin and root, and a complicated crown/root fracture involving the enamel, dentin, pulp and root.

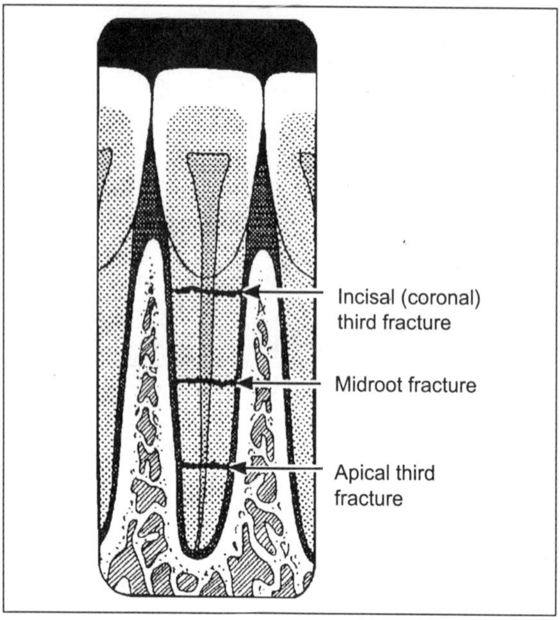

Figure 7-3: Root Fractures are usually classified by location of the fracture.

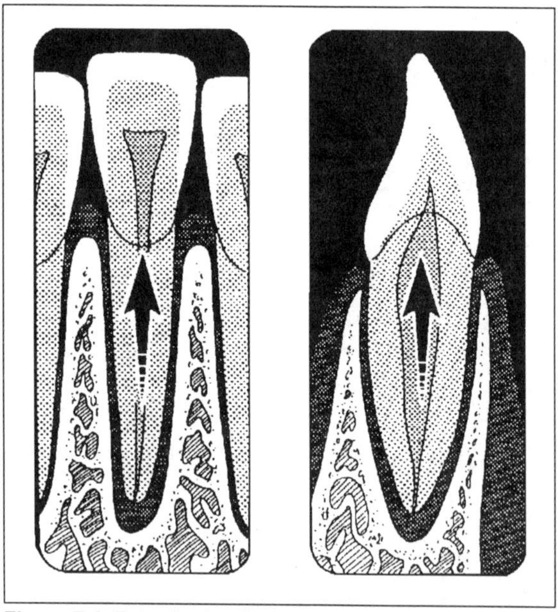

Figure 7-4: Extrusive luxation occurs when the tooth is forced partially out of the socket in an axial direction.

B. Non Displacement Tooth Injuries

Concussion injuries are those in which no tooth displacement occurs; that is, the tooth remains in its normal position. Typically, the injured tooth is not mobile, but is sensitive to percussion. ***Subluxation*** is an injury involving abnormal tooth mobility without evidence of displacement.

C. Displacement Tooth Injuries

Dental luxation means to displace or dislocate a tooth from the socket, either partially or totally. Many injury classifications use the term luxation as a broad general category that includes both nondisplacement and displacement injuries. The World Health Organization's classification is one such system. However, to minimize semantic confusion in this chapter, luxation will refer to displacement injuries, and the terms concussion and subluxation will refer to nondisplacement injuries. Hence, ***luxation*** is any injury that results in both abnormal mobility and displacement of the tooth. Luxation injuries are divided into four types. ***Extrusive luxation***, also referred to as ***partial avulsion***, is an injury in which the tooth is forced partially out of the socket in an axial direction, without root penetration of the alveolar wall (Figure 7-4). ***Intrusive luxation*** is an injury in which the tooth is forced apically and is usually accompanied by crushing or fracture of the apical portion of the alveolus (Figure 7-5). ***Lateral luxation***

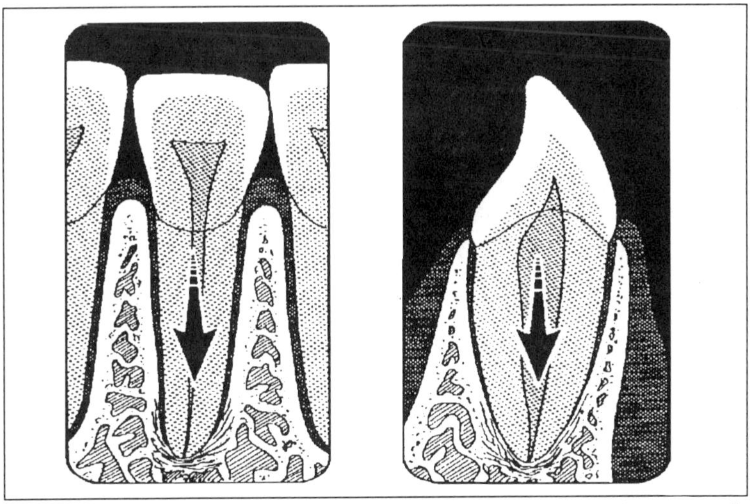

Figure 7-5: Intrusive luxation of a tooth compresses the periodontal ligament and vascular supply of the pulp and may crush the apical bone.

occurs when the tooth is displaced either facially, lingually, mesially or distally. This injury is frequently accompanied by damage to the alveolar wall secondary to root penetration or gross fracture (Figure 7-6). ***Complete luxation***, also known as ***complete avulsion*** or ***exarticulation***, results in the total removal of the tooth from the socket.

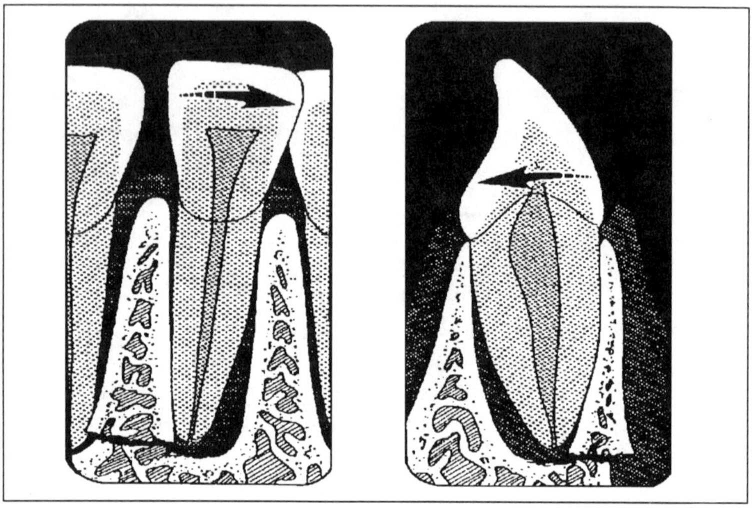

Figure 7-6: Lateral luxation occurs when the tooth is displaced in either a lingual, mesial, distal or facial direction. Fractures of the alveolus frequently accompany lateral luxation injuries.

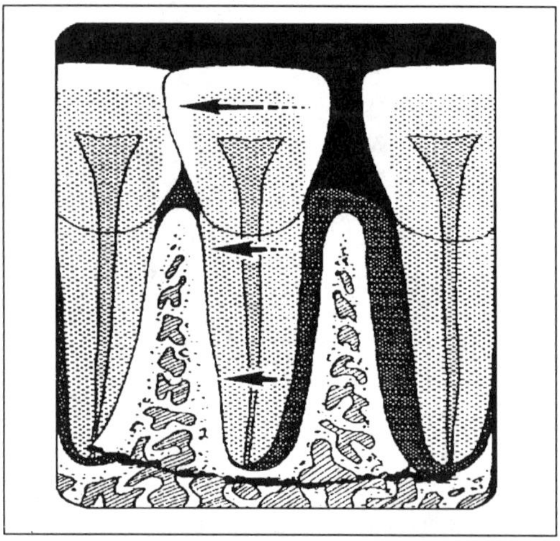

Figure 7-7: Fracture of an entire segment of the alveolar process.

D. Alveolar Fractures

Alveolar fractures may involve a block segment of the alveolar process (Figure 7-7) or just a wall of the socket, and are frequently associated with luxation injuries. Lateral luxations often fracture or penetrate the facial or lingual alveolar plate, while intrusive luxations generally involve a crushing, penetration or fracture of the socket's apical portion. More extreme fractures may involve the entire alveolar process or be associated with fractures of the maxilla or mandible.

Table 7-3: Crown Fracture Injuries

Type of Injury	Incidence	Description of injury	Immediate Treatment	%Developing Pulp Necrosis
Crown Fractures	Permanent Teeth 26 - 76% Primary Teeth 4 - 38%	See below	See below	See below
Uncomplicated Crown Fracture	No pulp exposure		Percussion, vitality & mobility tests and shade match	
Enamel Craze or Crack	10.5 - 12.5%	No loss of tooth structure. Small craze lines in enamel.	*Permanent & Primary teeth* No treatment required Follow-up in 6 - 8 weeks	0 - 3.5%
Enamel/Dentin	23 - 67%	Loss of enamel and/or Dentin	*Permanent & Primary teeth* *Enamel* No treatment required, or smooth rough egdes or restore. Follow-up in 6 - 8 weeks *Dentin* Cover dentin with calcium hydroxide within 24 hours & place restoration. Follow-up in 6 - 8 weeks	Enamel 1% Dentin 1 - 7%
Complicated	3.5 - 8%	Always exposes the pulp. Involves enamel, dentin & pulp	Percussion, mobility & vitality tests and shade match *Permanent vital teeth* Place a calcium hydroxide cap if <3 hours since injury, if >3 hrs, remove coronal 2mm of pulp & place calcium hydroxide & restoration. Pulpectomy if insufficient tooth structure remains Follow-up in 6 - 8 weeks *Primary teeth* Perform pulpotomy or place pulp cap Follow-up in 6 - 8 weeks	12 - 29% in mature teeth with a calcium hydroxide cap 0 - 6% in Immature teeth with calcium hydroxide cap

E. Soft Tissue Injuries

Fractures of an alveolar wall or the entire alveolar process are frequently associated with lacerations of the gingival tissues. Hence, when a laceration of the gingiva is found, the injury should prompt the examiner to look for a proximate alveolar fracture. Soft tissue penetration by teeth may also lacerate the lips, cheeks and tongue. The reader is referred to Chapter 6 for the management of such soft tissue injuries.

III. THE DIAGNOSIS AND TREATMENT OF DENTOALVEOLAR INJURIES

A. Uncomplicated Crown Fractures (Table 7-3)

Incidence

Uncomplicated crown fractures comprise 26 to 76% of all dentoalveolar injuries in permanent teeth and 4 to 38% in all primary teeth.

Diagnosis

The tooth with an uncomplicated crown fracture should be checked visually for small pulp exposures in cases where the dentin has been involved. In those instances when no tooth structure has been lost, the tooth should be examined by both direct and indirect light (including transillumination) to detect small, incomplete fractures. Radiographs should be taken to include a mesial and distal angulation of the injured tooth, and film holders should be used when possible to standardize the radiographic technique. It is important to look for evidence of root or alveolar fractures as well as changes in the width of the periodontal ligament. The size of the pulp chamber, the degree of root formation and the proximity of the pulp to the fracture should also be noted. An endodontic examination including thermal and electric vitality tests, percussion sensitivity and mobility, and a tooth shade should be recorded. The color can be determined by matching the tooth with the closest shade on a tooth color guide. Aside from the immediate diagnostic value, this information should be recorded for relative comparison at follow-up appointments.

Treatment

A tooth which shows only crazing requires no treatment in the immediate post-injury period, even though the tooth may be percussion sensitive and unresponsinve to vitality testing. However, at regular intervals tooth color, vitality, percussion sensitivity and mobility should be checked and compared to the initial values. Radiographs should also be taken using the same technique employed at the time of the trauma. Patients should be motivated to return at regular intervals, so that endodontic treatment can be instituted in a timely manner when necessary. Enamel fractures may also not require immediate post-injury care other than smoothing rough edges. Any needed restorative treatment can be deferred to a later time if necessary.

In contrast, dentinal fractures should be treated within 24 hours of the injury because treatment instituted beyond this time period is associated with an increased frequency of pulp necrosis. It has been shown that bacteria are capable of penetrating the larger dentinal tubules and this contamination has been implicated in ensuing pulpal inflammation. Local anesthesia may be necessary before placing a restoration if the exposed dentin is painful to the patient. Calcium hydroxide applied to the exposed dentin and covered with a composite resin is an acceptable immediate restoration. The composite may be constructed to final contours and finished if time, equipment and circumstances permit. If not, the composite may be applied in a thin covering over the calcium hydroxide to the etched surface of the enamel acting as a "composite bandage" until a final restoration can be completed. Temporary metal or acrylic crowns and glass ionomers may also be used as interim restorations. When the fractured portion of the tooth is available, some clinicians have used composite systems to rejoin the fractured segment to the tooth.

The prognosis for teeth which have sustained uncomplicated crown fractures is good. Teeth with injuries involving crazing or isolated enamel fractures are not likely to develop pulp necrosis. In clinical studies, the number of teeth that developed pulp necrosis following crazing injuries ranged between 0 to 3.5%, while pulp necrosis developed approximately 1% of the time in teeth with fractured enamel. The incidence of pulp necrosis with dentinal fractures is 1 to 7% and the frequency increases with longer periods of dentin exposure. Injured teeth which fail to dissipate the traumatic energy by fracturing, may sustain more damage to the periodontal ligament and the periapical neurovascular bundle than teeth that do fracture. In a study of uncomplicated dentinal crown fractures by

Zadik, no differences in the prognosis were found between teeth with immature apices and those with closed apices. Fifty percent of the teeth which gave a negative pulp response at the time of trauma (i.e., a nonvital response), required endodontic therapy within 3 months. However, of those teeth which gave an initial negative response, 30% had a positive response within 3 months. It should be reiterated here that, following trauma, an initial negative response to vitality tests is never sufficient grounds upon which to initiate endodontic treatment. Instead, follow-up examinations for these patients should be scheduled at regular intervals. Zadik found that pathologic indications of pulp necrosis usually developed within 4 months of the trauma. Similarly, Ravn reported that most teeth that developed pulp pathology with uncomplicated crown fractures did so within 6 months of the injury. Hence, follow up appointments should be scheduled within 3 to 4 months post-injury to assess patients with uncomplicated crown fractures.

Regarding primary teeth, McTigue advises against the routine performance of pulp vitality testing because the teeth respond unpredictably and because younger children often lack the ability to report reactions objectively. The treatment procedures for primary teeth with uncomplicated crown fractures are the same as those for the permanent dentition.

B. Complicated Crown Fractures (Table 7-3)

Incidence

It has been estimated that 3.5 to 8% of dentoalveolar injuries may be classified as complicated fractures of the crown.

Diagnosis

These injuries always result in an exposure of the pulp, although the exposures are sometimes very small and difficult to detect. Therefore, it is important to thoroughly clean the teeth, particularly where soft tissue bleeding could complicate the examination. The typical injury involves a pulp horn exposure when a corner of a tooth is fractured. Radiographs should include those taken for an uncomplicated crown fracture. It is important to note the stage of radiographic root formation because this finding will directly effect the tooth's treatment and prognosis. The periapical area should also be examined for evidence of pre-existing pathology such as a radiolucent periapical lesion.

When there is sufficient tooth structure remaining, a full range of endodontic tests should be conducted regardless of the time since the injury. These tests should include vitality, percussion sensitivity and mobility prior to anesthetizing the area for treatment. In addition, a shade should be taken. The exposed pulpal tissue should be carefully examined for evidence of necrosis, especially if a negative response is registered to vitality testing or if bleeding is not observed at the exposure site.

Treatment

There are five relationships between root maturity and the size of the pulpal exposure which will be covered. These relationships are as follows: 1) teeth with fully formed apices and small pulp exposures, 2) teeth with fully formed apices and large pulp exposures, 3) teeth with immature apices and small pulp exposures, 4) teeth with immature apices and large pulp exposures, and 5) teeth with necrotic pulps.

Direct pulp capping with calcium hydroxide is recommended by most authors in cases with small exposures of a vital pulp and a fully formed apex. It is desirable to cover the exposure with calcium hydroxide as soon after the trauma as possible. The calcium hydroxide must then be covered with a restoration such as temporary metal or acrylic crowns, glass ionomers or composites.

Teeth with large vital pulp exposures and fully formed apicies have been treated in several ways. Some authors recommend starting root canal treatment immediately by performing a pulpectomy, others suggest a pulpotomy and some recommend pulp capping. Regarding pulp capping, both Ravn and Cvek have demonstrated good success by removing 2mm of the pulp tissue and placing a direct cap of calcium hydroxide. In support of this approach, Cvek found that pathologic changes did not extend beyond 2mm from the exposed pulpal surface during the first 3 hours following pulp exposure. When a pulpotomy is performed, it should only be considered as an interim measure because of ensuing problems such as pulp necrosis and canal obliteration. If sufficient enamel and dentin have been lost in the injury, a pulpectomy is generally needed.

In teeth with incomplete root formation and vital pulps, a direct pulp cap with or without the removal of 2 mm of coronal pulp tissue is considered as the treatment of choice by many clinicians, regardless of the size of exposure. Endodontic apexification therapy with calcium hydroxide followed by final shaping and obturation is indicated should pulpal necrosis develop. Finally, complete endodontic therapy is the treatment of choice in permanent teeth with complete root formation and pulpal necrosis.

When sufficient tooth structure remains, the restoration of teeth with complicated crown fractures is probably best achieved with composites and glass ionomers, temporary acrylic or metal crowns as interim measures. Composites may serve as the final restoration in anterior teeth. Endodontic treatment in combination with orthodontic extrusion or periodontal crown lengthening may be indicated in cases where the fracture compromises the biologic crown width or is below the crestal bone.

Pulp capping carries a favorable prognosis as a means of maintaining tooth vitality, regardless of the size or duration of the exposure in teeth with either incomplete or complete root formation. In a study of 301 incisors, Ravn found the success rate for teeth with incomplete root formation to be 100%. In teeth with completely formed roots and apicies, the success rate dropped to 88%. Similarly, Andreasen noted that successful pulpal healing occurred in 71 to 88% of permanent teeth treated by direct calcium hydroxide pulp capping. A 96% success rate was reported by Cvek in a study using 60 anterior teeth with complicated crown fractures. These studies mainly involved patients under 21 years of age and there is little information on the prognosis of teeth in older adults that sustain similar injuries. However, it is thought that the prognosis for pulp capping is not as favorable in older patients because pulpal reparative capacity appears to decrease with age. In the immature tooth, 72% of pulps will heal following removal of the necrotic coronal portion and placement of calcium hydroxide.

In primary teeth, McTigue recommends a mummifying pulpotomy instead of pulp capping with calcium hydroxide. However, Andreasen states that pulp capping in primary teeth is an acceptable procedure.

Pulpectomy is the recommended treatment in cases involving necrotic pulps. At least three-fourths of the root should be present before a pulpectomy is considered, and it is suggested that instrumentation and filling be kept at least 1mm short of the apex to minimize the risk of injury to the permanent tooth.

C. Root Fractures (Table 7-4 & 5)

Root fractures may be divided into two categories, those which involve the crown and those that do not. Andreasen found that root fractures involved the crowns of permanent and primary teeth 5% and 2% of the time respectively. Root fractures limited to the enamel, dentin, and cementum are termed uncomplicated while those involving the pulp are classified as complicated. Fractures of the root and the crown usually occur with either oblique or vertically directed fractures. Root fractures occur in 0.5 to 7% of the dentoalveolar trauma cases involving the permanent teeth and in 2 to 4% of primary dentoalveolar trauma. Fractures of the root not involving the crown are usually horizontal or obliquely directed and are classified as either apical third, coronal third or mid-root fractures depending on their anatomical location.

Diagnosis

On examination it is important to explore all fracture lines with a dental explorer for mobility of any segment. Root fractures involving the crown usually retain the movable, fractured portion because of the soft tissue root attachments. With isolated root fractures, displacement of the coronal segment is more likely with coronal root fractures. Hence, the presence of coronal segment displacement is variable and is less likely as the fracture line moves apically. Bleeding from the gingival sulcus should also raise the examiner's index of suspicion for root fractures even in the absence of other detectable injuries. However, root fractures are frequently associated with other injuries such as alveolar fractures and lateral tooth luxations.

When a root fracture is suspected, Andreasen recommends occlusal and periapical radiographs to demonstrate fractures in the apical third and a conventional bisecting angle periapical radiograph to reveal cervical third fractures. If the examiner is uncertain of the fracture's location, both radiographs should be taken. Fractures are not detectable unless the central beam is directed within 15 to 20 degrees of the fracture's plane. Hence, when a fracture is suspected, it is recommended that two additional radiographs be taken to confirm the finding. One radiograph should be taken at an increased angle of 15 degrees and the other at a decreased angle of 15 degrees. Examiners should be aware that a single root fracture may radiographically appear as multiple fracture lines when the central beam is not parallel to the fracture. Also, radiographs taken immediately following an injury may not demonstrate the presence of a root fracture because the segments have not had time to separate. In such cases, subsequent radiographs taken a few days later can reveal the occult injury.

The value of pulp testing immediately after a root fracture injury occurs is controversial. Many authors suggest that pulp vitality tests not be done on the initial examination. Gerstein states that horizontal root fractures do not respond to vitality testing immediately after traumatic injury. However, Andreasen states that one of the key prognostic indicators of the type of root fracture healing is the pulpal response to vitality testing at the time of injury. A favorable hard tissue union between segments was usually found when the tooth initially tested vital. In addition to vitality testing, mobility must be checked and it is recommended that a color shade be taken on initial examination.

Table 7-4: Crown/Root Fractures

Type of Injury	Incidence	Description of Injury	Immediate Treatment	% Developing Pulp Necrosis*
Crown/Root Fractures	Permanent teeth 5% Primary teeth 2%	See Below	Percussion & vitality tests and shade match	See below
Uncomplicated crown/root fractures	No data available	Involve enamel, dentin, & cementum but not the pulp. Oblique or vertical in direction	Permanent Teeth Remove coronal segmental, place calcium hydroxide over dentin, provide restoration. Follow-up in 6 - 8 weeks Primary teeth Extract	No data available
Complicated crown/root fractures	3 - 5%	Involve enamel, cementum & pulp. Oblique or vertical direction	Permanent teeth Extract if >1/3 of clinical root involved. If < 1/3, pulpectomy & temporize. (May combine with surgical repositioning &splinting) Follow-up in 1- 2 weeks Primary teeth Extract	8.3% after direct cap with calcium hydroxide 4% after coronal 2mm of pulp is removed and a cap placed

*In general, the prognosis is more favorable when the apex is immature. Data obtained is in the age range of 9 - 18 years. No data is presently available for older ages.

Table 7-5: Root Fractures

Type of Injury	Incidence	Description of Injury	Immediate Treatment	% Developing Pathology
Root Fractures	Permanent teeth 0.5 - 7% Primary teeth 2 - 4%	Involves cementum, dentin & pulp. Oblique or horizontal in direction. Classified as coronal or apical 1/3 or midroot fractures. Sulcular bleeding may be present	Percussion, mobility & vitality tests, and shade match Permanent teeth Reposition coronal segment & rigidly splint 2 - 3 months regardless of fracture site. Verify repositioning with a radiograph. If fracture communicates with the gingival sulcus, extract coronal segment & perform pulpectomy on retained root. Follow-up in 3 weeks Primary teeth Extract teeth fractured in coronal 1/3. Splint apical 1/3 fractures if mobile otherwise, do not treat. Follow-up in 3 weeks. Treatment of midroot fractures is controversial.	20 - 44% develop pulp necrosis 22 - 60% undergo root resorbtion 40 - 60% undergo canal obliteration

Treatment

Before considering the treatment of teeth with root fractures, it is important to understand the types of healing that can occur. Healing following root fracture has been described by Andreasen as either by hard tissue union, connective tissue union, the interposition of bone and connective tissue or by nonunion with granulation tissue. The interposition of bone and connective tissue, however, represents a late component of connective tissue healing; therefore, only three types of healing will be discussed.

A hard tissue union consists of dentin in the innermost areas of the tooth and cementum peripherally, while connective tissue union is comprised of connective tissue from the periodontal ligament. Nonunion results from the interposition of granulation tissue secondary to an inflammatory reaction. Nonunion occurs when the integrity of the pulp and periodontal ligament are not preserved. These tissues are vital to the overall repair process following root fractures. Hard tissue union is the most desirable outcome in cases of root fracture followed by connective tissue union. The principal factors which influence the outcome in root fracture cases are: 1) the type of fixation, 2) the degree of luxation of the coronal segment, 3) the stage of root development (the age of the patient), and 4) the pulp vitality following injury. Of these factors, pulp vitality appears to be the single most important factor to the hard tissue union of the segments. When a tooth gives a vital response immediately after injury, it is more likely to result in hard tissue healing. Hard tissue union is also more likely in immature teeth (open apex), in teeth with less coronal mobility and when fixation is applied atraumatically. In addition, hard tissue union has not been found to occur in teeth with pre-existing restorations or periodontal disease. No relationship has been found between the type of healing and the interval of time from injury to reduction and fixation. Also, the location of the fracture in the coronal, middle or apical third has not been a determinant of the type of healing. Connective tissue union is more likely to occur following severe insult that results in lateral luxation of the coronal segment. Pre-existing dental restorations and periodontal disease and the use of traumatic fixation techniques also favor a connective tissue union.

Nonunion by granulation tissue is associated with traumatic fixation appliances, a mature apical foramen, increased mobility of the coronal segment and the administration of antibiotics at the time of the injury. Nonunion has not been found to occur in teeth with immature roots and open apicies.

Andreasen notes that following healing, hard tissue union is characterized by the close approximation of the segments with an indistinct fracture line radiographically, and by equal mobility of injured and non-injured teeth clinically. Connective tissue healing demonstrates a very

Table 7-6: Steps in Splint Application

- Select a method of stabilization (rigid or nonrigid)*
- Reposition injured components
- Clean blood and debris from teeth to be splinted
- Isolate teeth to be splinted (cotton rolls, gauze, etc.)
- Dry teeth
- Apply etching material to enamel (follow manufacturer's directions)
- Rinse etching material off teeth
- Apply unfilled resin to etched surfaces of abutment teeth
- Position splint (precurved orthodontic wire or monofilament nylon)
- Apply filled resin to abutment teeth and splint[+]
- Light polymerize
- Apply unfilled resin to etched surfaces of repositioned teeth
- Apply filled resin to repositioned teeth
- Light polymerize
- Disk any rough composite surfaces
- Verify repositioned components with a radiograph

* Rigid splinting for root fractures, alveolar fractures and avulsions > 1-2 hours old. Non rigid splinting for extrusive & lateral luxations and avulsions < 1 hour old.
[+] Composite resin by itself may serve as rigid splint.

distinct fracture line radiographically, with increased mobility of the injured tooth relative to non-injured teeth. Nonunion with granulation tissue is characterized by a very distinct radiolucent fracture line that extends into the alveolar bone on the radiograph with marked tooth mobility. Root resorption, which occurs in 60% of all root fractures within 1 year, may also be detected radiographically either along the fractured edges or at the apex of the tooth.

The initial treatment decision to be made is whether or not the injured tooth or teeth should be saved. Consideration must be given to such factors as the periodontal health and pre-existing caries of the injured tooth and other teeth in the mouth. Prosthetic consideration must be given to the relative value of retaining the tooth and to the desires of an informed patient. In general, teeth with complicated crown/root fractures in which the fracture involves more than one-third of the root should be extracted. A pulpectomy should be performed and the tooth temporized in those cases involving less than one-third of the root, and this may be combined with immediate surgical repositioning and rigid splinting or orthodontic repositioning. Once the decision has been reached to save a tooth with a horizontal or oblique root fracture, the treatment is the same regardless of whether the fracture occurs in the coronal, middle or apical third of the tooth. The area should be anesthetized, the segments reduced manually and the tooth rigidly splinted. When selecting a splinting technique, it is important to choose one which will cause the least trauma during application. A rigid, passive orthodontic wire applied with acid etch composite resin meets the requirements for firmly immobilizing a root fracture. The splint should extend at least two teeth beyond the fracture site on both sides for reliable stability (Table 7-6). Once the reduction and fixation has been completed, a radiograph should be taken to verify the position of the segments (Figure 7-8).

The exception to the aforementioned procedure is encountered in teeth with root fractures extending into the gingival sulcus. In these cases healing is complicated by bacterial contamination and a lack of alveolar support for the coronal segment. Most authors recommend extraction of the mobile coronal segment followed by endodontic treatment of the remaining portion. Periodontal crown lengthening or orthodontic extrusion are suggested to reproduce the biologic width and allow restorative treatment.

The recommended length of immobilization varies considerably but, in general, a period of 2 to 3 months is proposed by most authors. During this time, three week follow-up visits are recommended during which a full range of endodontic tests should be conducted including pulp vitality testing. If pulp necrosis develops during the period of immobilization,

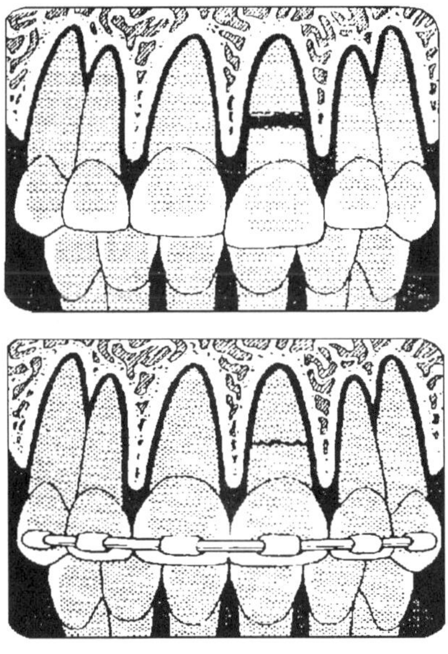

Figure 7-8: Horizontal root fracture of a central incisor prior to reduction and fixation (top). Reduction and fixation with orthodontic wire and acid etch composite resin (bottom). This type of fixation may also be used for alveolar fractures. Monofilament nylon should be used in place of orthodontic wire in cases of luxation injuries and complete avulsions, when there are no fractures of the teeth or bone.

Table 7-7: Nondisplaced Luxation Injuries

Type of Injury	Incidence	Description	Immediate Treatment	% Developing Pathology
Concussion	16.4% of all dentoalveolar injuries 28% of all luxation injuries	Injury to PDL without abnormal mobility or displacement. Does not fracture tooth structure. May occur in combination with other injuries.	Permanent teeth Percussion & vitality tests and shade match. Occlusal adjustment of involved teeth if indicated, otherwise no treatment. Follow-up in 6-8 weeks Primary teeth No treatment	Mature teeth 4.2% develop pulp necrosis & 5.8% undergo canal obliteration Immature teeth 0% develop pulp necrosis & 3.4% undergo canal obliteration
Subluxation	3.1% of all dentoalveolar injuries 35% of all luxation injuries	A more severe injury to the PDL with abnormal mobility but no displacement. sulcular bleeding may be present. Does not fracture the tooth structure. May occur with other injuries.	Permanent teeth Percussion & vitality tests and shade match. Occlusal adjustment of involved teeth and splint for 7-10 days to minimize pain if needed. Follow-up in 6-8 weeks unless splinted. Primary teeth No treatment	Mature teeth 15.1% develop pulp necrosis & 8.6% undergo canal obliteraion Immature teeth 0% develop pulp necrosis & 11.5% undergo canal obliteration

endodontic treatment should be initiated. Pulp necrosis usually occurs within the first two months following the injury, and is frequently limited to the coronal segment. When necrosis of the coronal segment develops, endodontic treatment should be confined to this segment without extending into the apical portion. Andreasen reported that root fractures heal by connective tissue union following root canal treatment of the necrotic coronal segment and that these teeth have a 90% success rate. When endodontic treatment is necessary, consideration should be given to increasing the period of splint immobilization to improve the type of fracture healing.

Regarding primary teeth, most clinicians believe that root fractures in the apical third should not be splinted, allowing the apical portion to resorb. However, controversy exists concerning the treatment of midroot fractures with some clinicians recommending splinting while others recommend extraction. Further, in such cases some authors suggest that the apical root segment be extracted while others feel that this therapy risks damage to the permanent tooth recommending that the apical segment remain undisturbed. If not removed, the residual root segment should be followed radiographically on subsequent visits until resorption is complete. Regarding fractures in the cervical third of primary teeth, there is reasonably good agreement that both segments should be extracted. Likewise, there is good agreement that primary crown fractures that extend to the root should be treated by extracting both segments.

D. Concussion and Subluxation (Table 7-7)

Incidence

Comparatively, concussion injuries are a milder type of injury resulting in less damage to the periodontal ligament and pulp. The combined frequency is estimated to be 3 to 16% of all dentoalveolar trauma.

Diagnosis

The visual examination for concussion and subluxation injuries should include a thorough cleaning of any debris from the surfaces of the teeth. The teeth should be dried and examined for evidence of fractures which would place the injury into another category. In neither of these types of injuries should there be any evidence of fractures or displacement; however, in some cases there may be slight hemorrhaging from the gingival sulcus because of injury to the periodontal ligament. Patients may report that the involved teeth are sore for both types of trauma.

A full range of endodontic tests should be conducted including pulp vitality, mobility, percussion sensitivity and color shade. Teeth which have sustained a concussion injury will usually have normal mobility, be sensitive to percussion and have a positive vitality response. In contrast, subluxated teeth will usually have increased mobility, be sensitive to percussion and 50% will not respond to vitality tests. These differences reflect the increased severity of the injury to the periodontal ligament suffered in subluxation injuries.

Treatment

Usually there is no immediate treatment required for teeth which have been either subluxated or concussed. If sufficient damage has occurred to the periodontal ligament, edema or hemorrhage in the apical tissues may place the tooth in hyperocclusion. When this occurs, a limited occlusal adjustment is indicated. Immediate pulpal therapy and tooth fixation are not necessary; however, endodontic tests should be conducted at the initial

Table 7-8: Displaced Luxation Injuries

Type of Injury	Incidence	Description	Immediate Treatment	% Developing Pulp Necrosis
Extrusive Luxation (Partial Avulsion)	1.9% of dentoalveolar injuries 8.3% of all luxation injuires	The tooth is displaced coronally out of the socket & is very mobile.	Permanent teeth Percussion & vitality tests and shade match Reposition manually or surgically. Splint non-rigidly 2-3 weeks. Occlusal adjustment if needed. Verify repositioning with a radiograph. Follow-up in 2-3 weeks. Primary teeth Extract	55% in mature teeth 9% in immature teeth
Lateral Luxation	19% of all luxation injuries	The tooth is displaced in the horizontal plane (lingual, facial, mesial or distal) May be very firmly positioned. Gingival laceration & alveolar fracture may be present.	Permanent teeth Percussion & vitality tests and shade match. Reposition manually or surgically. Splint non-rigidly for 2-3 weeks. If alveolus is fractured, splint rigidly 3-6 weeks. Adjust occlusion and suture lacerations if necessary. Verify repositioning with a radiograph. Follow-up in 2-3 weeks. Primary teeth may be re-positioned & splinted, allowed to re-align itself (if not interfering with occlusion) or extracted. The underlying permanent tooth must not be injured during treatment. Follow-up in 2 weeks if splinted.	77% in mature teeth 8.8% in immature teeth
Intrusive Luxation	3.9% of dentoalveolar injuries 9.5% of all luxation injuries	The tooth is displaced apically in the alveolus crushing the bone.	Permanent teeth Percussion test. Vitality & shade match if possible. Follow-up in 2 weeks Mature teeth - No treatment, await re-eruption or orthodontically extrude. Immature teeth - No treatment, await re-eruption. Primary teeth No treatment, await re-eruption	100% in mature teeth 62% in immature teeth

*includes the nondisplaced luxation injuires, concussion and subluxation

visit and at routine follow-up appointments. The prognosis for concussed teeth is generally favorable. Pulp necrosis occurs 4.2% of the time in mature teeth and not at all in immature teeth. In mature teeth, 3.4% undergo complete calcification of the root canal system. In contrast, subluxated teeth have a less favorable prognosis. Studies indicate that 15.1% of subluxated, mature teeth develop pulp necrosis and 8.6% undergo complete calcification of the canal. Very few immature teeth develop pulp necrosis and 11.5% undergo canal obliteration. Andreasen reported that pulp necrosis occurs within 3 months of concussion injuries and within 1 year following subluxation injuries. The two major predictors of pulp survival in these injuries are the stage of root development and the severity of the trauma. The earlier the stage of root development and the less severe the trauma the more likely the pulp is to survive.

Regarding primary teeth, no treatment is indicated at the initial visit for either concussion or subluxation injuries. Parents should be advised of the need to bring the child in for follow-up visits so that endodontic therapy or extractions are provided in a timely manner when indicated.

E. Luxation Injuries: Extrusive, Lateral and Intrusive (Table 7-8)

Incidence

In general, extrusive luxation injuries cause the least amount of damage to the pulp and periodontal ligament while intrusive luxations are the most damaging. Zadik reported that 3.9% of all traumatized teeth were intruded and 1.9% were extruded; however, Andreasen has reported that 2 to 31% of injured teeth were intruded. The incidence of lateral luxation injuries has been reported to be 19% of all luxation injuries.

Diagnosis

The visual inspection for luxation injuries should include a thorough cleaning of all tooth surfaces and soft tissue. Teeth should be examined for the presence of crown and root fractures which, if present, would indicate a combination injury. Lateral luxation injuries are evident from the displacement of the crown in a lingual, buccal, mesial or distal direction. Gingival lacerations and alveolar wall fractures frequently accompany lateral luxations and may be palpated through the soft tissue.

Extrusively luxated teeth, sometimes referred to as partial avulsions, will appear to be elongated compared to adjacent teeth because the teeth have been partially forced out of the socket. Intrusive luxation injuries push the tooth into the socket and as a result, the tooth will appear below the occlusal plane of adjacent teeth.

Intrusively luxated teeth are usually firm without mobility and the adjacent alveolar bone may be crushed, penetrated or fractured. In cases of severe intrusion, the tooth may actually be submerged below the gingiva giving the appearance of a complete avulsion. Occassionally, the apex of a maxillary tooth will penetrate into the nasal cavity causing epistaxis, which should prompt the examiner to look for this possibility. As with other types of dental injuries previously discussed, a full range of endodontic tests should be carried out prior to the use of a local anesthetic agent.

Specifically, percussion tests may be of added significance in differentiating extrusion and intrusion injuries. Compared to the percussion of a normal tooth, a dull sound may be heard when percussing extruded teeth while a metallic, solid sound characterizes intruded teeth. This distinction is most important in determining whether an erupting tooth has been intruded.

Radiographically, Andreasen reported that occlusal radiographs were best suited for revealing extrusive and lateral luxations. Intrusive luxation injuries were best disclosed by either occlusal or periapical radiographs. To insure maximum accuracy, periapical radiographs should be taken from mesial and distal angulations. Following the reduction of a luxated tooth, a final occlusal radiograph should be taken to verify positioning.

Treatment

Lateral and extrusive luxations should be treated by manually repositioning the tooth after anesthetizing the area. Repositioning generally requires more force than expected thus demanding that special attention be paid to the integrity of the buccal plate. As such, it is recommended that the practitioner grasp the crown of the luxated tooth with one hand using the other to stabilize the buccal and lingual walls of the alveolus. Prior to applying force, patients should be appraised of the procedure and the expected sensations. At times, reduction is prohibited by either hydrostatic pressure secondary to edema or from alveolar fragments. In such cases, surgical repositioning is necessary. The tooth should be carefully elevated and extracted, the socket irrigated, and the tooth repositioned, splinted and a pulpectomy performed. A full mucogingival flap may also be required for adequate debridement when there is an accompanying alveolar fracture. It is essential that periosteum cover the bone and as much bone be preserved as possible.

Some authors, however, suggest that lateral luxations not be manually repositioned at the time of injury in favor of orthodontic repositioning one week later. However, this approach is impractical in cases where the luxated tooth interferes with occlusion and when there is a concomittent fracture of the alveolar process. Alveolar fractures should be reduced within one hour of the injury to minimize the incidence of pulpal necrosis, which increases as time to treatment increases.

After the tooth has been repositioned, the position should be stabilized and the occlusion adjusted. Once repositioned, if the tooth is mobile but not loose in the socket, a splint may not be necessary. A splint is indicated if the tooth is loose in the socket or if an alveolar fracture is present. A splint should be chosen which can be applied with the least trauma to the injured dentition and which allows for some functional tooth movement unless an alveolar fracture is present. Splints retained by etched composite resin are atraumatic and are preferred to arch bars. The best prognosis is achieved with splints which allow for some functional movement rather than those which rigidly retain the tooth in position.

Non rigid splints have been shown to decrease the chances of replacement resorption (ankylosis). In contrast, however, Berude reported no differences in healing between rigid and functional splints in monkeys.

Rigid splints are indicated when there is an accompanying alveolar fracture. Splints should also be constructed to facilitate oral hygiene and allow for the conduction of vitality testing. Ideally, access should be maintained to the same area used for vitality testing before the splint was applied, so that accurate follow-up comparisons may be made. Antrim developed a splint of monofilament nylon bonded to the teeth with acid etched composite resin. This splint is hygienic and allows for physiologic movement of the repositioned tooth. When a more rigid splint is indicated, a passive, precurved, rectangular orthodontic wire can be used in place of nylon monofilament. A splint composed only of composite resin can also be used as a form of rigid fixation. When acid etch composite resin retained splints are indicated and one or more of the anchor teeth is a porcelain or metal crown, adhesives such as 4-META materials or silane couplers are indicated. These adhesives are used to treat the surfaces of crowned teeth, rendering them susceptible to composite bonding. Gingival lacerations, which frequently occur with lateral luxations, should be cleaned and sutured after teeth and bone have been repositioned and the splint applied.

Non-rigid splints should be removed in 2 to 3 weeks, while rigid splints for alveolar fractures should remain in place for 3 to 6 weeks. At the time of splint removal, the luxated teeth will still be considerably more mobile than the adjacent normal teeth. As such, care should be taken during splint removal to avoid further trauma to the injured teeth. The occlusion should be checked and adjusted if necessary and the patient should avoid chewing hard food for several days.

When the luxational injury involves the intrusion of teeth, the teeth should not be manually repositioned except in specific circumstances. For example, if the root is incompletely formed the tooth may be allowed to re-erupt or, in the case of teeth with complete root formation, the tooth can be orthodontically repositioned. Limited manual repositioning of intruded teeth with completed root formation is indicated when it is not possible to gain access for bonding orthodontic brackets or hooks. The orthodontic extrusion of intruded teeth should be accomplished within a few weeks because a high percentage of intruded teeth require endodontic treatment within three months of the injury. The stage of root formation is the single most important predictor of pulp necrosis following luxation injuries. The more complete the root formation, the greater the likelihood

Table 7-9: Displaced Luxation Injuries - Avulsion

Type of Injury	Incidence	Description	Immediate Treatment	% Developing Pathology
Complete Luxation (Avulsion)	0.5-16% of all dentoalveolar injuries	The tooth is displaced completely out of the socket.	<u>Permanent teeth out < 1 hour</u>: · Grasp tooth by crown only · Irrigate PDL if contaminated · Replant with gentle pressure · Irrigate socket if unable to replant · Splint nonrigidly for 1 week · Adjust occlusion if needed · Verify position with radiograph · Rx PCN 500 mg qid x 7 days · Tetanus evaluation · Follow-up in 1 week <u>Permanent teeth out >1-2 hours</u>:* · Remove PDL & pulp if stored dry · 20 minute soak in 2.4% sodium fluoride solution (pH 5.5) · Obturate canal with gutta percha · Replant with gentle pressure · Irrigate socket if unable to replant · Splint rigidly for 6 weeks · Adjust occlusion if needed · Verify position with a radiograph · Rx PCN 500 mg qid x 7 days · Tetanus evaluation · Follow-up in 2 weeks <u>Primary teeth</u>: Do not replant	100% develop pulp necrosis in mature teeth 72% develop pulp necrosis in immature teeth 74 - 96% develop progressive root resorption

*From Andreasen, *Essentials of Traumatic Injuries of the teeth*, 1990.

of pulp necrosis. Compared to lateral and extrusive luxation injuries, intrusive luxations more commonly result in pulpal necrosis. Nearly 100% of intruded teeth with completely formed roots are nonvital within 3 months following injury. The potential for pulp necrosis with lateral luxations is significantly decreased when the teeth respond positively to vitality tests at the time of injury.

Although it is desirable to treat luxation injuries in a timely manner, the length of time from the injury to treatment is not prognostically significant, except with alveolar process fractures. In such cases, an increase in pulpal necrosis has been shown when treatment is not rendered within the first hour following injury. The immediate manual or surgical repositioning of both lateral and intrusive luxations is associated with an increase in pulpal necrosis. However, lateral luxations may become fixed in position if repositioning is delayed. The potential sequela associated with the treatment and healing process in luxation injuries can include root resorption, canal calcification, loss of marginal alveolar bone and replacement resorption (ankylosis).

Regarding the primary dentition, luxation injuries may be the most serious of the dentoalveolar injuries because developmental deformities of the permanent tooth may result. Many of these developmental deformities are cosmetically unacceptable. Appendix 2 reviews the development and eruption chronology of primary and permanent teeth. Andreasen reported that developmental disturbances of the permanent dentition occur in 34% of extrusive luxations and in 69% of intrusive injuries. In the case of lateral and extrusive luxations, some authors recommend extraction of the primary teeth while others feel that splinting is indicated. In choosing an appropriate approach, the amount of root resorption and patient cooperation must be taken into account.

In general, extraction is the more likely choice in cases where the primary root is resorbing and the child is uncooperative. A space maintainer should be placed if the permanent tooth is not going to erupt soon after the primary is removed and where space maintenance is a concern. When primary incisors are extracted, space maintenance is not needed if the primary canines are intact.

Regarding intrusive luxation of primary teeth, the two recommended approaches are the same as those suggested in the permanent dentition: extraction and passive eruption. Some clinicians recommend extraction if the primary tooth is contacting the permanent tooth and re-eruption in the remaining cases. Ravn reported that 72% of the permanent teeth demonstrated developmental disturbances when intruded primary teeth were extracted, but when primary teeth were left to re-erupt, only 52% of the permanent teeth showed similar disturbances. Primary teeth will usually re-erupt in 2 to 6 months. If the intruded tooth is left to re-erupt during this time the patient must be followed monthly for signs of pulp necrosis and should it develop, extraction is recommended.

F. Complete Luxation (Avulsion) (Table 7-9)

Incidence

There is more in the literature about avulsed teeth and their treatment than on any other single subject in the area of dentoalveolar trauma. Complete luxation injuries account for 0.5 to 16% of dentoalveolar injuries in teeth with complete root formation and 7 to 13% of dentoalveolar injuries in teeth with incomplete root formation.

Diagnosis

In the diagnosis of avulsion injuries, it must be remembered that the prognosis worsens the longer a tooth is out of the socket. A standard thorough examination should therefore be modified to quickly address essential information such as:

1. Is the tooth damaged to the extent that it should not be replaced?

2. Will replacement of the tooth be of benefit to the patient?

3. Does the patient want to have the tooth replanted after being advised of potential follow-up treatment and costs?

A full examination and evaluation should be completed following replantation of the avulsed tooth. If the patient has not replanted the tooth it should be quickly inspected for root and crown fractures, the stage of root development and the presence of gross contamination. If the tooth is grossly contaminated it should be rinsed with sterile saline. A rapid overall assessment of the patient's oral hygiene and periodontal status will help determine the practicality and advisability of replanting the tooth. Radiographs should be taken in cases where teeth are missing but have not been located, suggesting the possibilities of avulsion, intrusion, ingestion or aspiration. Aspiration cases have been cited in which there were no clinical signs of aspiration, such as coughing. The diagnosis of alveolar fracture can be confirmed by radiographic examination; however, in the interest of time, routine radiographs should not be taken unless alveolar fracture is suspected clinically. A radiograph is indicated following replantation and splinting to verify the tooth position. Obviously, endodontic tests cannot be performed while the tooth is out of the socket and are not indicated following replantation. The tests are indicated on follow-up examinations on avulsed teeth with immature root formation and on neighboring teeth that have sustained injuries other than complete luxation.

Treatment

The steps shown in Table 7-9 may be followed on the initial visit and used as a quick reference in treating avulsions. These steps must be accomplished with speed and accuracy, so that the tooth is replanted as quickly as possible. One of the major factors in the long term success of replanted teeth is the health of the periodontal ligament. The longer a tooth is out of the socket the more likely it is to develop a necrotic periodontal ligament. Should a patient telephone the office before seeking emergency care for an avulsed tooth, the patient should be advised to replant the tooth immediately and then come to the office or clinic. If the patient cannot replant the tooth, it should be placed in milk, saline or in the patient's mouth for transportation. Milk has been shown to be the best media in which to transport avulsed teeth. Intraoral storage is the least favored method because the microorganisms and low osmolality of saliva have an overall adverse effect on the periodontal ligament. Also, because of the aspiration risk, this means of storage is contraindicated in children. Oddly, it has been observed that teeth replanted by patients and physicians have a more favorable prognosis than those replanted by dental professionals because dentists often delay replantation to perform unnecessary procedures.

When handling the tooth, it should be carefully held by the crown so that viable periodontal ligament fibers do not suffer further damage. It is also important to determine how long the tooth has been out of the mouth and how it was stored. If the tooth has been grossly contaminated with foreign material, it should be rinsed gently and quickly with sterile normal saline and examined for damage such as fractures. Drying of the PDL is a major factor in increasing root resorption following replantation and should be avoided. A tooth which has been dry for two or more hours will usually have a substantially necrotic periodontal ligament. Some clinicians state that the root surface should not be mechanically scrubbed, scaled or debrided irrespective of its contamination or state of dessication. However, Lindskog demonstrated in monkeys that the removal of the dried, necrotic periodontal ligament results in a slower destruction of the root by resorption than if the necrotic ligament was untouched. Tetanus prophylaxis should be reviewed if the tooth or socket were contaminated with debris and the patient should be referred for tetanus prophylaxis when indicated. These indications are listed in Appendix D.

It is generally not recommended to soak avulsed teeth in materials such as fluoride solutions; however, there are conflicting results concerning the use of fluoride. In particular, onc study reported that the immersion of avulsed teeth in 2% neutral sodium fluoride retarded the progression of resorption when the tooth was dry and out of the socket for two or more hours. Prior to replantation, Andreasen recommends immersing teeth which have been dried for longer than 1 to 2 hours in a solution of 2.4% sodium fluoride for 20 minutes after the pulp and PDL have been removed. Yet another study by Barbakow found no useful effects of fluoride application to the root surface of avulsed teeth. In a recent animal study, Cvek found that suspending teeth in a solution of doxycycline (1mg) and physiologic saline (20cc) for 5 minutes increased the frequency of pulp revascularization and decreased microorganisms in the pulpal lumen. Zanetta-Barbosa found that suspending teeth in a solution of adenosine triphosphate (ATP) for 5 minutes before replantation improves the healing. Removing part of the apex and/or the placement of an apical restoration is also to be avoided, as these procedures actually interfere with healing and will further delay reimplantation. It is thought that the effects of intracanal calcium hydroxide following replantation may actually be blocked by placing an apical restoration before replantation.

The socket should also be carefully examined before replantation and any alveolar fractures should be reduced before the tooth is inserted. If the pain threshold of the patient is low, a local anesthetic may be needed for reimplantation; however, this procedure may only serve to delay reimplantation and decrease the chances for a favorable prognosis.

To replant a tooth, it is slowly placed into the socket with firm steady pressure until the tooth is completely repositioned. Evacuation of the clot from the socket prior to replantation of the tooth is not usually necessary as this will only prolong the out-of-socket time. However, Andreasen demonstrated in monkeys that sockets in which the clots were removed by saline irrigation healed the same as sockets in which the teeth were replanted without clot removal. In contrast, Matsson reported that fewer cases of ankylosis developed in dogs when sockets were first irrigated with saline. Irrigation and/or exploration of the socket is indicated whenever the tooth cannot be reimplanted.

Once in position, the tooth should be splinted using the same principles discussed with luxation injuries. Similarly, a radiograph should be taken to verify the tooth position following splinting and the occlusion should be evaluated to insure minimal contact on the injured tooth. Endodontic treatment should be initiated in 7 to 10 days following replantation (Table 7-10) and should not be initiated at the time of injury, unless the tooth has been dried out of the mouth for longer than 1 to 2 hours. Studies have indicated that significantly more replacement and surface resorption result when any endodontic treatment is performed at the initial emergency visit, as compared to deferring endodontic therapy to a follow-up appointment. Delaying replantation to place calcium hydroxide in the canal is not recommended for this reason.

Andersson reported that when endodontic treatment was accomplished within 3 weeks of replantation, minimal inflammatory resorption occurred. In cases where endodontic therapy was delayed beyond 3 weeks, there was a higher incidence of inflammatory resorption in younger patients, but not in older patients. Some clinicians recommend delaying endodontic treatment beyond this 3 week window in teeth with immature roots because a small percentage (18%) of these teeth revascularize. However, there is a real risk that inflammatory resorption may destroy much of the root within a few months with this approach. Follow-up appointments should be scheduled within 7 to 10 days following replantation, at which time the canal should be cleaned, shaped and filled with a calcium hydroxide paste. Calcium hydroxide is the recommended filling material because it has been shown to arrest or decrease inflammatory root resorption. After the endodontic treatment with calcium hydroxide has been completed, the

Table 7-10: Follow-up Endodontic Treatment for Avulsed Teeth

Mature Apex out of Mouth < 1-2 Hours

- 7-10 days post injury
  Extirpate pulp
  Clean & shape root canal system
  Place calcium hydroxide
  Remove splint (after endodontic treatment)
  Adjust occlusion if needed
  Take a radiograph

- 6 weeks post injury
  Replace calcium hydroxide
  Take a radiograph

- 2-3 month intervals
  Replace calcium hydroxide if resorbed
  Take a radiograph

- 1 year post injury
  Obturate canal with gutta percha

Immature Apex out of mouth < 1-2 Hours

- 7-14 days post injury
  Check pulp vitality
  Take a radiograph

- 2 week intervals
  Check pulp vitality
  Take a radiograph at periodic 2 week intervals

- Institute calcium hydroxide therapy if tooth
  becomes necrotic or resorbtion is detected

splint should be removed as atraumatically as possible. The occlusion should be re-checked for prematuraties on the injured tooth. The next appointment should be scheduled 6 weeks later, during which, Gerstein recommends replacement of the calcium hydroxide. Following this appointment, the patient should then be seen at 2 to 3 month intervals for the first year. At one year following the injury, the tooth may be obturated with a permanent filling material and followed at six month intervals thereafter. Radiographs of the avulsed teeth and neighboring teeth that may have also been damaged should be taken at all follow-up appointments.

The American Association of Endodontics does not recommend the routine use of antibiotics in cases of complete luxation, and a recent study by Cvek showed that the systemic administration of doxycycline did not improve pulpal revascularization. However, other authors recommend the routine use of antibiotics, usually penicillin 500 mg qid, for 7 to 10 days following reimplantation. Andreasen states that the use of antibiotics to decrease inflammatory resorption is justified and recommends 1 million units (0.6 gm) of penicillin immediately followed by 2 to 4 million units

(1.2 - 2.4 gm) four times daily for four days. Hammarstrom found no inflammatory resorption in monkeys that had been given systemic dehydrostreptomycin and benzylpenicillin for six days following replantation; however, replacement resorption was still evident. Likewise, the use of intracanal antibiotics has also been shown to prevent inflammatory resorption.

Regarding the prognosis of reimplanted, avulsed teeth, it has been shown in animal studies that only 18% revascularize. Bacterial contamination has been proposed as the major reason for failure. Also, inflammatory and replacement resorption are the primary sequela encountered. Occurring 74 to 96% of the time, resorption is directly related to the length of time the tooth is out of the socket and the method used to store the tooth prior to reimplantation. In general, the shorter the out-of-socket time, the better the prognosis. It has been found that teeth replanted within 15 minutes of avulsion have a favorable prognosis showing little progressive root resorption, and that teeth reimplanted within 10 minutes show no progressive root resorption. Regardless of the length of extra oral time, initial root resorption and minor areas of ankylosis occur within one week of the injury. The prognosis of this sequela is improved when endodontic treatment with calcium hydroxide is completed within 3 weeks of the injury. In addition, the use of intracanal antibiotics also appears to hold promise for decreasing inflammatory resorption.

The stage of root formation is also an important factor regarding the development of pulp necrosis. In general, the more mature the root development, the worse the prognosis for pulpal revascularization. Thirty minutes is considered the maximum time a tooth with an open apex can be out of the socket without developing pulpal necrosis. Andreasen found that avulsed teeth with immature roots healed in 74 to 94% of the cases when proper endodontic therapy was performed.

Finally, the age of the patient is a factor in the prognosis of reimplanted teeth. Andersson found that teeth in younger patients that were reimplanted with a necrotic PDL, and had been out of the socket for one hour became ankylosed and resorbed within 3 to 7 years. Older patients, however, retained the same teeth for a considerably longer time. In summary, the key factors in evaluating the prognosis of avulsed teeth are:

1. The health of the periodontal ligament, as determined clinically by the time the tooth is out of the socket and the storage media in which the tooth was transported.
2. The stage of root development.
3. The age of the patient.
4. The time elapsed between the injury and the initiation of root canal therapy.

Regarding avulsed primary teeth, Andreasen reported that developmental disturbances of the permanent dentition occurred in 52% of the cases where a primary tooth was avulsed, even though it was not reimplanted. The recommendation is not to reimplant avulsed primary teeth because of delayed eruption and developmental disturbances in the succedaneous permanent tooth. When indicated, a space maintenance appliance should be inserted to prevent space loss and subsequent crowding problems in the permanent dentition.

G. Alveolar Fractures Associated with Dentoalveolar Injuries

(Table 7-11)

Dentoalveolar injuries involving bone have been divided into 4 categories by Andreasen: 1) Comminution of the alveolar socket that occurs from intrusive luxation injuries producing a crushing type of fracture, 2) fractures of the buccal or lingual walls of the socket, seen with lateral luxations, 3) fractures of the alveolar process resulting in mobility of an entire segment of teeth and bone, and 4) fractures of the mandible and maxilla. The first three types will be described in this chapter, while maxillary and mandibular fractures are discussed in Chapter 8.

Table 7-11: Alveolar Fractures

Type of Injury	Incidence	Description	Immediate Treatment	% Developing Pathology
Alveolar Fracture	5 - 9%	A fracture of the supporting bone which usually occurs in conjunction with other dentoalveolar injuries but may occur alone. Often noted when an entire segment of teeth move in response to pressure on a single tooth.	Permanent teeth: ·Reposition segments ·Splint rigidly for 3-6 weeks ·Verify position with a radiograph ·Suture laceration if present ·Repair injuries to ·Follow-up in 3 weeks Primary teeth: ·Reposition segments ·Usually do not need to splint, if needed splint rigidly for 2-3 weeks ·Verify position with a radiograph ·Suture lacerations if present ·Repair injuries to teeth ·Follow-up in 2-3 weeks All alveolar fractures should be reduced within 1 hour following injury. Pulp necrosis rapidly increases >1 hour.	75% develop pulp necrosis 15% undergo canal obliteration 11% undergo progressive root resorption

Diagnosis

Fractures of the alveolar process can occur alone, but are usually associated with luxation injuries and/or root fractures. Mobility of a bone segment is a common finding and is typically evident when the mobility of a single tooth is checked and several teeth move simultaneously. Alveolar fractures can usually be detected by palpation and in displaced segmental injuries are often accompanied by gingival lacerations.

Fractures of the alveolar process may be confirmed by using standard radiographic techniques. When the facial wall is involved, a supplementary lateral film is often helpful. Because root fractures often accompany alveolar fractures, distinguishing the two can be difficult, especially with superimposition of the fracture lines. In such cases, radiographs taken from different angles will show a fracture line does not change position on the root if there is only a root fracture. However, when there is an alveolar fracture superimposed on the root surface the fracture line will change position. Because teeth in close proximity to an alveolar fracture may have been traumatized, a full range of endodontic tests should be conducted on these teeth prior to the administration of local anesthetics.

Treatment

Fractures of an entire alveolar segment are usually reduced following the administration of a local anesthetic agent, by manually repositioning the involved teeth into proper arch alignment. Fractures of the socket wall associated with lateral luxation injuries are reduced in a similar fashion; however, the buccal or lingual plate may be displaced and locked into place by overlapping the remainder of the alveolar bone. In these cases it is necessary to simultaneously apply apical pressure on the alveolar plate and on the coronal portion of the tooth to disengage the fractured alveolus. When attempts at repositioning are unsuccessful, the wound should be irrigated and debrided. If repositioning continues to fail then a full thickness flap is needed to allow thorough irrigation and debridement with the aid of visual inspection. Care should be taken to avoid separating any bony segments from their periosteal attachment. If the fractured segments of alveolar bone have all or most of the periosteum intact the bone should be repositioned and preserved. Sequestration of alveolar bone is not a frequent complication, especially when the periosteum is uninjured. However, small sequestra without periosteal attachment should be removed in most cases. If there are teeth requiring extraction in the area of an alveolar fracture, the extractions should be delayed until the alveolar fracture has healed.

A rigid splint should be applied to immobilize alveolar fractures, which is in contrast to the semi-rigid splints recommended for luxation injuries.

A rectangular orthodontic wire placed with acid etched composite resin or a splint made entirely of composite resin are ideal for this purpose. Most clinicians recommend that alveolar fractures be immobilized for 3 to 6 weeks with a follow-up examination scheduled in 2 to 3 weeks to evaluate tooth vitality. After 3 to 6 weeks, the splint is removed and tooth vitality is rechecked again. There is little information in the literature concerning the appropriate timing of endodontic therapy in relation to alveolar fractures except that the therapy should not be initiated until pulpal necrosis is confirmed. Other clinicians advocate an endodontic approach similar to that already discussed for complete luxation injuries.

In a study of dental complications following alveolar fractures in humans, Andreasen found that 75% of the teeth developed pulp necrosis, 15% of the canals underwent complete calcification, 11% had root resorption and 13% lost marginal supporting bone. Teeth were more likely to develop pulp necrosis when splinting was delayed beyond 1 hour from the time of injury; hence, as with avulsion injuries, it is important to minimize the time from injury to fixation.

Regarding maxillary and mandibular fractures, healthy teeth along the fracture line should be preserved to establish occlusion and serve as anchors. Antibiotic coverage (Penicillin 500mg qid) for at least one week is generally recommended when teeth are in the line of such a fracture.

In a recent study by Oikarinen, it was found that 64% of the teeth in the line of a mandibular fracture developed pulp necrosis when the fracture line passed through the apex of the tooth. When the fracture line went through the alveolar septal bone, 20% of the teeth developed pulp necrosis. Finally, when the mandibular fracture extended through the lateral periodontal ligament space, 15% of the teeth developed pulpal necrosis. Age was also found to effect the prognosis of teeth in the line of a jaw fracture, as older patients developed pulpal necrosis more frequently than did younger patients.

Regarding the primary teeth, fractures of the alveolar socket wall should be reduced manually but usually do not require splinting because of rapid bony healing in children. However, segmental fractures in children should be reduced and splinted for 2 to 3 weeks. The diet should be restricted to soft food for 2 weeks in either case.

References

Alling C., Osbon D., *Maxillofacial Trauma*. Philadelphia: Lea & Febiger, 1988.

Andreasen J.O., Andreasen F.M., *Essentials of Traumatic Injuries to the Teeth*. Copenhagen: Munksgaard, 1990.

Andreasen F.M., Andreasen J.O., Bayer T., "Prognosis of root-fractured permanent incisors - prediction of healing modalities." *Endod Dent Traumatol*. 5 (1989): 11-22.

Andreasen F.M., "Pulpal healing after luxation injuries and root fracture in the permanent dentition." *Endod Dent Traumatol.* 5 (1989): 111-131.

Andreasen F.M., "Histological and bacteriological study of pulps extirpated after luxation injuries." *Endod Dent Traumatol.* 4 (1989): 170-181.

Andreasen F.M., Zhijie Y., Thomsen B.L., "Relationship between pulp dimensions and development of pulp necrosis after luxation injuries in the permanent dentition." *Endod Dent Traumatol.* 2 (1986): 90-98.

Andreasen F.M., "Transient apical breakdown and its relation to color and sensibility changes after luxation injuries to teeth." *Endod Dent Traumatol.* 2 (1986): 9-19.

Andreasen F.M., Vestergaard Pedersen B., "Prognosis of luxated permanent teeth - the development of pulp necrosis." *Endod Dent Traumatol.* 1 (1985): 207-220.

Andreasen F.M., Andreasen J.O., "Diagnosis of luxation injuries: The importance of standardized clinical, radiographic and photographic techniques in clinical investigations." *Endod Dent Traumatol.* 1 (1985): 160-169.

Andreasen J.O., Schwartz O., "The effect of saline storage before replantation upon dry damage of the periodontal ligament." *Endod Dent Traumatol.* 2 (1986): 67-70.

Andreasen J.O., "Challenges in clinical dental traumatology." *Endod Dent Traumatol.* 1 (1985): 45-55.

Andreasen J.O., Kristerson L., "The effect of limited drying or removal of the periodontal ligament." *Acta Odontol Scand.* 39 (1981): 1-13.

Andreasen J.O., "The effect of excessive occlusal trauma upon periodontal healing after replantation of mature permanent incisors in monkeys." *Swed Dent J.* 5 (1981): 115-122.

Andreasen J.O., "Effect of extra-alveolar period and storage media upon periodontal and pulpal healing after replantation of mature permanent incisors in monkeys." *Int J Oral Surg.* 10 (1981): 43-53.

Andreasen J.O., "The effect of pulp extirpation or root canal treatment on periodontal healing after replantation of permanent incisors in monkeys." *J Endod.* 7(6) (1981): 245-252.

Andreasen J.O., Kristerson L., "The effect of extra-alveolar root filling with calcium hydroxide on periodontal healing after replantation of permanent incisors in monkeys." *J Endod.* 7(8) (1981): 349-354.

Andreasen J.O., *Traumatic injuries of the teeth.* 2d ed, Copenhagen: Munksgaard, 1981.

Andreasen J.O., "Analysis of pathogenesis and topography of replacement root resorption (ankylosis) after replantation of maturė permanent incisors in monkeys." *Swed Dent J.* 4 (1980): 231-240.

Andreasen J.O., "The effect of removal of the coagulum in the alveolus before replantation upon periodontal and pupal healing of mature permanent incisors in monkeys." *Int J Oral Surg.* 9 (1980): 458-461.

Andreasen J.O., "A time-related study of periodontal healing and root resorption activity after replantation of mature permanent incisors in monkeys." *Swed Dent J.* 4 (1980): 101-110.

Andreasen J.O., "The effect of splinting upon periodontal healing after replantation of permanent incisors in monkeys." *Acta Odont Scand.* 33 (1975): 313-323.

Andreasen J.O., "Treatment of fractured and avulsed teeth." *J Dent for Child.* 1 (1971): 29-48.

Andreasen J.O., "Fractures of the alveolar process of the jaw." *Scand J Dent Res.* 78 (1970): 263-272.

Andersson L., Boding I., "Avulsed human teeth replanted within 15 minutes - a long-term clinical follow-up study." *Endod Dent Traumatol.* 6 (1990): 37-42.

Andersson L., Bodin I., Sorensen S., "Progression of root resorption following replantation of human teeth after extended extraoral storage." *Endod Dent Traumatol.* 5 (1989): 38-47.

Andersson L.; Lindskog S.; Blomlof L.; Hedstrom KG.; Hammarstrom L., "Effect of Masticatory stimulation on dentoalveolar ankylosis after experimental tooth replantation." *Endod Dent Traumatol.* 1 (1985): 13-16.

Andersson L.; Blomlof L.; Lindskog S.; Feiglin B.; Hammarstrom L., "Tooth ankylosis clinical radiographic and histological assessments." *Int J Oral Surg.* 13 (1984): 423-431.

Antrim D.D., "A functional splint for traumatized teeth." *J Endod.* 8(7) (1982): 328-331.

Bakland L.K., Christiansen E.L., Strutz J.M., "Frequency of dental traumatic events in the etiology of temporomandibular disorders." *Endo Dent Traumatol.* 4 (1988): 182-185.

Barbakow F.H.; Cleaton-Jones P.E.; Austin J.C.; and Vieira E., "Healing of replanted teeth following topical treatment with fluoride solutions and systemic admission of thyrocalcitonin: a histometric analysis." *J Endod.* 7(7) (1981): 302-398.

Barnett F., Rabie G., Tronstad L., "Long-term splinting of maxillary incisor with intra-alveolar root fracture." *Endo Dent Traumatol.* 4 (1988): 99-103.

Bender I.B., Freedland I.B., "Clinical considerations in the diagnosis and treatment of intra-alveolar root fractures." *JADA.* 107 (1983): 595-600.

Berude J.A.; Hicks M.L.; Jerome M.S.; Sauber J.; and Li S.H., "Resorption after physiological and rigid splinting of replanted permanent incisors in monkeys." *J Endod.* 14(12) (1988): 592-600.

Birch R., Rock W.P., "The incidence of complications following root fracture in permanent anterior teeth." *Br Dent J.* 160 (1986): 119-122.

Blomlof L.; Lindskog S.; Andersson L.; Hedstrom K.G.; and Hammarstrom L., "Storage of experimentally avulsed teeth in milk prior to replantation." *J Dent Res.* 62(8) (1983): 912-916.

Camp J.H., "Recommended guidelines for treatment of the avulsed tooth." *J Endod.* 9(12) (1983): 413-420.

Cvek M.; Cleaton-Jones P.; Austin J.; Kling M.; Lownie J.; and Fatti P., "Effect of topical application of doxycycline on pulp revascularization and periodontal healing in reimplanted monkey incisors." *Endod Dent Traumatol.* 6 (1990): 170-176.

Cvek M.; Cleaton-Jones P.; Austin J.; Kling M.; Lownie J.; and Fatti P., "Pulp Revascularization in reimplanted immature monkey incisors - predictability and the effect of antibiotic systemic prophylaxis." *Endod Dent Traumatol.* 6 (1990): 157-169.

Cvek M.; Cleaton-Jones P.E.; Austin J.C.; and Andreasen J.O., "Pulp reactions to exposure after experimental crown fractures or grinding in adult monkeys." *J Endod.* 8(9) (1982): 391-397.

Cvek M., "A clinical report on partial pulpotomy and capping with calcium hydroxide in permanent incisors with complicated crown fracture." *J Endod.* 4(8) (1978): 232-237.

Dumsha T., Hovland E.J., "Pulpal prognosis following extrusive luxation injuries in permanent teeth with closed apexes." *J Endod.* 8(9): 410-412.

Garcia-Godoy F., "A classification for traumatic injuries to primary and permanent teeth." *J Pedodont.* 5(4) (1981): 295-297.

Gerstein H., *Techniques in clinical endodontics.* Philadelphia: WB Saunders Company, 1983.

Hammarstrom L., Blomlof L., Lindskog S., "Dynamics of dentoalveolar ankylosis and associated root resorption." *Endod Dent Traumatol.* 5 (1989): 163-175.

Hammarstrom L.; Blomlof L.; Feiglin B.; Andersson L.; and Lindskog S., "Replantation of teeth and antibiotic treatment." *Endod Dent Traumatol.* 2 (1986): 51-57.

Jacobsen I., Kerekes K., "Long-term prognosis of traumatized permanent anterior teeth showing calcifying processes in the pulp cavity." *Scand J Dent Res.* 85 (1977): 588-598.

Kling M., Cvek M., Mejare I., "Rate and predictability of pulp revascularization in therapeutically reimplanted permanent incisors." *Endod Dent Traumatol.* 2 (1986): 83-89.

Kopel H.M., Johnson R., "Examination and neurologic assessment of children with oro-facial trauma." *Endod Dent Traumatol.* 1 (1985): 155-159.

Kristerson L., Andreasen, J.O., "Influence of root development on periodontal and pulpal healing after replantation of incisors in monkeys." *Int J Oral Surg.* 13 (1984): 313-323.

Lindskog S.; Pierce A.M.; Blomlof L.; and Hammarstrom L., "The role of the necrotic periodontal membrane in cementum resorption and ankylosis." *Endod Dent Traumatol.* 1 (1985): 96-101.

Matsson L., Klinge B., Hallstrom H., "Effect on periodontal healing of saline irrigation of the tooth socket before replantation." *Endod Dent Traumatol.* 3 (1987): 64-67.

Matsson L.; Andreasen J.O.; Cvek M.; and Granath L., "Ankylosis of experimentally reimplanted teeth related to extra-alveolar period and storage environment." *Pediat Dent.* 4(4) (1982): 327-329.

Nasjleti C.E., Castelli W.A., Caffesse R.G., "The effects of different splinting times on replantation of teeth in monkeys." *Oral Surg.* 53(6) (1982): 557-566.

Oikarinen K., Lahti J., Rasutia A.M., "Prognosis of permanent teeth in the line of mandibular fractures." *Endod Dent Traumatol.* 6 (1990): 177-182.

Oikarinen K., "Functional fixation for traumatically luxated teeth." *Endod Dent Traumatol.* 3 (1987): 224-228.

Oikarinen K., Kassila O., "Causes and types of traumatic tooth injuries treated in a public dental health clinic." *Endod Dent Traumatol.* 3 (1987): 172-177.

O'Neil D.W.; Clark M.V.; Lowe J.W.; and Harrington M.S., "Oral trauma in children: a hospital survey." *Oral Surg Oral Med Oral Pathol.* 68 (1989): 691-696.

O'Riordan M.W., Curt S.R., Doerr S.E., "Treatment of avulsed permanent teeth: an update." *JADA.* 105 (1982): 1028-1030.

Oswald R.J., Harrington G.W., Van Hassel H.J., "A postreplantation evaluation of air-dried and saliva-stored avulsed teeth." *J Endod.* 6(5) (1980): 546-551.

Peterson L.J., *Contemporary Oral and Maxillofacial Surgery.* St. Louis: CV Mosby Company, 1988.

Pinkham J.R., *Pediatric dentistry infancy through adolescence.* WB. Philadelphia: Saunders Company, 1988.

Ravn J.J., "Follow-up study of permanent incisors with complicated crown fractures after acute trauma." *Scand J Dent Res.* 90 (1982): 363-372.

Ravn J.J., "Follow-up study of permanent incisors with enamel fractures as a result of an acute trauma." *Scand J Dent Res.* 89 (1981): 213-217.

Ravn J.J., "Follow-up study of permanent incisors with enamel-dentin fractures after acute trauma." *Scand J Dent Res.* 89 (1981): 355-365.

Ravn J.J., "Follow-up study of permanent incisors with enamel cracks as a result of acute trauma." *Scand J Dent Res.* 89 (1981): 117-123.

Ravn J.J., "Developmental disturbances in permanent teeth after intrusion of their primary predecessors." *Scand J Dent Res.* 84 (1976): 137-141.

Remeikis N.A., Stroner W.F., "Inflammatory resorption: intreated, arrested, prevented." *Endod Dent Traumatol.* 5 (1989): 292-297.

Rock W.P., Grundy M.C., "The effect of luxation and subluxation upon the prognosis of traumatized incisor teeth." *J Dent.* 9(3) (1981): 224-230.

Rock W.P.; Gordon P.H.; Friend L.A.; and Grundy M.C., "The relationship between trauma and pulp death in incisor teeth." *Brit Dent J.* 136 (1974): 236-239.

Schindler W.G., Gullickson D.C., "Rationale for the management of calcific metamorphosis secondary to traumatic injuries." *J Endod.* 14(8) (1988): 408-412.

Stanley H.R., Laskin J., Broom C.A., "Moistness, more than temperature variation, prevents autolysis of pulp tissue in avulsed teeth." *J Endod.* 9(9) (1983): 360-367.

Tronstad L.; Trope M.; Bank M.; and Barnett F., "Surgical access for endodontic treatment of intruded teeth." *Endod Dent Traumatol.* 2 (1986): 75-78.

Zachrisson B.U., Jacobsen I., "Long-term prognosis of 66 permanent anterior teeth with root fracture." *Scand J Dent Res.* 83 (1975): 345-354.

Zadik D.; Fuks A.; Eidelman E.; and Chosak A., "Traumatized teeth: two-year results." *J Pedodont.* 4(1) (1979): 116-123.

Zadik D., Chosack A., Eidleman E., "The prognosis of traumatized permanent anterior teeth with fracture of the enamel and dentin." *Oral Surg.* 47(2): 173-175.

Zanetta-Barbosa D., Carvalho A.C.P., "Effect of brief storage in ATP solution on periodontal healing after replantation of teeth in rats." *Endod Dent Traumatol.* 6 (1990): 193-199.

Wei H.Y., *Pediatric dentistry: total patient care.* Philadelphia: Lea and Febiger, 1988.

8 Facial Fractures

B. D. Tiner, D.D.S., M.D.

INTRODUCTION

The management and treatment of maxillofacial injuries requires a thorough knowledge of anatomy, physiology and biomechanics. Additionally, since fractures of the facial skeleton are diagnosed primarily by clinical and radiographic findings, the clinician should possess the diagnostic skills to properly evaluate maxillofacial trauma patients. Patients suffering facial fractures frequently have injuries to other areas of the body and a complete evaluation of the entire patient is always indicated prior to definitive treatment of any maxillofacial injury.

The goal in the management of facial fractures is to return the patient, as close as possible, to his pre-injury level of function and appearance. This is achieved by applying the basic principles of bony fragment reduction and immobilization to allow healing of the fracture to occur.

I. INITIAL MANAGEMENT AND EVALUATION

Fractures of the facial skeleton arc commonly accompanied by a variety of other bodily injuries which can be life-threatening. As such, these injuries often require immediate attention. The initial assessment of the maxillofacial trauma patient should follow the ABC's of trauma management: Airway, Breathing and Circulation.

The presence of an adequate airway may be quickly assessed by observing and listening for signs of air exchange. Cyanosis, wheezing, snoring and the use of accessory muscles are suggestive of ventilatory difficulty. When obstruction of the airway is noted, the oral cavity should be checked for any potential obstruction that can be immediately removed or suctioned from the oro-pharynx such as dentures, avulsed teeth, foreign debris, vomitus or blood. Displaced, bilateral fractures of the mandibular condyles or parasymphysis can result in hypopharyngeal airway obstruction secondary to retrodisplacement of the tongue and mandible. Simple jaw thrust, chin lift maneuvers or stabilization of the anterior mandible will usually open the airway.

All maxillofacial trauma patients are assumed to have a cervical spine fracture until proven otherwise. Hence, any unnecessary movement of the neck to improve an airway should be avoided until a clinical and radiographic examination of the cervical spine is accomplished. Additional measures that may aid in establishing an airway are the placement of a soft nasopharyngeal airway in conscious patients or an oropharyngeal airway in unconscious patients. Should these measures fail to provide an adequate airway, endotracheal intubation is usually indicated. Emergency tracheostomy outside of the operating room is almost never indicated in the acute management of trauma patients due to the technical difficulties and the high probability of patient morbidity and mortality.

Once an adequate airway is secured, the patient's ventilatory effort should be assessed. Visual inspection of the chest for symmetrical expansion and auscultation of the chest bilaterally for breath sound equality are important respiratory evaluations. Potential problems from chest wall trauma include flail chest, tension pneumothorax, hemothorax and pericardial tamponade.

Paradoxical chest wall motion with breathing and crepitus upon chest palpation are suggestive of a flail chest. Injury to the underlying lung, usually from multiple rib fractures, frequently results in hypoxia. Treatment of flail chest includes judicious intravenous fluid management, adequate oxygenation and ventilation, and lung re-expansion when necessary.

A tension pneumothorax occurs when air enters the pleural space and accumulates through a flap-valve type mechanism. This allows air to enter, but not leave, and both the pleural space and the lung become compressed. Unilateral absence or a decrease in breath sounds, hyperresonance of the chest, distended neck veins, tracheal deviation to the opposite side and cyanosis are all classic signs of a tension pneumothorax. Treatment consists of placing a 12 to 16 gauge needle into the second intercostal space in the midclavicular line to decompress the affected hemithorax. This converts the tension pneumothorax to a pneumothorax. A large thoracotomy tube is then placed at the fifth or sixth intercostal space in the midaxillary line to evacuate the pleural space.

In a hemothorax, the lung collapses and blood, along with air, accumulates in the pleural cavity. Hemothorax is treated by placing a large thoracotomy tube to decompress the chest and by restoring and maintaining intravascular volume with intravenous fluids. A thoracotomy is frequently necessary to identify and repair the source of bleeding.

Pericardial tamponade occurs when blood fills the pericardium, which limits cardiac contractility and, thereby, impairs cardiac output. Classic signs of pericardial tamponade are distended neck veins, muffled heart sounds, hypotension and a narrowed pulse pressure. The recommended treatment is the evacuation of blood from the pericardial sac with a 16 to 18 gauge over-the-needle catheter, termed pericardiocentesis. All of the aforementioned injuries are considered life-threatening and can severely impede the exchange of oxygen. As such, all trauma patients are candidates for supplemental oxygen therapy to improve tissue oxygenation.

The third component of trauma management is an intact circulation. The hemodynamic stability of the patient can be evaluated by assessing the level of consciousness, observing the skin color, palpating the pulse and determining the blood pressure. Hypotension, pallor, a rapid thready pulse and a decreased level of consciousness are signs of circulatory volume depletion. The presence of a pulse at various bodily sites can provide a rough estimate of the blood pressure. For example, a systolic pressure of at least 80 mm Hg is necessary for a radial pulse to be palpable, a systolic pressure of 70 mm Hg is required for femoral pulse palpability, and a systolic pressure of at least 60 mm Hg is needed to palpate a carotid pulse. Any exsanguinating hemorrhage sites should be identified and immediately controlled once the airway is secure. Direct digital pressure or pressure packs are the best methods for halting rapid blood loss. Pneumatic splints can also be helpful in controlling extremity or intra-abdominal bleeding. The use of tourniquets and hemostats are not advised in the uncontrolled emergency room setting. Intravenous fluid therapy should be instituted as soon as possible after the initial ABC assessments.

All trauma patients should have at least two large gauge (16 or larger) peripheral intravenous catheters inserted and volume replacement initiated with a balanced salt solution. The fluid of choice for initial volume replacement should be close to the composition of extra-cellular fluid, containing physiologic quantities of sodium, potassium, and chloride (i.e., Lactated Ringer's). An initial fluid challenge of 1 to 2 liters is given as rapidly as possible for adult patients, while a bolus of 20 cc/kg is recommended in pediatric patients.

II. HISTORY AND PHYSICAL EXAMINATION

After the initial ABC's of trauma management have been addressed, a complete history and physical examination is performed looking for additional injuries that were not identified in the initial survey. If possible, a detailed history should be obtained from the patient concerning how, when and where the injury occurred. Additional details about the mechanism of injury and whether loss of consciousness occurred are also important determinants. In many cases, secondary to either a loss of consciousness or a decreased level of consciousness, information should be obtained from witnesses, family members or emergency medical technicians. Finally, a complete past medical history including allergies, medications and tetanus immunizations is obtained.

The physical examination is performed in a systematic fashion using a head-to-toe approach. Studies have shown that over 70% of patients involved in motor vehicle accidents suffer a head injury. In examining the head, great care must be exercised until a cervical spine injury is ruled out. In cases of known cervical spine injuries, the neck is immobilized. The scalp, skull and face are inspected and palpated for lacerations, contusions, abrasions and contour deformities. An otoscopic examination of the ears is performed looking for either the presence of blood or cerebrospinal fluid in the external auditory canal, or blood behind the tympanic membrane (hemotympanum), all of which are suggestive of a basilar skull fracture. Ecchymotic areas behind the ear overlying the mastoid (Battle's sign) are also suggestive of a basilar skull fracture. The eyes are examined for the presence of blood in the anterior chamber (hyphema), lens dislocation and for gross visual acuity. Extraocular movements, pupil size, and the pupil's reactions to light and accomodation are also noted. A fundoscopic examination is needed to assess possible damage to the retina, macula and optic disc. A brief neurologic exam should be performed to evaluate the function of cranial nerves II-XII. Cranial nerves II, III, IV and VI can be assessed simultaneously during the eye examination (visual acuity, extra-ocular movements and pupillary reaction to light). Cranial nerve V function can be evaluated by assessing sensation to the skin of the face (sensory) and the muscles of mastication (motor). The function of cranial nerve VII can be evaluated by testing the muscles of facial expression. A finger snap or a ticking watch held near each ear is a quick way to assess cranial nerve VIII function. Cranial nerves IX and X can be assessed simultaneously by checking for a gag reflex and soft palate motion. Shrugging the shoulders against resistance is indicative of cranial nerve XI function. The function of cranial nerve XII can be assessed by tongue movement. Any noted deficits of cranial nerve function should be recorded.

The examination of the chest begins with inspection for obvious injuries such as rib fractures, paradoxical chest wall motion (flail chest), lacerations and puncture wounds. Identification and quick intervention are critical, since approximately 25% of all trauma deaths are secondary to injuries of the thorax. Auscultation of the lung fields to check for equal and bilateral breath sounds is important. The heart is auscultated for murmurs, friction rubs and other abnormal sounds. Bowel sounds heard upon auscultation of the chest may be indicative of a traumatic diaphragmatic hernia. The examination of the back and thoracic spine complete this portion of the physical examination.

Examination of the abdomen requires a high index of suspicion to identify abdominal injuries. The abdomen should first be inspected for distension, ecchymosis, lacerations or evidence of penetrating trauma. All four quadrants of the abdomen are then auscultated for the presence or absence of bowel sounds. The absence of bowel sounds is indicative of an ileus that is frequently secondary to peritoneal irritation. Tenderness and guarding with palpation and percussion of the abdomen suggest an injured viscus. When either a high suspicion of abdominal injury exists following completion of the physical examination or unexplained hypotension is present, then a diagnostic peritoneal lavage (DPL) is indicated. To accomplish this, a small catheter is inserted into the peritoneal cavity through a small incision just inferior to the umbilicus. Approximately 1000 cc of Ringer's lactate is introduced and then withdrawn. The DPL is considered positive if laboratory analysis of the lavage fluid shows greater than 100,000 RBC's per cubic mm, 500 WBC's per cubic mm, an amylase greater than 400 units or the presence of bile or feces.

Examination of the extremities begins with inspection for contusions, lacerations and obvious fractures, remembering that femoral, pelvic and humerus fractures can be a source of significant blood loss. Additionally, the assessment of the neurologic and vascular status of the extremities in trauma patients is critical. An absent peripheral pulse suggests vascular compromise, which requires further evaluation and intervention to prevent significant morbidity. As in the head and neck examination, the motor and sensory neurologic function of the extremities should be assessed and any deficits recorded.

The physical examination is completed with a thorough neurologic examination. Any lateralizing signs, such as the weakness or paralysis of an extremity, or the presence of abnormal reflexes should be noted. The patient's level of consciousness and pupillary response to light are re-evaluated and any change from the initial assessment recorded. Patients who have suffered head and facial trauma should be examined for cerebrospinal fluid leaks. CSF rhinorrhea or CSF otorrhea are frequently seen with LeFort fractures or basilar skull fractures. The double-ring test is a quick method used to detect cerebrospinal fluid. A drop of unclotted blood is placed on a piece of filter paper or linen and observed for separation into a central area of blood and a clear peripheral ring. The clear halo is characteristic of cerebrospinal fluid. A glucose level can also be obtained on the CSF. Normally this level is 20 mg less than the blood glucose level. The glucose level should be determined within two hours of the injury to avoid misleadingly low levels caused by glycolysis.

Definitive care of facial fractures should be delayed in most cases until all of the appropriate consultations with surgical subspecialties have been obtained and any indicated special studies such as CT scans, MRI's or angiograms have been completed. The use of analgesics preoperatively should be limited, if possible, to non-narcotic analgesics.

Narcotic analgesics administered to acutely injured patients will sedate and obtund these patients and make an accurate neurologic assessment difficult, if not impossible. Appropriate antibiotic therapy should be initiated in the emergency room, especially if open fractures are present. Soft tissue lacerations and abrasions should be cleaned and dressed with antibiotic ointment until definitive care is obtained. Finally, a coordinated treatment plan is formulated and appropriate referrals are made based on the injuries present.

III. RADIOGRAPHIC EVALUATION

Once the physical examination is completed, a radiographic survey is performed to provide additional diagnostic information. The extent of the radiographic examination depends on the clinical findings and the suspicion of an underlying injury. In facial trauma patients, radiographs can confirm the clinical diagnosis, provide additional information and more accurately define the extent of the injuries incurred. The radiographic examination may include a CT of the head and facial bones or plain films of the skull, facial bones, cervical spine, chest, abdomen (KUB) and extremities. An intravenous pyelogram (IVP) may also be indicated when hematuria is present or bladder or kidney injuries are suspected. In all cases, it is important to obtain a sufficient number of radiographic views to adequately assess all areas involved. In addition, the importance of high quality radiographs cannot be overemphasized from a medicolegal standpoint. Specific recommendations for radiographs, based on fracture type, are included within the following discussions.

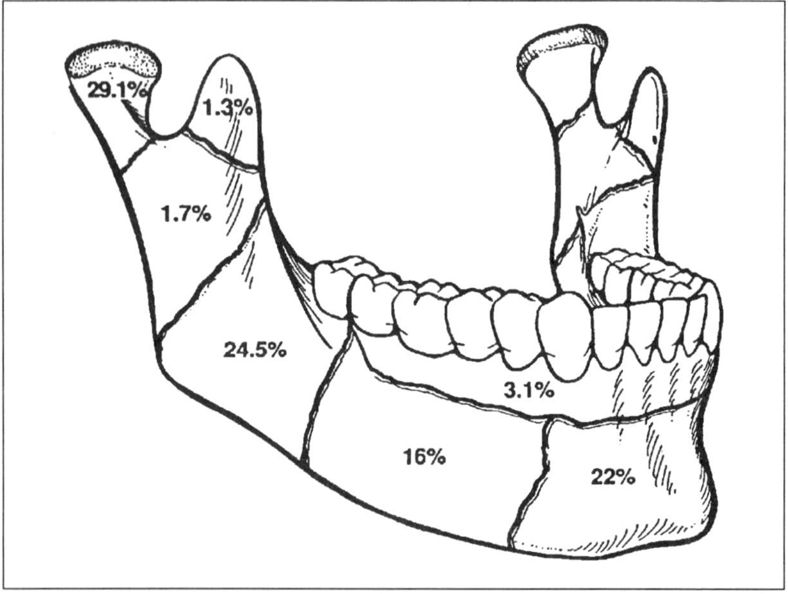

Figure 8-1: Diagram of anatomic distribution of mandibular fractures. From Olson RA, et al., *J Oral Maxillofac Surg.* 40 (1982): 23.

IV. MANDIBULAR FRACTURES

Fractures of the mandible are common facial injuries occurring twice as frequently as midfacial fractures and account for approximately two-thirds of all facial fractures. The nasal bones are the only bones of the facial skeleton that are fractured more frequently.

The major causes of mandibular fractures are motor vehicle accidents and interpersonal altercations. Other causes include falls, sports trauma, work-related accidents, gunshot wounds, third molar surgery and central pathologic lesions of the mandible. The majority of mandible fractures occur in young males with a peak incidence between the ages of 20 and 29 years.

A. Classification

Mandibular fractures may be classified according to the location, the severity and the direction of the fracture with the probability for secondary displacement. Fracture descriptions based on anatomic location are arbitrarily divided into seven categories (Figure 8-1). ***Condylar*** process fractures include all fractures of the condyle and condylar neck above the level of the sigmoid (mandibular notch). A ***coronoid*** process fracture runs from the sigmoid notch to the anterior border of the ramus. ***Ramus*** fractures occur between the angle of the mandible and the sigmoid notch. An ***angle*** fracture extends from the region of the mandibular second or third molar to the inferior border of the mandible in the region of the angle formed by the junction of the body and the posterior border of the ramus. ***Body*** fractures occur between the canine teeth and the angle of the mandible. Fractures of the ***symphysis*** are confined to the area between the mandibular canines. Finally, fractures of the ***alveolar process*** involve the bony structures above the level of the mental foramen, and are usually more limited or segmental in nature.

When fractures are classified according to severity, determinants include the condition of the bony fragments at the fracture site and whether there is communication with the skin or oral cavity. ***Greenstick*** fractures are incomplete where one side of the cortex is broken and the other side is bent, resembling a partially broken green stick. A ***simple*** fracture is complete through both cortical plates and can damage overlying soft tissues, but there is no communication between the fracture and the skin or oral cavity. Unlike simple fractures, ***compound*** fractures have a break in the overlying skin or mucosa providing direct communication of the bony fragments with the external environment. All mandibular fractures that occur through an alveolus of a tooth are considered compound. ***Comminuted*** fractures result when the bone is splintered, crushed or left in

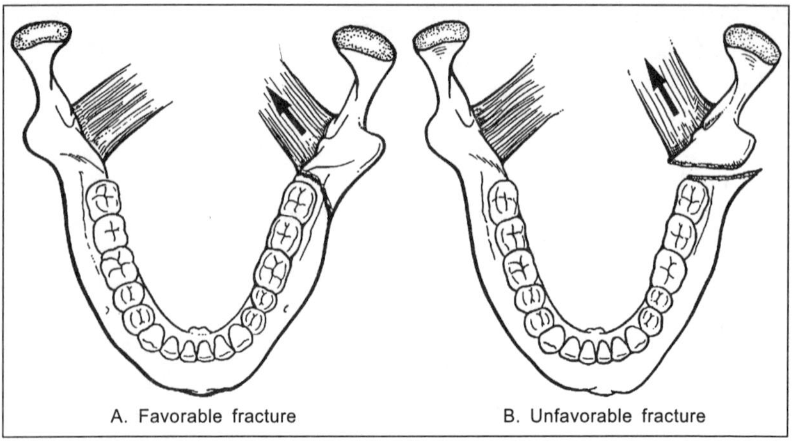

Figure 8-2: Vertical Favorable and Unfavorable Mandibular Fractures.

multiple segments from high impact injuries such as gun shot wounds. These fractures may be simple or compound.

Mandibular fractures are also classified as favorable or unfavorable depending on the direction of fracture and the probability of secondary displacement from muscle pull proximal and distal to the fracture (Figure 8-2). A fracture is considered ***favorable*** if the angulation of the fracture and the muscle pull tend to resist further displacement of the fracture. In contrast, the angulation of the fracture and the muscle pull result in the secondary displacement of the fractured segments with ***unfavorable*** fractures (Figure 8-3). These three classification schemes are useful in planning the definitive treatment of mandibular fractures.

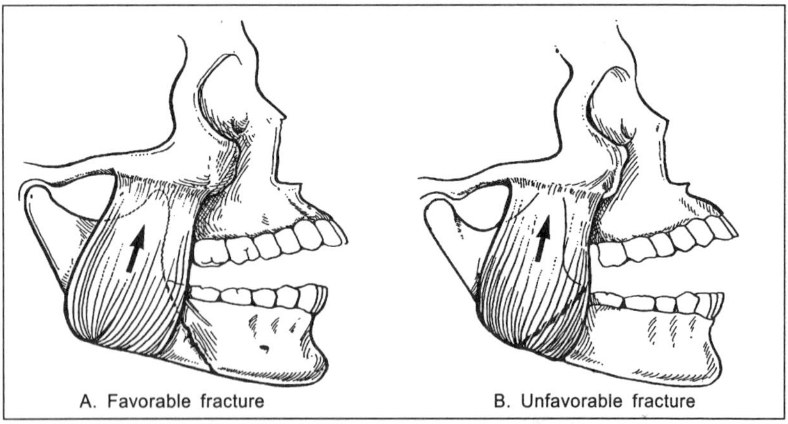

Figure 8-3: Horizontal Favorable and Unfavorable Mandibular Fractures.

B. Diagnosis

The clinical findings in fractures of the mandible can vary considerably depending on anatomic location and severity. The physical examination begins with an extraoral and intraoral inspection for contour deformities (asymmetries), swelling, ecchymosis (especially in the floor of the mouth), hematomas, lacerations, mucosal tears, excessive salivation and malocclusion.

A systematic bimanual palpation of the mandible follows, beginning in the area of the condyle and progressing inferiorly over the mandible. This is accomplished in a bilateral fashion moving from extraoral to intraoral while searching for a break or step defect in the cortex, crepitus or segmental mobility. Point tenderness over the fracture site will aid in localization of the fracture, and any pain from speaking, swallowing or opening and closing the mouth should be noted. Crepitus may also be elicited as the

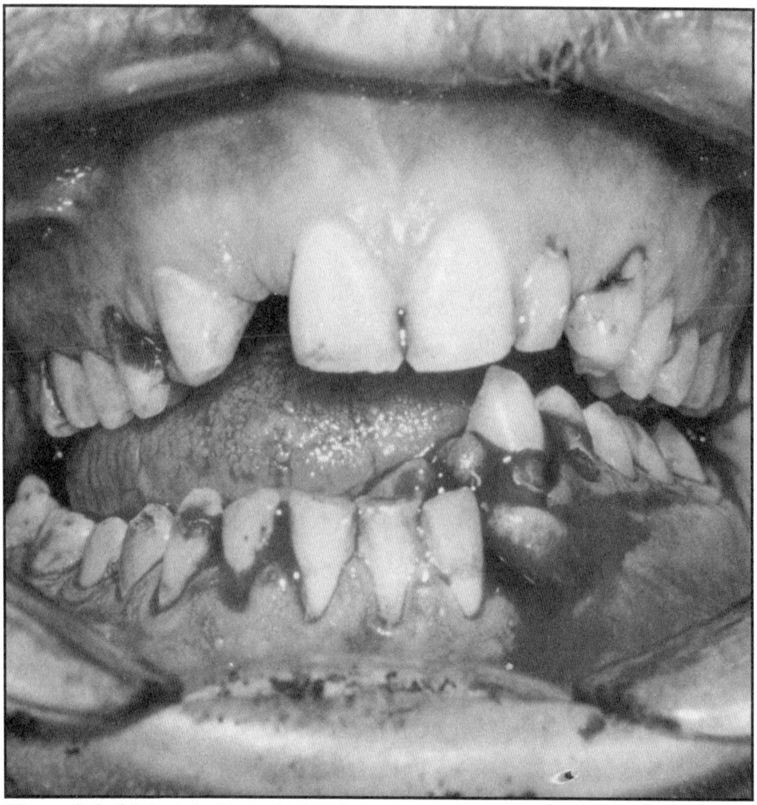

Figure 8-4: Clinical photograph showing gross malocclusion in a left mandibular parasymphysis fracture.

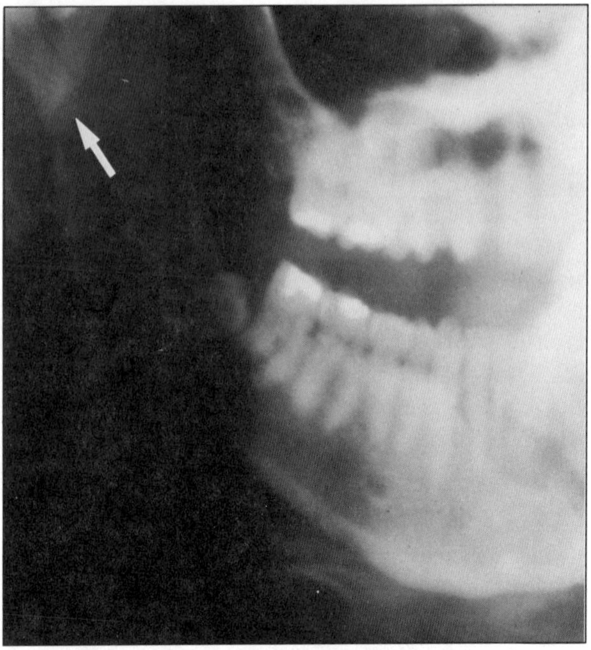

Figure 8-5a: Panoramic view demonstrating fractures of mandibular condyle and parasymphysis.

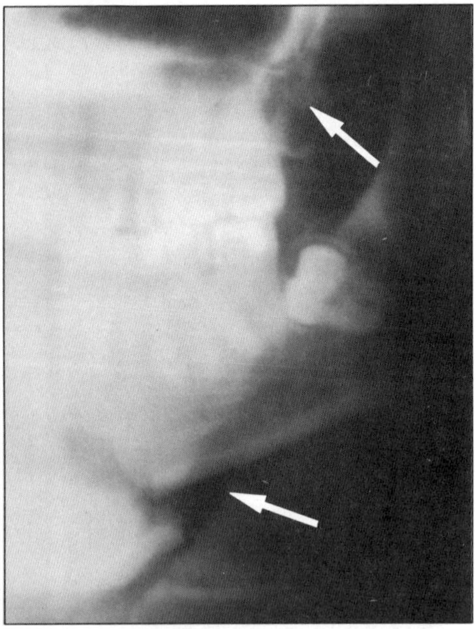

Figure 8-5b: Same as above.

bony fragments move against each other during palpation or attempted movement of the mandible. Abnormal mobility of the mandible, such as deviation, is a frequent finding in unilateral fractures. Deviation is ipsilateral with attempted opening or protrusion of the mandible because of lateral pterygoid muscle dysfunction on the side of injury. However, the most reliable finding in the diagnosis of mandibular fractures in dentate patients is the presence of a malocclusion. Even a minimally displaced fracture will cause patients to complain of an altered bite. When a malocclusion is present, the wear facets on the teeth should be evaluated to assess the patient's occlusion prior to injury. Typical malocclusions include a contralateral open bite with a unilateral subcondylar fracture and an anterior open bite with bilateral subcondylar fractures. Abrupt changes in the occlusal plane are characteristic of body and parasymphyseal fractures and should also be recorded (Figure 8-4).

Fractures of the mandibular angle and body frequently result in damage to the inferior alveolar nerve. When this occurs, patients may complain of unilateral dysesthesia or anesthesia of the lower lip, chin and mandibular teeth. Any sensory deficits should be noted and recorded prior to definitive treatment of the fracture.

The radiographic survey for suspected mandibular fractures can include a variety of views. A ***panoramic*** view can be used as an initial screening film and is probably the best view for overall diagnosis (Figure 8-5a, b). The ***lateral oblique*** view is good for visualizing the mandible from the first bicuspid area to the condyle region, while the ***postero-anterior*** (PA) views of the mandible are utilized for general appraisal for all areas except the condylar region. The condylar head and neck are best visualized with a ***Towne's*** or ***reverse Towne's*** view. This view eliminates the superimposition of the mastoid and zygoma over the condylar neck region. Basilar and occipital skull fractures, as well as nasal septal fractures, may be revealed by the Towne's projection. ***Occlusal*** views are the most reliable diagnostic films when fractures of the symphysis are suspected, and ***periapical*** films are useful for assessing the roots of teeth and alveolar fractures. To diagnose fractures from the radiographs, practitioners should scrutinize the cortical outline of the mandible looking for fracture lines and irregular contours.

C. Treatment

Early reduction and immobilization of mandibular fractures should be accomplished as soon as the patient's overall medical condition permits definitive treatment. When quick definitive treatment is not possible, temporary stabilization is indicated to increase the patient's comfort level.

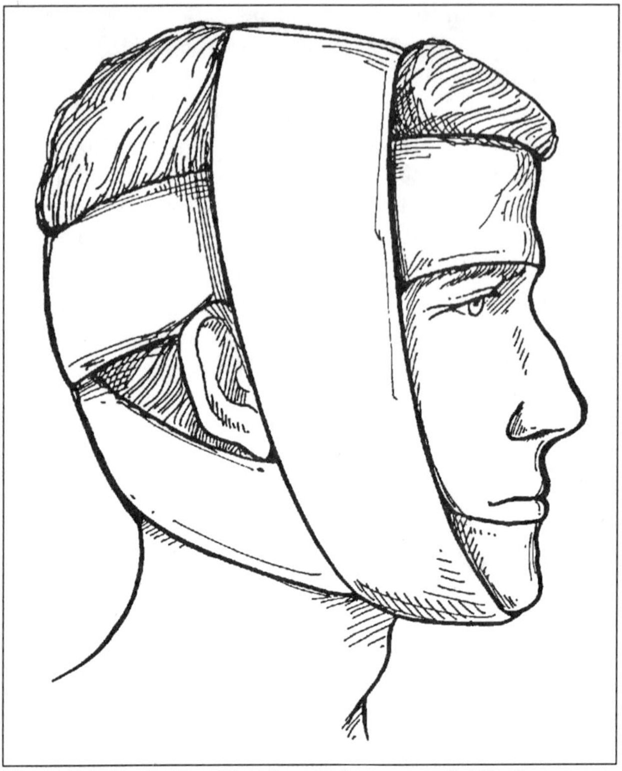

Figure 8-6: Barton head bandage for temporary stabilization of mandible fractures.

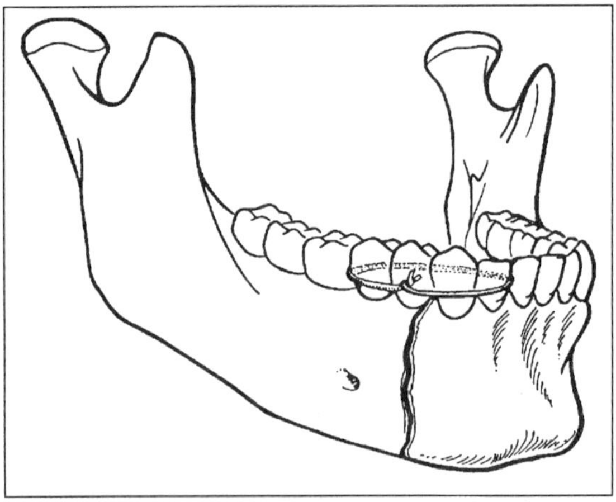

Figure 8-7: Bridal wire for temporary stabilization of mandibular fractures.

This can be achieved with a Barton head bandage (Figure 8-6), intraorally with the application of an arch bar or bridal wire (Figure 8-7) in dentate patients, or the circummandibular wiring of a denture in edentulous patients. The treatment alternatives for the definitive management of mandibular fractures are numerous. However, the common treatment objectives are the realignment of the bony fragments into an acceptable anatomic relationship and the maintenance of this position until bony healing occurs.

Teeth in the line of fracture that may aid in stabilization of the bony fragments should generally be retained. However, in the judgement of the clinician, teeth that are likely to cause complications in the postoperative period should be removed. Mobile teeth or teeth attached to a small segment of fractured alveolar bone should be adequately stabilized by wiring them to adjacent teeth or the arch bar.

Placement of the maxillary and mandibular teeth into the preinjury occlusal relationship is critical prior to attempting any type of fracture

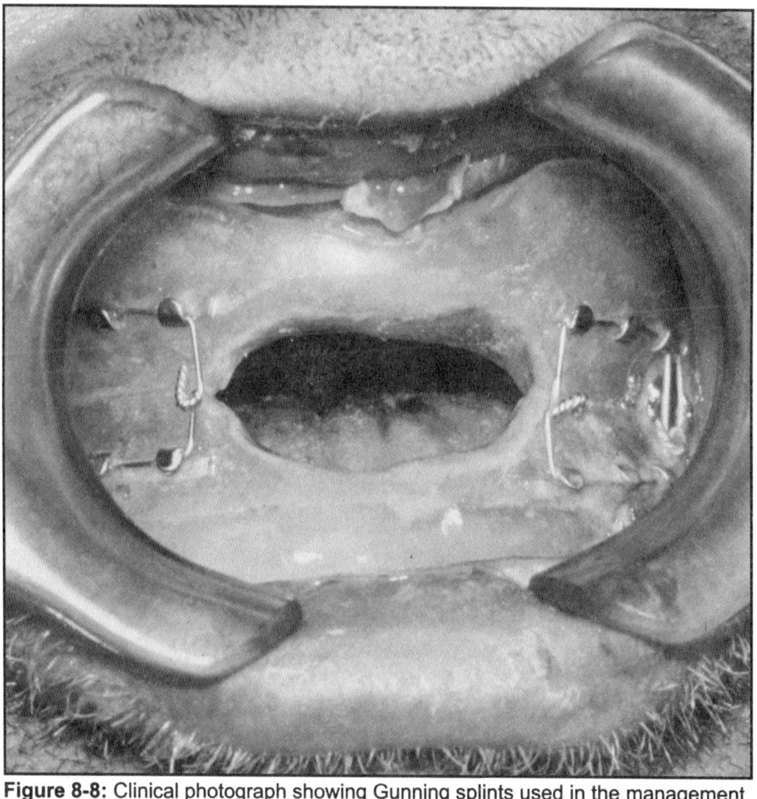

Figure 8-8: Clinical photograph showing Gunning splints used in the management of edentulous mandibular fractures.

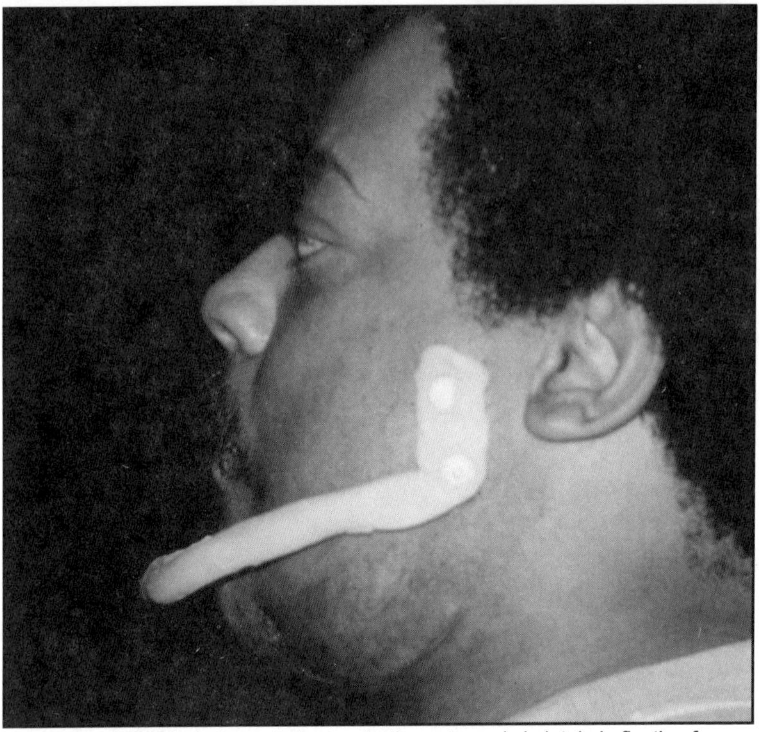

Figure 8-9: Clinical photograph demonstrating extraoral skeletal pin fixation for management of a mandibular fracture.

reduction. This is most commonly achieved with the ligation of Erich arch bars to the maxillary and mandibular teeth, followed by wiring of the arch bars together. Wiring of the teeth together into a normal occlusal relationship is known as maxillomandibular fixation (MMF) or intermaxillary fixation (IMF). Mandibular fractures treated solely with the application of arch bars and MMF (equivalent to a cast in extremity fractures) are termed ***closed reductions***. By definition, fractures reduced by a closed method do not require direct visualization of the fracture site.

In edentulous patients, the closed reduction of a mandibular fracture can be accomplished using the patient's existing dentures or by fabricating Gunning splints (Figure 8-8). In either case, the mandibular prosthesis is secured to the mandible with circummandibular wiring. The maxillary prosthesis is secured to the maxilla with threaded K-wires, bone screws or circumzygomatic suspension wires. Maxillomandibular fixation is then achieved by wiring the prostheses together.

In severely comminuted mandibular fractures and certain edentulous fractures, extraoral skeletal pin fixation (Joe Hall Morris appliance) is quite useful. This method involves the placement of two large bone-embedded screws on each side of the fracture. While the fracture is held in a reduced position, a cold cure acrylic bar is fabricated to connect the screws and permit stabilization of the fracture (Figure 8-9). This appliance has the advantage of stabilizing a comminuted fracture without surgically disrupting the multiple small fragments.

In pediatric patients with mandible fractures, an occlusal or lingual splint is desirable, considering the problems associated with maxillomandibular fixation in children (Figure 8-10). Placing arch bars on deciduous teeth is complicated by the ongoing processes of resorption and exfoliation.

Considerations for the ***open reduction*** of a mandible fracture include the location of the fracture, the degree of displacement and mobility, the presence of associated midface fractures and the probability of segment displacement secondary to muscle pull. By definition, an ***open reduction*** involves direct exposure and visualization of the fracture site through a surgical incision or pre-existing laceration. An open reduction is indicated in unfavorable fractures occurring posterior to the last natural tooth where a muscle pull can cause displacement of the proximal segment. Mandible fractures that accompany midface fractures should also be considered for open reduction so that a stable occlusion can be established and maintained while treating the midface fractures.

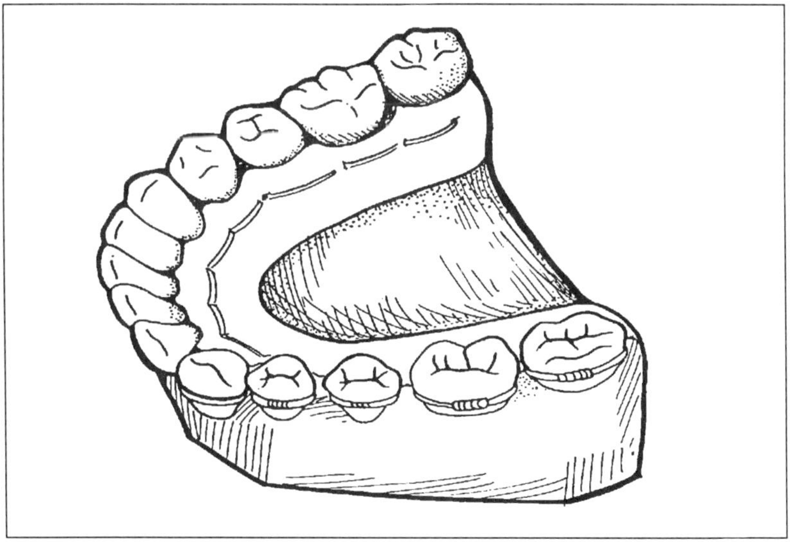

Figure 8-10: Mandibular lingual splint fixated to the teeth with ligature wires. In deep bite occlusions, the lingual splint may be the only treatment option available.

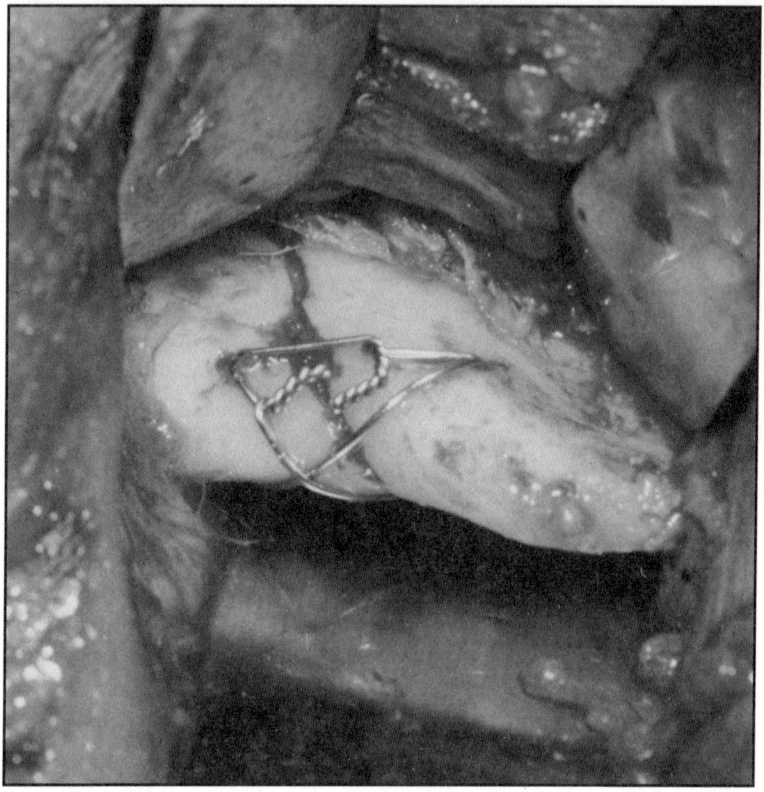

Figure 8-11: Clinical photograph showing open reduction and internal wire fixation of mandibular body fracture.

While the majority of condyle fractures can be treated by closed reduction, there are instances when open reduction is preferred. Absolute indications for open reduction include displacement of the condyle into the middle cranial fossa, invasion by a foreign body (i.e., gunshot wound), lateral extracapsular displacement of the condyle and the inability to obtain an adequate occlusion by a closed reduction. In selected cases, open reduction is also indicated in edentulous patients with bilateral condylar fractures and in bilateral condylar fractures associated with comminuted midface fractures.

When performing an open reduction, a closed reduction with arch bars and maxillomandibular fixation is first needed to place the mandible into a normal occlusal relationship with the maxilla. Direct surgical access to the fracture site is then accomplished either through an intraoral or extraoral incision or through an existing laceration. Most symphysis and parasymphysis fractures can be approached via an intraoral degloving incision. An extraoral approach is the most versatile for fractures of the body and angle, and allows for fixation of the segments with transosseous wires, bone plates, bone screws or mesh at the inferior mandibular border.

Internal fixation of fractures has been accomplished for decades using interosseous wires (Figure 8-11). However, during the last decade, rigid fixation with bone plates and/or bone screws has gained widespread popularity and has become the treatment of choice for many clinicians in the management of facial fractures (Figure 8-12). The use of rigid fixation eliminates or greatly reduces the need for postoperative maxillomandibular fixation and enhances postoperative nutrition, oral hygiene, speech and overall patient management.

There are a variety of frequently occurring complications associated with the treatment of mandibular fractures including osteomyelitis, wound infections, malocclusion, nerve injuries, nonunion or malunion, loss or damage to teeth, ankylosis, trismus and hypertrophic scarring. The informed consent prior to surgical management of mandibular fractures should include a frank and detailed discussion of these potential complications.

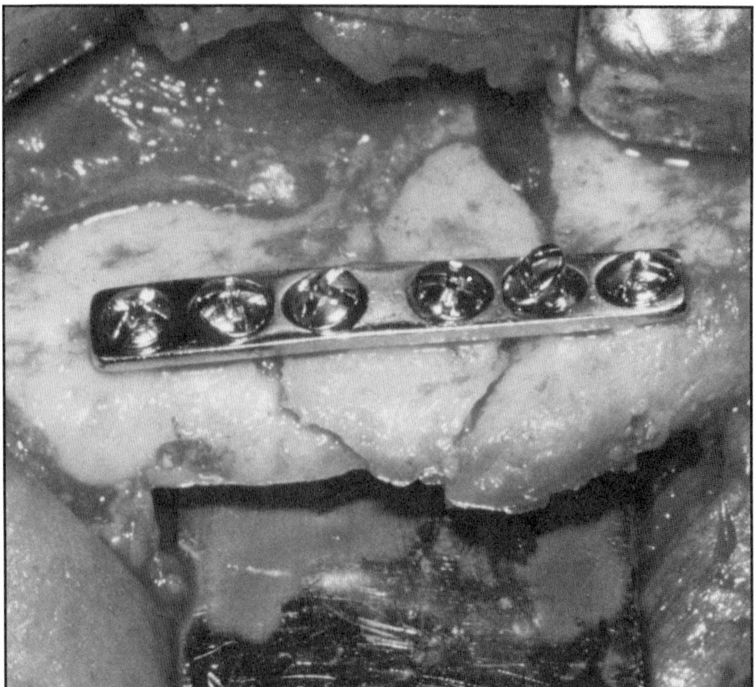

Figure 8-12: Rigid internal fixation of a comminuted mandibular fracture.

V. MAXILLARY FRACTURES

Fractures of the maxilla are less common than mandibular fractures, occurring in a ratio of approximately 1 to 4. Depending on the study cited, motor vehicle accidents account for 50 to 70 % of maxillary fractures. The greatest incidence of maxillary fractures occurs in the 20 to 30 year age group, with men outnumbering women 3 to 1. In 1901, Rene LeFort of Paris determined the areas of structural weakness in the maxilla by experimentally producing maxillary fractures in a series of 35 cadavers. From these findings, LeFort published a classification of maxillary fractures that still bears his name today (Figure 8-13).

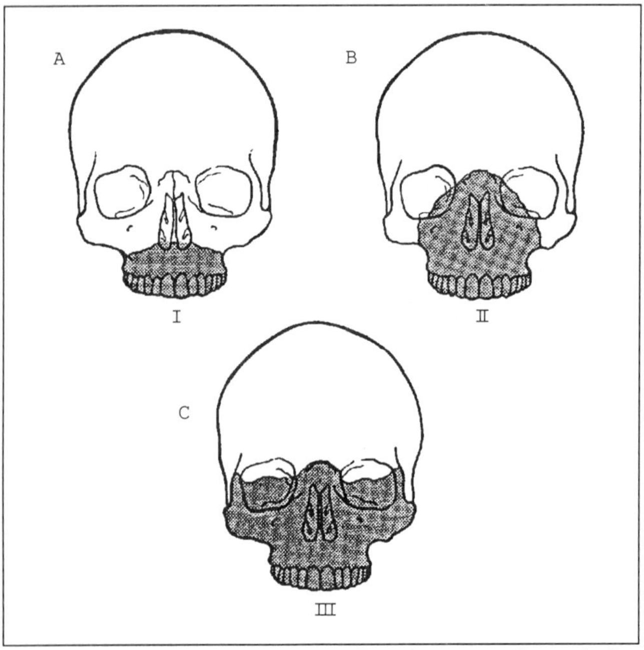

Figure 8-13: Maxillary fractures. A. LeFort I (transverse fracture). B. LeFort II (pyramidal fracture). C. LeFort III (craniofacial separation).

A. Classification

The most common type of maxillary fracture is the ***LeFort I*** fracture, which occurs above the level of the apices of the teeth and runs transversely through the maxilla. The fracture involves the alveolar process, the walls of the maxillary sinuses, the palate and the pterygoid processes. The ***LeFort II (pyramidal)*** fracture physically resembles a pyramid in its general outline. The fracture begins in the nasal bones and frontal processes of the maxilla and passes laterally and inferiorly through the lacrimal bones, the inferior orbital rims and the orbital floors near the zygomaticomaxillary suture. The fracture then continues posteriorly along the lateral wall of the maxilla, through the pterygoid plates into the pterygomaxillary fossa. A ***LeFort III*** (***craniofacial disjunction***) fracture occurs when sufficient horizontal forces are applied to the midface to cause complete separation of the facial bones from the cranial base. The fracture occurs through the zygomaticofrontal, frontomaxillary, nasofrontal sutures, the orbital floors, and the ethmoid and sphenoid sinuses. In the nose, the cribriform plate is frequently comminuted, resulting in dural tears and cerebrospinal fluid leaks from the nose (CSF rhinorrhea).

In many cases, patients suffer combinations of maxillary fractures in a unilateral or bilateral fashion. Maxillary fractures can be further complicated by a sagittal fracture of the maxilla and hard palate (midpalatal suture), resulting in sagittal separation of the maxilla into two halves. The clinical findings in maxillary fractures can vary considerably depending on the type, intensity, and direction of the trauma. High speed motor vehicle accidents tend to produce more severe displacement and comminution of the facial bones. Less traumatic forces, such as fists or minor falls, produce fractures with less fragmentation and displacement. Unlike mandibular fractures, muscle pull plays only a minor role in the displacement of maxillary fractures. Fractures extending into the pterygoid plates allow the pterygoid muscles to displace the fractured maxilla inferiorly and posteriorly, producing the classic open bite with dish face elongation of the midface.

B. Diagnosis

The clinical examination should follow a systematic approach beginning with inspection for hematomas, edema, ecchymosis, contour deformities (asymmetries) and bleeding from the nose or conjunctiva. All of these findings are suggestive of maxillary fractures. Intraorally, tears in the palatal mucosa or palatal ecchymosis are suggestive of a sagittal fracture of the hard palate and maxilla. Horizontal maxillary fractures with downward and posterior displacement of the proximal segment will produce a malocclusion (anterior open bite) secondary to premature contact of the posterior teeth. Impacted fractures of the maxilla also produce a malocclusion. Bilateral bimanual palpation of the orbital rims, nasal bones, zygomatic arches, zygomas and the intraoral prominences of the maxilla is performed to identify the type and extent of the maxillary fracture.

Crepitus, segment mobility and steplike defects on palpation are suggestive of underlying fractures.

To determine the level of the maxillary fracture, the anterior portion of the maxilla is grasped with the thumb and forefinger of one hand while the opposite hand palpates the facial skeleton. LeFort I fractures will reveal movement of the palate and alveolar process of the maxilla. If a sagittal fracture of the palate is also present, the two halves of the maxilla may move independently on palpation. Patients with LeFort II fractures will demonstrate movement at the nasofrontal junction and the medial portion of the inferior orbital rims with manipulation of the anterior maxilla. Manipulation of a LeFort III fracture will reveal movement of the entire midface, demonstrating separation and movement at the nasofrontal and frontozygomatic sutures, as well as the zygomatic arches.

The radiographic examination of patients with suspected maxillary fractures is obtained to confirm the findings of the clinical examination. The ***Waters'*** or ***stereo Waters'*** view provides the most diagnostic information with the least amount of superimposition of structures for assessing maxillary fractures. This view shows the nasal septum, the lateral nasal walls, the lateral walls of the maxillary sinus, the orbital rims, the maxillary sinuses, as well as the nasofrontal, frontozygomatic and frontomaxillary suture lines with minimal superimposition and distortion. The Waters' view is the best single view for confirming fractures of the maxilla, the maxillary sinus, the orbital floors, the inferior orbital rims, the zygomas and the zygomatic arches. ***Maxillary occlusal*** films (superior-inferior or superior-inferior oblique projections) are useful for evaluating suspected sagittal fractures of the maxilla and hard palate. Other useful plain films include the ***posteroanterior*** (PA) view of the maxilla, the ***lateral nasal*** projection, and the ***lateral skull*** projection. The PA view shows the lateral walls of the maxillary sinuses and may demonstrate displacement of nasal septum fractures. Fractures of the nasal bones, the anterior nasal spine and the frontal processes of the maxilla can be demonstrated with a lateral nasal projection. The lateral skull view is excellent for showing anterior open bites that result from the downward and posterior displacement of horizontal maxillary fractures.

Computed tomography (CT) is also useful in assessing fractures of the maxilla, orbits, zygomas and nasal bones. Secondary to soft tissue edema and the superimposition of overlying structures, fractures of the midface are often difficult to evaluate with plain films. CT scans of the midface will delineate hard and soft tissues and avoid the problem of superimposition. CT is also helpful in evaluating the optic canal and in identifying soft tissue changes, especially in the retrobulbar and periorbital areas.

C. Treatment

The treatment goals for maxillary fractures are to return to pre-injury levels of masticatory function, re-establish the proper occlusion and restore appearance by correcting resultant facial deformities. The initial therapeutic step is to re-establish a normal occlusal relationship by placing the maxilla into proper occlusion with the mandible. Arch bars are ligated to the maxillary and mandibular teeth and the patient is placed in maxillomandibular fixation. This accurately establishes the position of the maxilla and is the key for reducing maxillary fractures. Any coexisting mandibular fractures should first be reduced and immobilized before treating a maxillary or midface fracture. In edentulous patients, existing dentures or fabricated surgical Gunning splints can be used to index the mandible to the maxilla and assist in re-establishing the occlusal vertical dimension.

Most LeFort fractures can be adequately treated by a closed reduction with arch bars and maxillomandibular fixation. However, should additional stabilization be required, suspension wiring to stable bones above the fracture site may be used. Possible locations for dropping suspension wires include stable zygomatic arches, infraorbital rims, zygomatic processes of the frontal bone and the pyriform rims. The suspension wires may be attached to the maxillary arch bar, an occlusal splint or to the mandible. These wires prevent inferior displacement of the maxilla caused by attempted opening of the mandible while in maxillomandibular fixation. Caution is advised when suspension wires are used to prevent shortening of the midface, occlusal canting and retrodisplacement of the maxilla. The suspension wires are usually removed 4 to 6 weeks after placement.

LeFort I fractures that remain unstable following a closed reduction may be treated by an open reduction through an intraoral approach. Direct interosseous wires or mini bone plates are used for fixation of the fracture after a satisfactory reduction has been accomplished. The wires and miniplates are usually placed on the pillars of the midface (zygomatic buttresses and pyriform rims) to take advantage of the thicker and stronger bone in these areas. Open reduction of unstable LeFort II and LeFort III fractures is performed by reduction and stabilization at the infraorbital rims, zygomaticofrontal suture regions, or both. The infraorbital rim is approached through a transconjunctival incision or a subciliary incision in a skin crease of the lower eyelid, 2 to 3 mm inferior to the lid margin. Access to the zygomaticofrontal area is obtained through a lateral brow incision or an upper eyelid blepharoplasty incision. Mini bone plates or direct interosseous wires are used to stabilize the fractures after adequate reduction has been obtained (Figure 8-14).

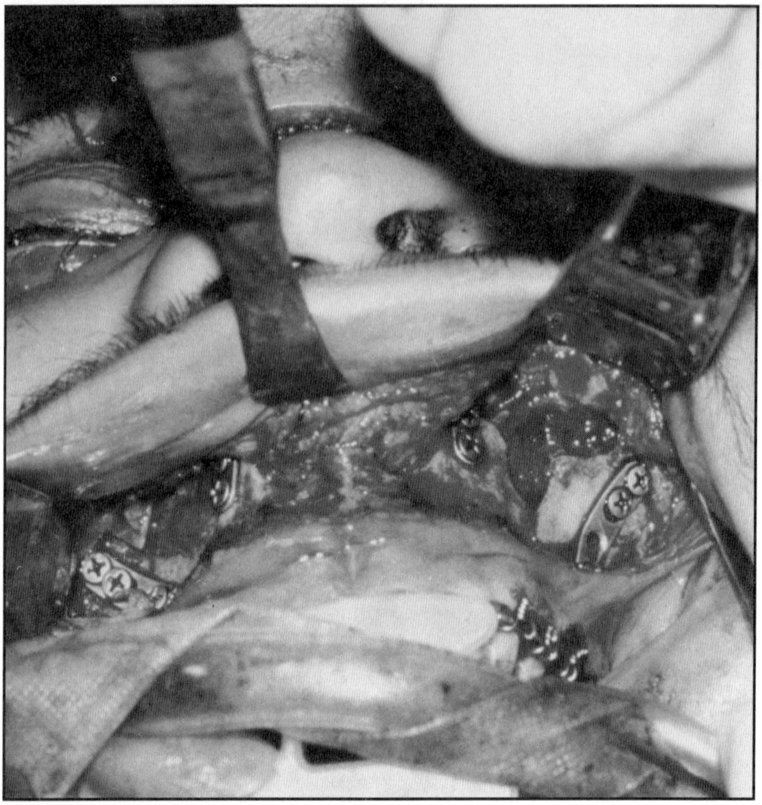

Figure 8-14: Rigid internal fixation of a LeFort I fracture. Bone plates placed at the zygomatic buttress and pyriform rim areas bilaterally.

The treatment of midface fractures with skeletal stabilization devices, such as head frames, has been limited by the widespread use of open reduction with mini bone plates. Indications include severely comminuted fractures that are not amenable to adequate reduction and stabilization by normal techniques, severely impacted or malunited fractures that require constant anterior traction for a satisfactory reduction, and LeFort fractures with maxillary continuity defects.

Complications related to the treatment of maxillary fractures include malunion, malocclusion, ectropion, vertical shortening of the face, dishface deformity and infection. Most of the significant complications of maxillary fracture treatment arise from either the failure to initially re-establish the pre-injury occlusion or from not recognizing the full extent of the injury and deformity.

VI. NASOORBITAL ETHMOID (NOE) COMPLEX FRACTURES

A. Classification

Fractures of the nasal skeleton, medial orbital walls, and interorbital area are difficult to manage and often result in significant functional and cosmetic problems. Hence, a team approach and appropriate consultation are required to successfully manage these injuries. These fractures may present with a variety of patterns including nasofrontal separation and comminution, ethmoid fractures, extensive medial orbital wall fractures, medial orbital rim fractures and disruption of the medial canthal ligaments. NOE fractures are usually produced by high velocity trauma, the most common etiology being motor vehicle accidents.

B. Diagnosis

Potential clinical signs and symptoms can include gross edema, periorbital ecchymosis, lacerations and a flat nasal bridge. Unilateral or bilateral telecanthus from disruption of the medial canthal ligament attachments is a significant finding. Additional findings associated with NOE fractures include enophthalmos, proptosis, dystopia, anosmia, nasal obstruction, subcutaneous emphysema, subconjunctival hemorrhage and blindness. With disruption of the cribriform plate, cerebrospinal fluid rhinorrhea may also be noted.

The radiographic survey for NOE fractures includes both plain films and CT scans. An ***axial CT scan*** is the study of choice because it provides information about medial orbital wall displacement and orbital volumetric changes. A ***coronal CT*** may be useful for assessing the extent of the fracture into the orbital floor, and the ***Waters'*** view will show fractures of the orbital rim. Finally, an ***underexposed lateral*** view is best for assessing the nasal bones and demonstrating transverse nasal fractures.

C. Treatment

The goals in the treatment of NOE fractures are as follows: 1) disimpaction, reduction and fixation of the nasal bones to the frontal bones, 2) repositioning or reconstruction of the medial orbital walls, 3) reattachment of the medial canthal ligaments, 4) restoration of lacrimal apparatus function, and 5)

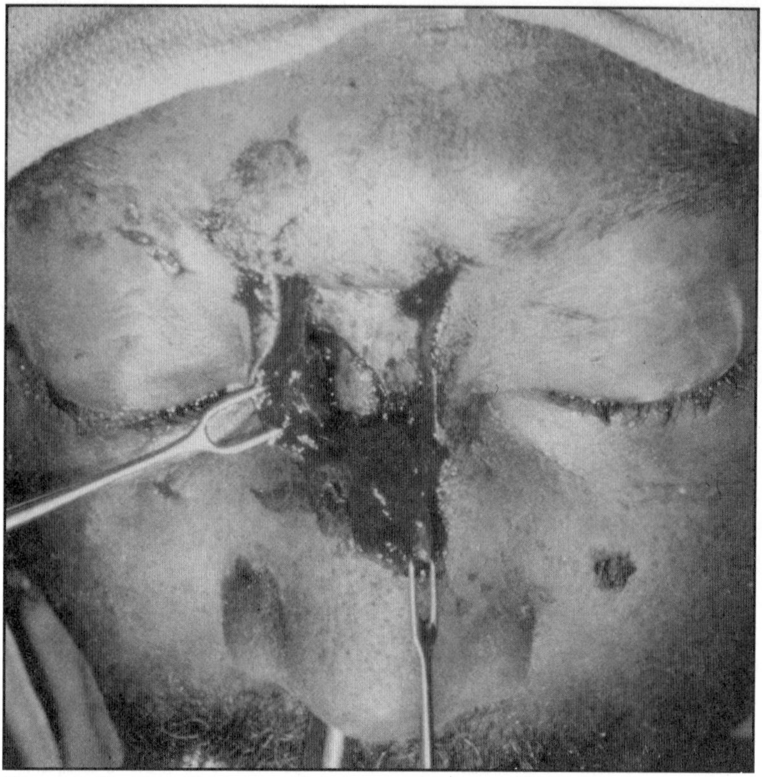

Figure 8-15: Open sky approach for accessing nasoorbital ethmoid complex fractures.

adequate reduction of the nasal bones and alignment of the nasal septum. Occasionally these objectives can be accomplished with closed reduction and manipulation of the nasal bones followed by crossnasal splinting. When nasal bones are comminuted with disruption of the medial canthal attachments, an open reduction of the nasal bones, medial and infraorbital rims, and medial orbital wall is usually indicated. Access to NOE fractures can be obtained through any existing lacerations, by an open sky approach (Figure 8-15), via curvilinear incisions at the medial aspect of the nasal bridge or by using a bicoronal flap (Figure 8-16). Fractures of the infraorbital rim are exposed through a subciliary incision and stabilized with bone plates or interosseous wires (Figure 8-17). Depending on the size and the degree of comminution, the remaining fractures can be plated or wired. If reconstruction of the medial orbital wall is necessary, an outer table cranial bone graft is harvested and inserted after reducing the orbital contents from the nasal cavity. The graft is stabilized with a wire or plate to a stable

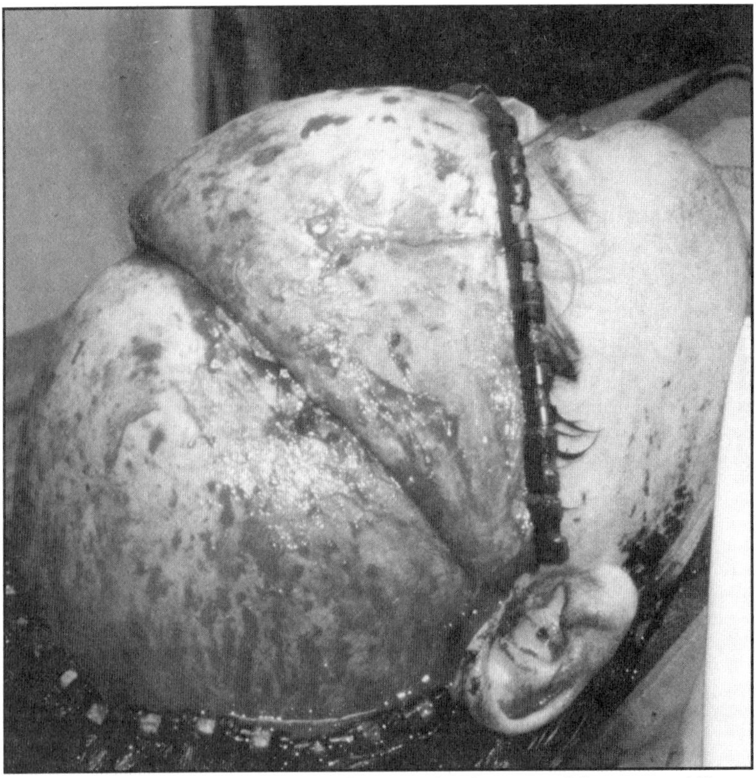

Figure 8-16: Bicoronal flap approach for accessing fractures of the upper midface and nasoorbital ethmoid complex.

area on the frontal bone. When nasal bridge reconstruction is needed, a cranial bone graft cantilevered to the nasal dorsum may be useful. The bone graft is secured to the glabellar area with bone screws.

To reattach medial canthal ligaments, the ligaments are identified, repositioned, and wired to a stable portion of the nasal process of the frontal bone. Securing the anterior limb of the medial canthal ligament is the most important part of this repair, since the functional reattachments of the posterior limb and Horner's muscle depend on this step.

Complications arising from the treatment of NOE fractures usually occur secondary to a poor understanding of the original fracture. Inadequate stabilization of the fractures, incorrect reattachment of the medial canthal ligaments and failure to reconstruct the medial wall of the orbit are common causes of complications. These complications include epiphora, dystopia, enophthalmos, telecanthus, widening and flattening of the nasal bridge, and dacrocystitis.

VI. ORBITOZYGOMATIC FRACTURES

Due to their prominent positions, the zygoma and zygomatic arch are highly susceptible to injury. Fractures of these bones may be isolated or may be combined with other midfacial injuries. The zygoma, also known as the malar bone, is a quadrilateral with four processes that articulate with the frontal, temporal, maxillary, and sphenoid (greater wing) bones. Hence, the commonly used term, "tripod fracture", is a misnomer in describing an orbitozygomatic fracture. These fractures should be considered quadrapod fractures with the fourth site of fracture, the zygomaticomaxillary buttress, representing the key to understanding and managing orbitozygomatic fractures. This buttress is critical because it provides structural support to the zygoma and acts as a direct antagonist to masseter muscle pull. In turn, the zygoma serves as a strong buttress between the maxilla and cranium through its' articulations.

The most common cause of orbitozygomatic and zygomatic arch fractures is an assault from a fist or club. Males outnumber females by as much as 4 to 1 with the peak incidence occurring in the 20 to 30 age group in males, and the 30 to 40 age group in females. Other frequent causes of these fractures include motor vehicle accidents and falls.

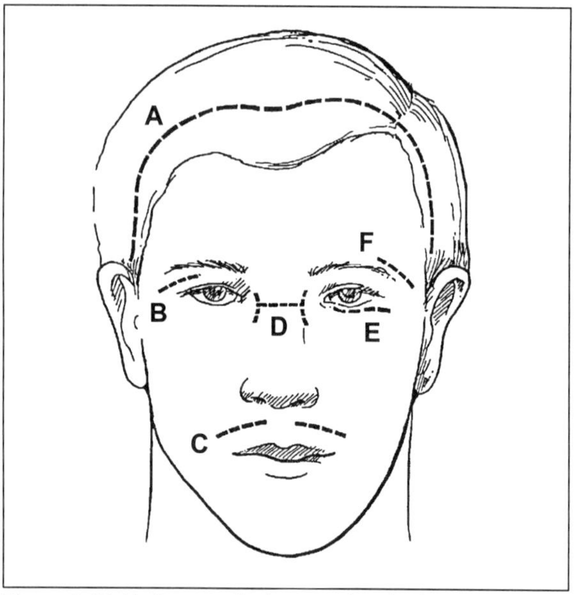

Figure 8-17: Various surgical approaches for fractures of the upper and middle face. (A) Bicoronal. (B) Upper lid blepharoplasty. (C) Buccal vestibule. (D) Open-sky. (E) Subciliary. (F) Lateral eyebrow.

A. Classification

In 1961, Knight and North developed a classification of zygomatic fractures based on a study of 120 such fractures. A ***Group I*** or ***no significant displacement fracture*** is defined as a radiographically discernible fracture without clinical evidence of displacement. ***Group II*** or ***zygomatic arch fractures*** are fractures caused by direct trauma over the zygomatic arch causing buckling of the arch in a classic angular deformity. There are three fracture lines in the middle and at each end of the zygomatic arch, resulting in two fracture segments. In ***Group III*** or ***unrotated body fractures***, the injury is usually caused by a direct blow over the zygomatic prominence with fracture and displacement of the zygoma into the maxillary antrum. The zygoma is usually displaced posteriorly, medially, and slightly inferiorly resulting in flattening of the cheek. A ***Group IV*** or ***medially rotated body fracture*** is caused by a blow to the zygomatic prominence, above the horizontal axis of the zygoma. The force produces posterior, inferior and medial displacement of the fracture. When the patient is viewed from the front, the zygoma appears to be rotated counterclockwise on the left and clockwise on the right. This group of zygomatic fractures has two subdivisions: ***type A***, in which there is forward displacement at the zygomatic prominence, and ***type B*** characterized by inward displacement at the zygomaticofrontal suture. ***Group V*** or ***laterally rotated body fractures*** are usually caused by blows below the horizontal axis of the zygoma, resulting in medial and posterior fracture displacement. When the patient is viewed frontally, the zygoma appears to be rotated clockwise on the left and counterclockwise on the right. This group of zygomatic fractures also has two subdivisions. ***Type A*** is characterized by upward displacement of the fracture at the infraorbital margin, while ***type B*** describes an outward displacement of the fracture at the zygomaticofrontal suture. ***Group VI*** or *complex fractures* include cases with additional fracture lines across the main fractured segment.

B. Diagnosis

The clinical examination usually reveals the classic signs and symptoms of zygomatic arch and zygoma fractures. Trismus and pain with mandibular movement, especially lateral excursions to the affected side, are suggestive of zygomatic arch fractures (Figure 8-18). Other arch fracture findings may include dimpling over the region of the arch or point tenderness with either intraoral or extraoral palpation. Regarding zygoma fractures, the clinical signs may be obscured by edema, hematomas and lacerations. If the patient is examined immediately following injury, inspection may

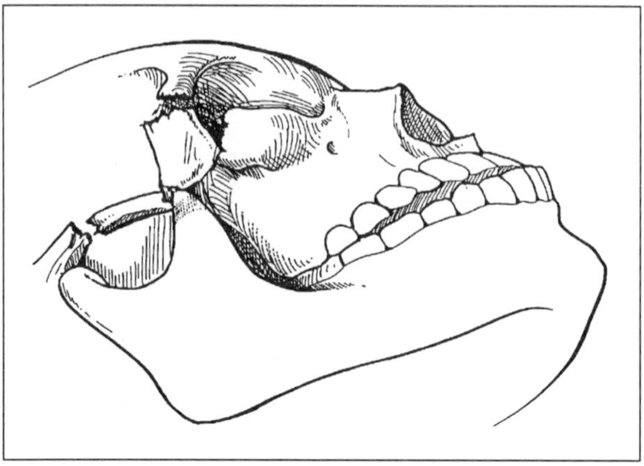

Figure 8-18: Mandibular coronoid process impingement from a depressed zygomatic arch fracture.

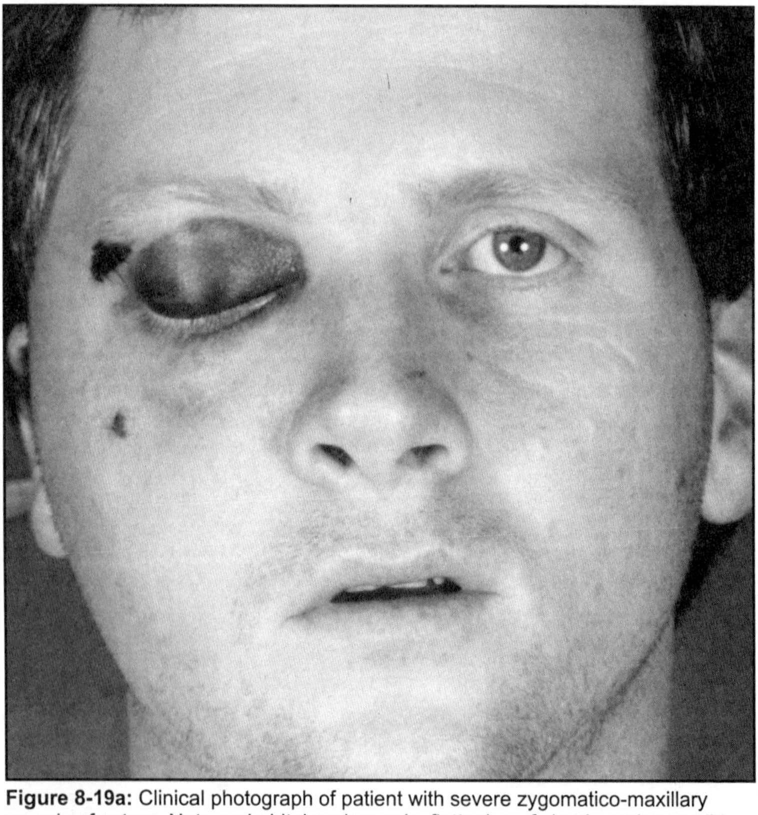

Figure 8-19a: Clinical photograph of patient with severe zygomatico-maxillary complex fracture. Note periorbital ecchymosis, flattening of cheek, and upper lid ptosis.

reveal flatness of the cheek, enophthalmos, retraction of the lower lid, unilateral epistaxis, ecchymosis of the lids, conjunctiva and sclera (Figure 8-19). Comparative bimanual palpation of the facial skeleton may reveal step defects in the inferior and lateral orbital rims. Intraoral palpation of the lateral and anterior walls of the maxilla is needed to identify any irregularities in the area of the maxillary buttress. Paresthesia or anesthesia along the distributions of the infraorbital, zygomaticotemporal and zygomaticofacial nerves often accompanies orbitozygomatic fractures. When the orbital floor is disrupted, the extraocular muscles may be entrapped and the patient may complain of diplopia. Upward gaze diplopia is usually secondary to entrapment of the inferior rectus or the inferior oblique muscles. Diplopia that is present in all fields of gaze commonly results from periorbital edema rather than muscular entrapment.

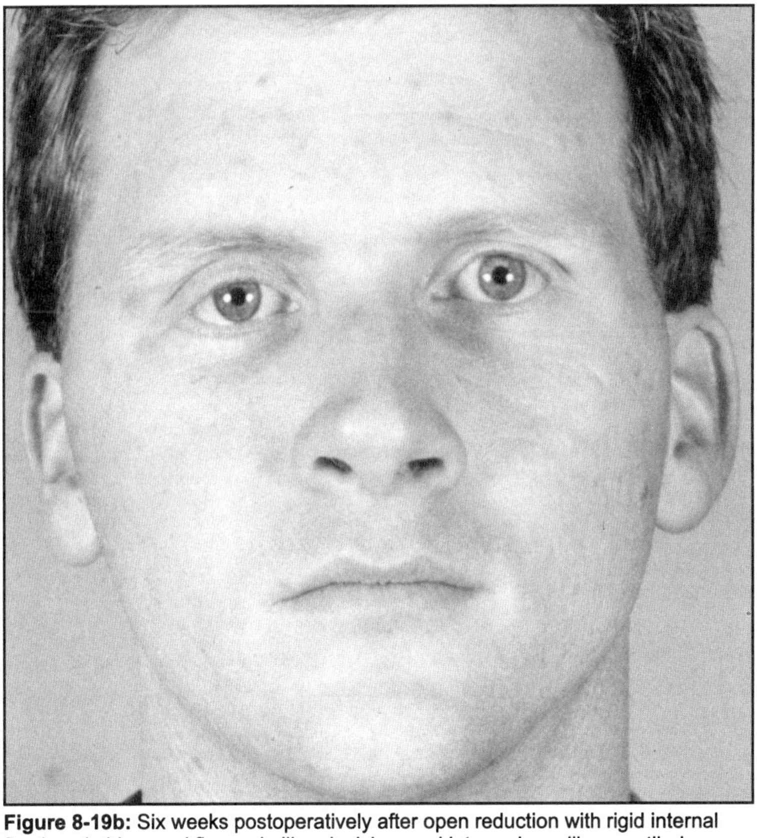

Figure 8-19b: Six weeks postoperatively after open reduction with rigid internal fixation via bicoronal flap, subciliary incision, and intraoral maxillary vestibular incision.

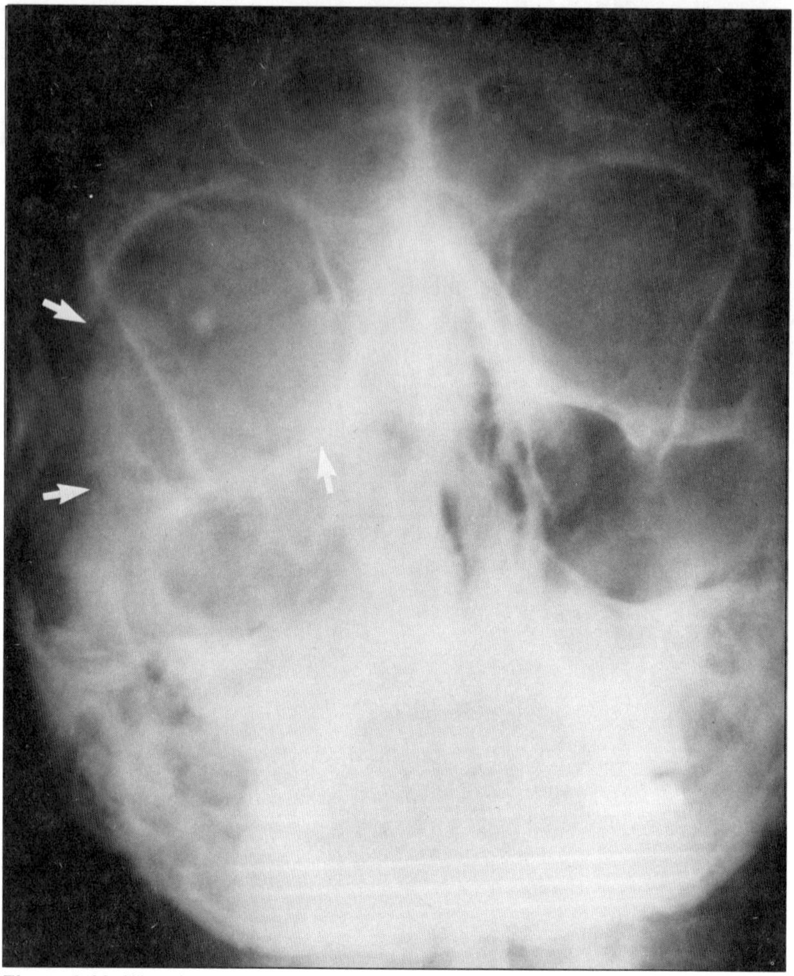

Figure 8-20: Water's view showing severe fracture and displacement of zygomaticomaxillary complex.

Ocular injuries that can accompany orbitozygomatic fractures include hyphema, lens dislocation, rupture of the globe, retinal detachment and vitreous hemorrhage. Prior to definitive treatment of these injuries, it is important to obtain an ophthalmologic consultation to formally assess visual acuity and ocular function.

The radiographic survey for zygomatic arch and orbitozygomatic fractures includes **PA** and ***lateral skull*** films for general appraisal. A ***Waters'*** view is the most useful plain film for evaluating the zygomas, the inferior and lateral orbital rims and the maxillary sinuses (Figure

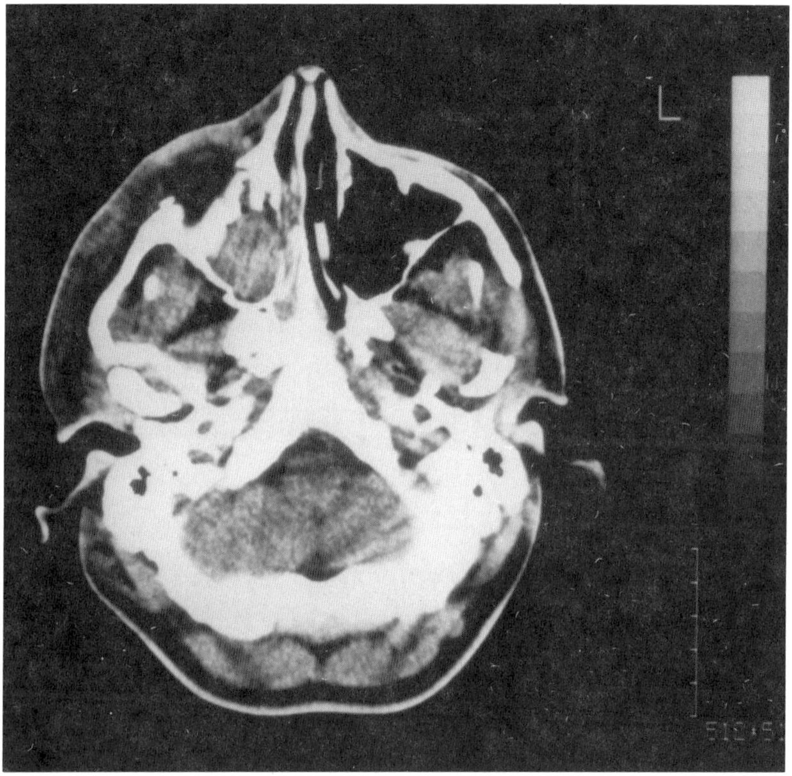

Figure 8-21: CT scan showing severe zygomaticomaxillary complex fracture.

8-20). The ***submentovertex*** view is useful for evaluating the zygomatic arches and to identify posterior displacement of the zygomas. A ***CT scan*** provides the most information in assessing the extent of orbitozygomatic fractures and in confirming the clinical diagnosis. CT scans permit accurate evaluations of the optic canals, ocular muscles, orbital hematomas, the extent of orbital floor fragmentation and the herniation of orbital contents (Figure 8-21).

C. Treatment

The treatment of depressed zygomatic arch fractures involves elevating and contouring the arch by placing a malar elevator medial to the collapsed segment. Both intraoral and extraoral approaches can be used to reduce these fractures. Extraoral methods include the Gilles' (temporal) and the

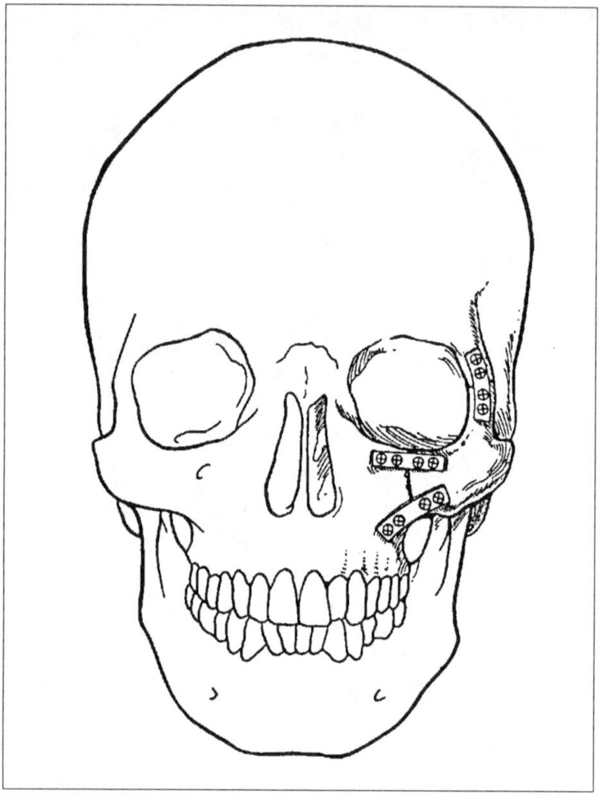

Figure 8-22: Recommended three point fixation for zygomatic complex fractures.

lateral brow approaches. Intraorally, a 1.5 cm incision is made in the buccal vestibule above the maxillary molar teeth to gain access to the depressed arch. Elevation of the depressed fracture will eliminate impingement on the coronoid process of the mandible and improve mandibular range of motion.

Unstable orbitozygomatic fractures are best managed by direct exposure of the infraorbital rim, the frontozygomatic suture area, the orbital floor and the zygomaticomaxillary buttress. The infraorbital rim and orbital floor are approached by a transconjunctival or a subciliary incision, while the frontozygomatic area is accessed by a lateral brow or upper eyelid blepharoplasty incision. Direct exposure of the buttress is obtained by means of an intraoral buccal sulcus incision. Fractures of the zygomaticomaxillary buttress will allow the body of the zygoma to rotate downward and inward from unopposed masseter muscle pull. Following manipulation and reduction of the zygoma, the infraorbital rim, the frontozygomatic suture line and the zygomaticomaxillary buttress are stabilized

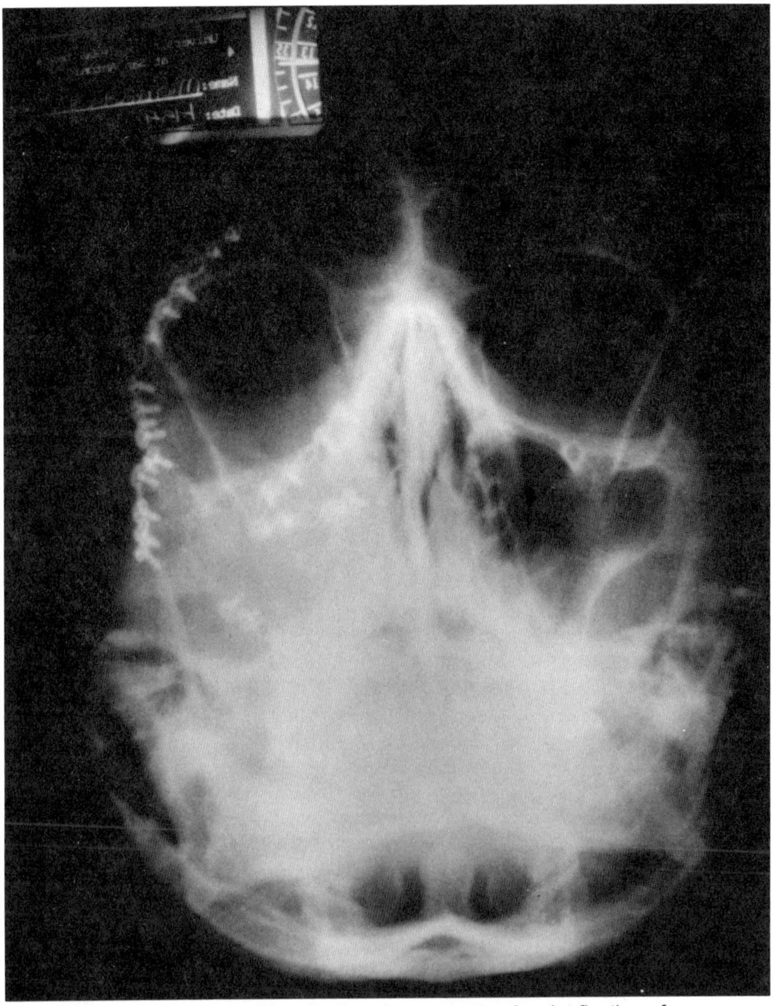

Figure 8-23: Postoperative Water's view demonstrating 3 point fixation of zygomaticomaxillary complex fracture (infraorbital rim, zygomatic buttress, and zygomaticofrontal suture area).

with mini bone plates or direct interosseous wires (Figure 8-22). Three point fixation of the zygoma at these 3 sites will prevent downward rotation of the zygomatic body and late depression of the zygomatic prominence, with resulting cheek flatness (Figure 8-23). While the orbital floor is exposed, herniated orbital contents are retrieved from the maxillary sinus and identifiable lacerations of the periorbital periosteum are repaired. Orbital floor defects can be reconstructed with autogenous cranial or iliac bone grafts, cartilage, freeze-dried bone or alloplastic materials, such as Silastic sheeting.

The most common cause of residual deformity following facial fractures is inadequate treatment of orbitozygomatic fractures. Persistent flattening of the cheek, trismus and diplopia are indicative of inadequate reduction or fixation of these fractures. The most serious complication in the management of orbitozygomatic fractures is blindness secondary to either aggressive antral packing, an expanding orbital hematoma or inadequate surgical access. Additional complications can include persistent infraorbital paresthesia, sinusitis, ectropion, enophthalmos, epiphora, oroantral communications and extrusion of orbital floor implants.

References

Adekeye E.O., "The pattern of fractures of the facial skeleton in Kaduna, Nigeria." *Oral Surg Oral Med Oral Pathol.* 49 (1980): 491.

Alling C.C., Osbon D.B., *Maxillofacial Trauma.* Philadelphia: Lea & Febiger, 1988.

Alpert B., "Complications in the treatment of facial trauma." *Oral Maxillofac Surg Clin North Am.* 2 (1990): 171.

Dingman R.O., Natvig P., *Surgery of Facial Fractures.* Philadelphia: W.B. Saunders, 1964.

Donoff R.B., *Massachusetts General Hospital Manual of Oral and Maxillofacial Surgery.* St. Louis: C.V. Mosby, 1987.

Ellis E., El-Attar A., Moos K.F., "An analysis of 2067 cases of zygomaticoorbital fracture." *J Oral Maxillofac Surg.* 43 (1985): 417.

Ellis E., Moos K.F., El-Attar A., "Ten years of mandibular fractures: An analysis of 2137 cases." *Oral Surg Oral Med Oral Pathol.* 59 (1985): 120.

Jackson I.T., Classification and treatment of orbitozygomatic and orbitoethmoid fractures." *Clin Plast Surg.* 16 (1989): 77.

Gruss J.S., Phillips J.H., "Complex facial trauma: The evolving role of rigid fixation and immediate bone graft reconstruction." *Clin Plast Surg.* 16 (1989): 93.

Kelly D.E., Harrigan W.F., "A survey of facial fractures: Bellevue Hospital, 1948-1974." *J Oral Surg.* 33 (1975): 146.

Kruger E., Schilli W., *Oral and Maxillofac Traumatology.* Vol 1. Chicago: Quintessence Publishing Co., 1982.

Olson R.A.; Fonseca R.J.; Zeitler D.L.; and Osbon D.B., "Fractures of the mandible: A review of 580 cases." *J Oral Maxillofac Surg.* 40 (1982): 1982.

Peterson L.J.; Ellis E.; Hupp J.R.; and Tucker M.R., *Contemporary Oral and Maxillofacial Surgery.* St. Louis: C.V. Mosby, 1988.

Ruskin J.D., Tu H.K., "Integrated management of the maxillofacial trauma patient with multiple injuries." *Oral Maxillofac Surg Clin North Am.* 2 (1990): 15.

Waite D.E., *Textbook of Practical Oral and Maxillofacial Surgery.* 3rd ed. Philadelphia: Lea & Febiger, 1987.

Zide M.F., Kent J.N., "Indications for open reduction of mandibular condyle fractures." *J Oral Maxillofac Surg.* 41 (1983): 1983.

9 Temporomandibular Disorders

Michael T. Montgomery, D.D.S.

Ernest B. Luce, D.D.S.

Temporomandibular Disorders (TMD) is a term applied to a group of musculoskeletal problems affecting the muscles of mastication and/or the temporomandibular joints. It is reported that 10% of the population suffer from these problems, which are commonly acute, but can be chronic. The disorders can also be associated with trauma such as motor vehicle accidents (MVAs) and fisticuffs. As such, these patients are frequently encountered in acute care settings. The signs and symptoms typify those of other musculoskeletal disorders including arthralgia, myalgia, joint sounds and limitations in range of motion. These manifestations are also common to facial fractures, therefore, care must be taken in the differential diagnosis. The presence of TMD is defined by patient self-report (history), a clinical examination and at times, radiographs. Treatment generally consists of patient education and palliation. The intent of this chapter is to review T-M Disorders from anatomy through treatment, focusing on acute maladies likely to be encountered by the acute care practitioner.

I. ANATOMICAL REVIEW

Muscles of mastication are the muscles most commonly affected in TMD and include those muscles responsible for opening and closing the mandible. Knowledge of the muscles' positions is essential for recognizing appropriate pain location and in performing a palpation examination. The **closing muscles** are most commonly affected and include the temporalis, masseters and medial pterygoids (Figure 9-1). The temporalis muscle originates in the temporal fossa and inserts on the coronoid process. The masseter muscles originate on the zygomatic arches and insert on both the lateral surface of the coronoid process and on the inferior border of the mandible. The medial pterygoid muscle complements the masseter muscle on the medial surface of the mandibular ramus, originating on the lateral pterygoid plates and inserting on the medial surface of the inferior mandibular border. The medial pterygoid and masseter muscles form a sling around the ramus and posterior body of the mandible. The muscle responsible

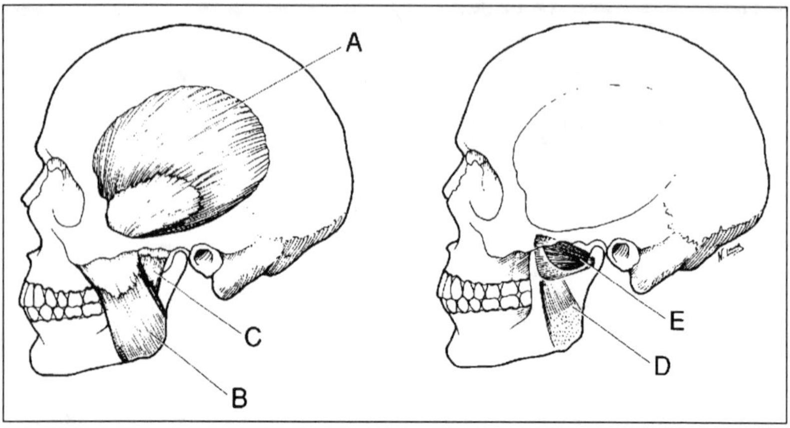

Figure 9-1: Muscles responsible for closing and excursive mandibular movements. Saggital skull views illustrating the anatomical positions of the following muscles: A - temporalis, B - superficial masseter, C - deep masseter, D - medial pterygoid, E - lateral pterygoid.

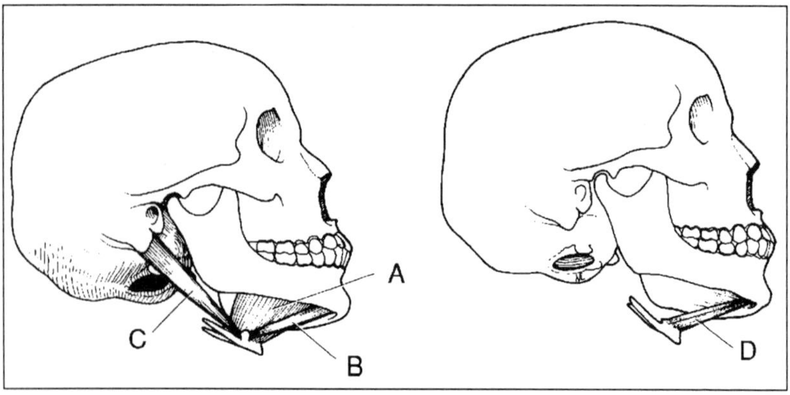

Figure 9-2: Muscles responsible for mandibular opening. Oblique skull views illustrating the anatomical positions of the following muscles: A - mylohyoid, B - anterior belly of the digastric, C - posterior belly of the digastric, D - geniohyoid.

for translation of the mandible is the inferior belly of the lateral pterygoid, which originates on the greater wings of the sphenoid and inserts on the anterior surface of the condyles. Bilateral contraction produces protrusion of the mandible, while ipsilateral contraction results in lateral movement of the mandible away from the side of muscle contraction.

The superior belly of the lateral pterygoid originates on the greater wing of the sphenoid and inserts into the capsular ligament. This muscle contracts during the final closing stages of the mandible, which is thought to stabilize the articulation by maintaining slight pressure between the condyle, disk and eminence. The superior belly of the lateral pterygoid muscle does not play a significant role in disk translation, which had been assumed in the past. The **opening muscles** are less commonly affected and include the muscles in the floor of the mouth; specifically, the anterior and posterior digastrics, mylohyoid, geniohyoid and infrahyoid muscles (Figure 9-2). Finally, the **anterior and posterior neck muscles** are often symptomatic, however, the relationship of neck pain to TMD is presently unclear. It appears that most of the neck pain is secondary

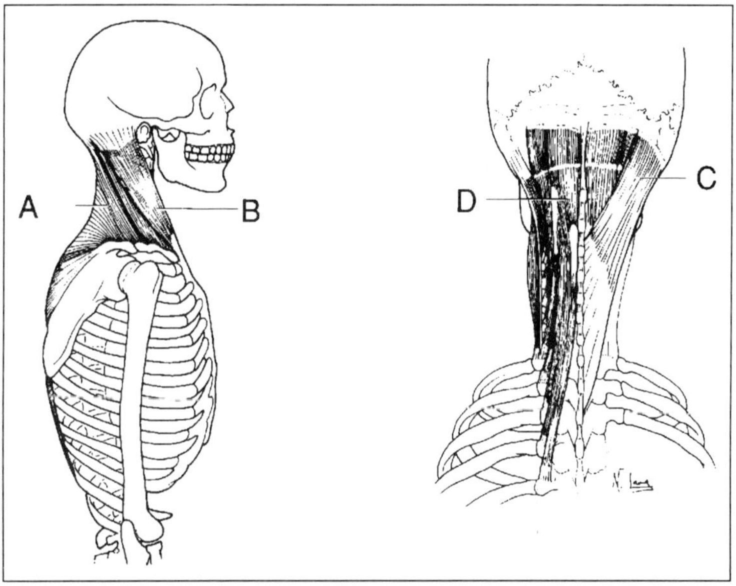

Figure 9-3: Anterior and Cervical Neck Muscles. Saggital and posterior skull views illustrating the anatomical positions of the following muscles: A - trapezius, B - sternocleidomastoid, C - splenius capitus, D - semispinalis capitus.

to concurrent, though unrelated, cervical dysfunction in most patients. Commonly affected neck muscles include the cervical muscles, the trapezius and the sternocleidomastoids (Figure 9-3).

The **temporomandibular joint** (TMJ) consists of the mandibular or glenoid fossa, the articular eminence and the condyle (Figure 9-4). Wide variations in anatomic appearance exist between patients reflecting differences in genetic inheritance and functional demands. As such, the practitioner must exercise caution against interpreting this variability as pathology. The **fossa** is located in the squamous portion of the temporal bone between the external auditory meatus and the articular eminence. The roof is thin, approximately 1 mm thick and nonstress bearing. The fossa has posterior and medial vertical walls (lips) that help limit condyle movement in these directions. The fossa, eminence and condylar head are covered with fibrous connective tissue that overlaps the fibrocartilage. Anterior to the fossa is the **articular eminence**, which represents the medial root of the zygomatic arch. The distal slope of the eminence is the region of articulation with the disk and the condyle when the patient's teeth are occluded in centric occlusion (maximal intercuspation). The condyle is the articulating terminus of the mandible. Sagittally, the **condyle** has a characteristic sigmoid shape, while in the transverse plane, the medial and lateral poles are two sites of disk attachment.

The **disk** consists of sagittally oriented collagen fibers in a biconcave shape (Figure 9-4). The intermediate zone is the site of articulation between the condyle and eminence that is bound anteriorly by a thickening, termed the anterior band, and posteriorly by a similar thickening, termed the posterior band. These thickenings in the disk define the area of articulation and keep the disk positioned on the condylar head during movement. Anteriorly, the disk attaches to the capsular ligament and minimally to the superior belly of the lateral pterygoid muscle. Medially and laterally, the disk attaches to the medial and lateral poles of the condylar head. Posterior to the posterior band, the disk evolves into the **retrodiskal tissue**. This tissue consists of loose elastic connective tissue that is richly innervated and vascularized. This composition is starkly contrasted with the disk, which is essentially avascular and uninnervated. The retrodiskal tissue attaches to the condylar neck, capsular ligament and fossa. The disk divides the joint space into superior and inferior cavities that are lined by synovium. The synovial fluid produced by this tissue provides lubrication to assist the joint in movement and supplies nutrients and biologically active proteins to the disk. The superior joint space is the larger of the two spaces and is the place of translatory articular movement between the disk and the eminence. The inferior joint space is the site of rotational articulatory movement between the disk and the condylar head.

The capsular and temporomandibular ligaments limit condylar movement (Figure 9-4). The capsular ligament envelops the condylar head by attaching to the rim of the fossa and to the condylar neck, just beneath the condylar head. The temporomandibular ligament attaches to the zygomatic arch and to the lateral condylar neck, limiting lateral condylar movement.

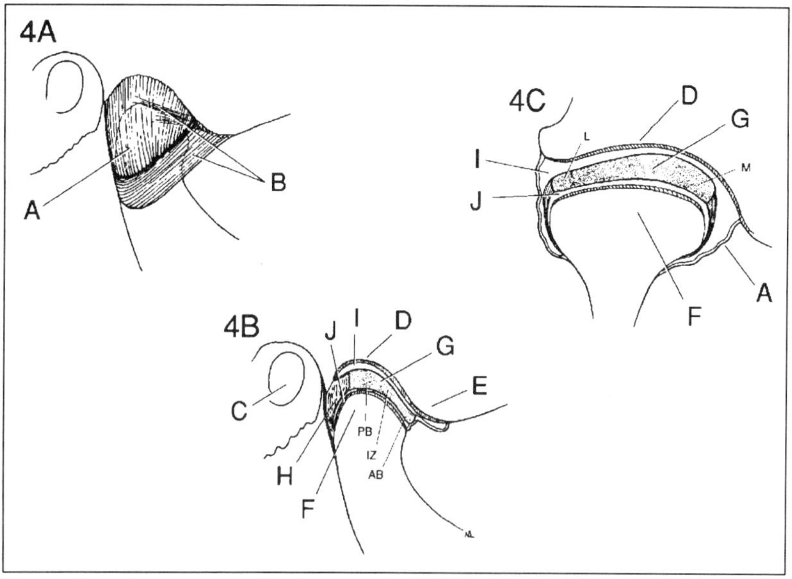

Figure 9-4: Temporomandibular Joint. **4A** - Saggital view illustrating the major joint ligaments: A - capsular, B - temporomandibular. **4B** - Saggital view illustrating intraarticular anatomy: C - external auditory meatus, D - glenoid fossa, E - articular eminence, F - condyle, G - disk (AB=anterior band, IZ=intermediate zone, PB=posterior band), H - retrodiskal tissue, I - superior joint space, J - inferior joint space. **4C** - Frontal view of joints illustrating the following structures: A - capsular ligament, D - glenoid fossa, F - condyle, G - disk with medial (M) and lateral (L) pole attachments, I - superior joint space, J - inferior joint space.

Movement of the condyle involves rotational and translatory motions. The condyle rotates around a horizontal axis in the condylar head or neck, while translation is the sagittal movement from the fossa to the height of the eminence. These motions occur simultaneously from the centric occlusal position when a patient opens or closes their mouth. [A pure rotational movement of the condyle occurs only along the posterior border path for the first (approximately) 25 mm of opening. Therefore, a pure rotational movement will only exist during initial opening from a retruded occlusal position. As such, the concept of a pure rotational movement is artificial and not to be confused with the initial condylar movements (simultaneous rotation and translation) from an intercuspal position. This point is important to comprehend, as it implies that any interpositional appliance (orthotic) used in the treatment of TMD will result in condylar translation and, therefore, alter the occlusion. Practitioners have assumed that flat plane orthotics will not alter the occlusion because the condyle is simply rotating and not translating, unaware that this assumption is based on originating the movement from a retruded contact

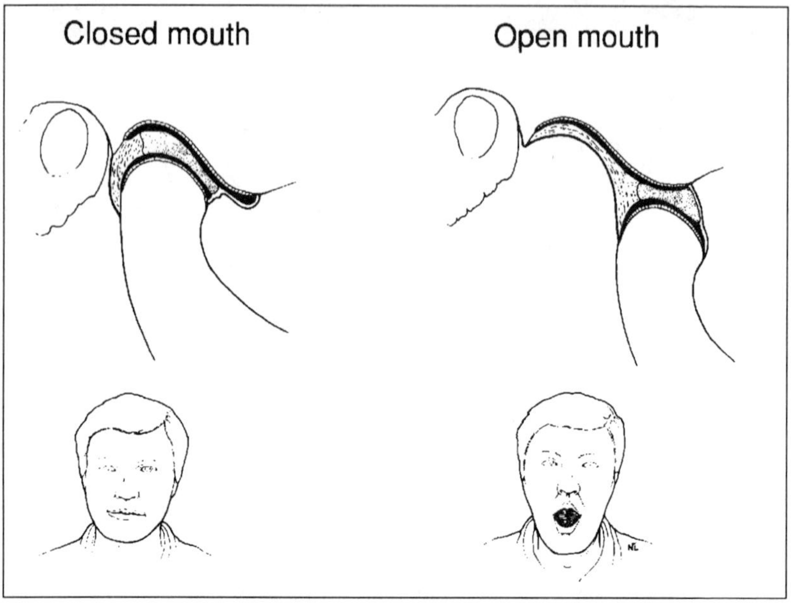

Figure 9-5: Normal Joint Biomechanics. Closed Mouth - disk is interposed between the condyle and the articular eminence in an anterior-superior direction. Open Mouth - disk is now superior to the condylar head having translated anteriorly and rotated in a counterclockwise direction.

position.] The articular lips on the fossa, the articular ligaments and the orientation of the muscles determine the direction and extent of condyle movement. Condylar movement essentially occurs in an anterior-posterior direction accompanied by slight lateral movement. With the teeth together (centric occlusion), the disk is located in an anterior-superior direction relative to the condylar head. As the mouth opens and the condyle translates, the disk rotates posteriorly around the condyle, remaining interposed between the condylar head and the eminence. Thus, with the mouth fully open, the disk is now superior to the condylar head (Figure 9-5). Translation of the disk along with the condyle is thought to principally depend on disk anatomy, while the posterior rotation of the disk results from the elastic fibers in the retrodiskal tissue. Disruption of either the disk's anatomy or attachments is believed to cause incoordination between the condyle and the disk, resulting in disk displacement. Histologic studies have shown that the composition of the retrodiskal tissue changes with age, rendering this tissue less resistant to injury and less capable of adaptation. Such changes include a decrease in vascularity and elasticity of the retrodiskal tissue. These changes may partially explain why persistent intra-articular disorders are more common in older patients. The neuromuscular control of mandibular movement is determined by central cortical input in conjunction with afferent peripheral receptors in the joints, muscles and teeth (periosteum and periodontal ligament).

The location of an intra-articular injury is partially determined by the previously described anatomical relationships. The orientation of the lateral pterygoid muscle pulls the condyle in an anterior and medial direction, and places greatest strain on the lateral pole disk attachment. Also, the disk is thinner laterally than medially and the lateral pole attachment lacks the support of a fossa lip, unlike the medial attachment. This, coupled with the ability of the condyle to move laterally (and not medially) suggests that soft tissue intra-articular injuries will most likely occur either at the lateral pole attachment or in the retrodiskal tissue. This projection has been confirmed by surgical and postmortem findings. Displacement of the disk is associated with stretching or tearing of disk attachments, resulting in an enlargement of the inferior joint space. This finding has been confirmed by TMJ arthrography.

II. SIGNS AND SYMPTOMS

Some combination of either headaches, jaw pain, ear pain, neck and shoulder pain, trismus or deviations in mandibular movement, muscle palpation tenderness, jaw locking, and joint sounds constitute the presence of TMD. A complete listing of TMD signs and symptoms is provided in Table 9-1. The signs and symptoms can be unilateral or bilateral, and the pains may be intermittent (most common) or constant. Defining the presence of TMD can be difficult as it is unclear how many signs and symptoms are needed for a positive diagnosis. However, because this is a musculoskeletal disorder affecting the jaw joints and/or the muscles of mastication, TMD pain should occur on these regions and be exacerbated with mandibular movement or function. This symptom may deserve the designation of a pathognomonic finding. Epidemiologic data reports that 70-80% of the population may report one or more signs and symptoms, yet it is estimated that only a fraction of this population (10%) may be diagnosed with TMD. The disorder predominantly affects women (9:1) and the incidence is uniform across all age groups, except in the very young (<10 years old) and in the very old (>70 years old). The typical patient is a female aged 20 to 40 years old. Explanations for the female predilection have included gender differences in health utilization as well as other behavioral and psychological gender distinctions. However, recent investigations into intra-articular estrogen receptors and the effects of estrogen on inflammatory cell mediators may explain the gender difference on a physiological basis.

Table 9-1: TMD Signs and Symptoms

Sign or Symptom	Distinguishing Features	Intra-articular (IA) or Extra-articular (EA)	How Diagnosed
Headache	temporal region; dull; like tension headache	both	self-report
Jaw Pain	sharp or dull; sides of face; increased with jaw movement	IA	self-report; palpation
Ear Pain	sharp or dull; associated with jaw pain; represents referred pain	IA	self-report
Neck/Shoulder Pain	anterior and posterior cervical; represents associated cervical dysfunction; increased with neck movement	both	self-report; palpation
Trismus	opening less than 35-40 mm; associated with; adhesions or DDNR	IA	self-report; meas. vert opening
Deviation	usually ipsilateral; associated with DDNR	IA	observation
Deflection	usually ipsilateral; associated with DDWR	IA	observation
Joint Sounds			
-Clicking/Popping	discrete, sudden sound; indicates DDWR	IA	auscultation
-Crepitus	harsh, grating sound; indicates DJD	IA	auscultation
Muscle Palpation Tenderness	muscles of mastication; especially the masseter and temporalis	both	palpation
Locking			
-Open	wide opening in a hypermobile joint; reducible	IA	self-report
-Closed	DDNR; may be reducible but stabilization is difficult	IA	self-report
Gross Occlusal Changes	intra-articular tumor, condylar head erosion; DJD; developmental growth disorders	IA	observation
Sleep Disruption	bruxism, depression, nocturnal pain	both	self-report
Dietary Restrictions	hard, chewy foods; foods requiring wide opening	both but mainly IA	self-report
Bruxism/Attrition	a.m. pain; sleep disruption; acknowledged by sleep partner	both	self-report

TMD pain is typically a dull ache, however, sharp components may be described with an intra-articular disorder. The associated **headache** is commonly located in the temporal region, although it can be generalized. The pain is not associated with paresthesias, visual disturbances or nausea and is not paroxysmal in onset or remission. The headache's character resembles that of muscle contraction or tension headaches. The association of a headache with TMD is determined by patient report and the occurrence of the headache with other TMD signs and symptoms. **Jaw pain** is typically located preauricularly and is usually described as sharp. This pain can be elicited with mandibular movements (e.g., wide opening or eating) and during a palpation examination. The pain is thought to result from intra-articular inflammation and/or edema. **Ear pain** is generally associated with the jaw pain and is thought to represent referred pain secondary to the ear's close proximity to the joint. As such, TMD patients generally do not have an otitis or any identifiable ear pathology (i.e., otoscopic and palpation examinations are typically negative for pathosis). Other ear symptoms reported by TMD patients include stuffiness, tinnitus, hearing loss and itching; however, the validity and relationship of these complaints to TMD is unclear. Attempts to determine a pathophysiologic relationship between ear symptoms and TMD have been unconvincing to date.

As with ear pain, the relationship of **neck and shoulder pain** to TMD is poorly understood. Anterior neck, cervical and trapezius pain can be common complaints and are verifiable on palpation examination. However, it appears that most of the neck pain is secondary to cervical dysfunction that is unrelated to the TMD. This conclusion is based on the inconsistency of onset between neck pain and other TMD complaints, and the observation that the neck pain is more often exacerbated by cervical movement than by mandibular movement. **Joint sounds**, either clicking (popping) or crepitus (grating) are also common TMD complaints. The incidence of these signs is dependent upon the method by which they are recorded. For example, epidemiologic studies report that clicking, recorded by palpation, occurs 30% of the time in the TMD population, compared to 15% in the normal population. If a stethoscope is used to record the joint sounds, the aforementioned figures are doubled. This data also points out that although clicking is more common in TMD patients, this sound is compatible with health, and occurs in a sizable frequency in the normal population. The clicking sound predictably (80% correlation) results from disk displacement with reduction. This means that the disk is displaced anteriorly (and medially), requiring the condyle to jump onto the disk (reduction) with translation during mandibular opening (Figure 9-6). In contrast, crepitus is an uncommon finding that is predictably (90% correlation) associated with the presence of degenerative joint disease (DJD) or osteoarthritis (Figure 9-8). This sound results from either a perforation in the disk or retrodiskal tissues or, less commonly, from calcifications in these soft tissues. The friction of hard tissue contact during mandibular movement produces this harsher, grating sound. Both of the aforementioned joint sounds can be detected by palpation or stethoscope examinations.

Additional potential signs of TMD include: the inability to move the mandible through a full range of motion (**trismus**), jaw locking, deviation and deflection of the mandible to one side on opening. Normal ranges of mandibular movement are 35 to 55 mm of vertical opening and 6 to 12 mm of lateral movement. Trismus can occur secondary to muscle splinting or contracture, but most commonly results from adhesions and/or disk displacement within the joint(s). The presence of trismus can be determined by patient report and by measurement of the patient's range of mandibular movements. The significance of trismus is defined by the resultant functional limitations, whereby, an opening of 30 mm requires therapeutic attention only if thc patient is dysfunctional as a result. **Deviation and deflection** of the mandible to one side are also associated with intra-articular disorders. Deflection refers to the momentary deviation of the mandible on opening that is seen with disk displacement with reduction (Figure 9-6). In this condition, condylar translation is briefly impeded, causing the mandible to deviate to the affected side (ipsilateral). As the disk is recaptured on opening, the mandible swings back to the midline. In contrast, with deviation the mandible does not return to the midline with further opening, remaining deviated at maximal opening. This sign is associated with disk displacement without reduction, in which an anteriorly displaced disk is not recaptured with maximal mandibular opening (Figure 9-7).

Locking refers to the sticking of the jaw in either the open or closed positions. This problem is typically momentary, as patients are able to manipulate their jaws and restore movement. Sometimes, however, patients are unable to reduce their jaws and acute treatment is needed. Open locking is thought to result from mechanical displacement of the condylar head anterior to the eminence. Prerequisites for open locking include a hypermobile joint (stretched ligaments) that allows the condylar head to translate beyond the eminence and become stuck. Mild contracture of the closing muscles, especially the temporalis, may help maintain this locked relationship. Open locking generally occurs with activities requiring wide opening, such as yawning. Closed locking is the acute manifestation of disk displacement without reduction, in which the condyle is unable to recapture the disk. The posterior band remains anterior to the condyle with maximal opening producing trismus, pain, ipsilateral deviation and diminished contralateral

lateral movement. **Bruxism**, the clenching or grinding of one's teeth either nocturnally or diurnally, is a frequently reported TMD observation. Grinding will produce an audible sound that can be confirmed by a sleep partner, while clenching is silent and, therefore, a more occult activity. Bruxism is both a sign/symptom and a potential cause for TMD, appears to occur intermittently through one's life and is common in children. However, the presence of the activity itself is not synonymous with TMD. Also, the behavior appears to be stress-related, as research has shown that anxiety can induce or exacerbate the activity. Nocturnal bruxism can be identified by pain in the morning upon wakening, confirmation by a sleep partner or nocturnal awakenings because of pain. Identifiers for diurnal bruxism include patient awareness and a diurnal pain pattern. Accelerated tooth wear patterns (attrition) and hypertrophy of the masseter muscles are additional signs attributed to bruxism.

Sleep disruption refers to the frequent difficulty in either getting to sleep or staying asleep. This problem may be associated with bruxism activity or may be a manifestation of depression. The relationship of this problem with depression will depend on the presence of other signs of depression (i.e., changes in appetite, diminished self-worth, malaise etc.). Bruxism-related sleep disruption may be signaled by the awareness of TMD pain or facial muscle stiffness upon wakening.

Finally, with respect to exacerbators and alleviators of TMD, symptoms should worsen with mandibular movement or with functions such as eating, yawning and extended talking. Thus, **dietary restrictions** are common in TMD patients and sufferers cannot chew gum or eat hard or chewy foods (meat, uncooked vegetables, apples) without exacerbating their pain. Periods of increased anxiety such as the death of a loved one, problems with interpersonal relationships, marital strife, financial problems, re-locating, job discord and educational pressures may also worsen the condition. TMD is not exacerbated by changes in head position, neck movement or light touch. The improvement of TMD pain is typically seen with simple analgesics, rest, the limitation of oral activities and with thermal applications such as moist heat (noticed in the shower or sauna) or cold. In most cases, TMD pain is not of a sufficient magnitude to require oral or parenteral narcotic analgesics.

III. CLASSIFICATION SCHEME AND PATHOPHYSIOLOGY

TMD disease classification schemes are plentiful and diverse. Unfortunately, most schemes are based on clinical impressions that lack scientific validation, and purport a refinement that exaggerates our present level of understanding. As such, most classification schemes entail a lengthy list

Table 9-2: TMD Classifications

Entities	Distinguishing Clinical Features
Extra-articular	
1-Myalgia with or without capsulitis	pain in facial muscles and TMJ without signs of a more serious intra-articular problem
2-Fibromyalgia (systemic)	generalized myalgias and arthralgias; sleep disruption; stress/anxiety
Intra-articular	
1-Capsulitis or synovitis alone	discreet TMJ tenderness; may be accompanied by trismus and difficulty occluding teeth; no myalgia; can mimic a condylar fracture
2-Disk displacement with reduction (DDWR) A- without locking	clicking/popping is pathognomonic; may be accompanied by capsulitis or myalgia
B- with locking	may indicate a transition to DDNR
3-Disk displacement without reduction (DDNR)	
A- acute	characteristic constellation of signs and symptoms including sudden trismus, ipsilateral deviation, no joint sound and decreased contralateral movement
B- chronic	minimal to imperceptible decreases in mandibular movements and deviation; diversity of joint sounds; difficult diagnosis; detailed history is critical; imaging may be needed for diagnosis
4-Degenerative joint disease (DJD)	crepitus is pathognomonic; may be accompanied by episodic trismus, capsulitis, myalgia and occlusal changes (e.g., open bite); older patients

of disorders that are deceptively impressive. For the purpose of acute disease triage, the authors propose a simplified categorical scheme to facilitate referral and treatment decisions. This scheme will modestly abridge the recently proposed TMD classification of Truelove, et al., 1992. This classification was selected because it attempts to base the disease delineators on scientific understanding which limits the resulting classification possibilities. The classification proposed for this text divides TMD into intra-articular, extra-articular and combination disorders (Table 2).

The **extra-articular disorder** is the most prevalent type of TMD and is comprised of myalgia of the muscles of mastication, which may also include the neck and shoulder muscles. The estimated incidence of this disorder is 90% of all TM Disorders, as **myalgia** is also present with most intra-articular problems. The myalgia is thought to result from myositis secondary to muscle injury, splinting or overuse. Because the involved muscles are generalized throughout the sides of the head and neck, the associated pain complaints include headaches, facial pain, and, on occasion, neck and shoulder pain. Jaw pain and related ear pain may also be present, however, these symptoms signal the presence of intra-articular inflammation, rather than myositis. Technically, this would represent a combination disorder, though such a distinction is unnecessarily burdensome and therefore, simple accompanying intra-articular inflammation (capsulitis or synovitis) will be included under myositis. On clinical examination, these patients will have muscle and, perhaps, joint palpation tenderness. However, signs of an intra-articular disorder, such as locking, trismus, deviation and painful joint sounds should not be present. It is important to note that if joint sounds are present, they are unrelated to the patient's pain and dysfunction. Therefore, the presence of joint sounds, in and of themselves, does not signify the presence of disease. Joint sounds are considered a contributor to the TMD problem when they are associated with the production of pain, locking or significant trismus. This recommendation is based on the frequency of joint sounds in the normal population, the disparity between the onset of joint sounds and pain in most patients, and the documented ability to relieve symptoms without alleviating joint sounds. The latter point is supported by treatment outcomes of both nonsurgical and surgical therapies, in which patient improvement appears unrelated to the relief of joint sounds. Some classification schemes divide myalgia into subgroups according to the degree of symptomatology (more and less symptomatic) or relative to the number of muscles involved. However, in the acute care setting, this distinction is less meaningful.

Uncommonly, head and neck myalgia is a component of a systemic myalgic condition known as **Fibromyositis or Fibromyalgia**. This disorder represents an ill-defined rheumatologic disease which is typically diagnosed when other, well defined musculoskeletal disorders cannot be identified in the presence of systemic myalgia and arthralgia. Specifically, Fibromyalgia exists when a patient exhibits pain in three or more joints for a period of three months, which cannot be attributed to a recognized rheumatologic disorder. Although such a patient is uncommonly encountered, the reader should be aware of this disorder and inquire about systemic musculoskeletal pain to avoid making an inappropriate diagnosis. Simply stated, a patient with Fibromyalgia will have myalgia characteristic of TMD, as well as systemic arthralgia/myalgia, sleep disruption and anxiety.

Intra-articular disorders generally refer to various disk displacement entities, adhesions and chronic inflammation that cannot be tolerated by the host. Implied in this definition is the assumption that none of the disk displacement disorders are pathologic unless accompanied by intra-articular pain and/or dysfunction. The simplest intra-articular disorder is intra-articular inflammation, termed **capsulitis** or **synovitis**. Isolated intra-articular inflammation commonly occurs following external head and neck trauma. Manifestations include discreet preauricular tenderness that may be accompanied by trismus and an inability to occlude one's teeth. The source of the inflammation is trauma to the retrodiskal tissue, presumably from sudden compression (condyle impaction) or tensile forces (stretching), resulting in intra-articular edema. Disk displacement refers to the anterior and medial displacement of the disk secondary to tearing or stretching of the disk-hard tissue attachments. Most commonly, the injury occurs in either the retrodiskal tissue or in the lateral condylar pole attachment. The disk is anteriorly and medially displaced because of the directional pull of the lateral pterygoid muscle. This mechanical displacement is preceded by structural changes in the disk that predispose the disk to injury. For example, it appears that morphologic changes in the disk impair the disk's ability to maintain its relationship to the condyle during mandibular movement. The morphologic changes create incoordination between the condyle and the disk, and set the stage for a stretching or tearing injury to the disk attachments. Also, recent research on cell mediators within the joints suggests that intra-articular injury and the release of inflammatory mediators may impair the host's adaptive response by altering tissue fiber type. The resulting fiber type is less capable of withstanding intra-articular forces, thus, predisposing the host to further injury or perpetuating an existing injury. It is this author's opinion that our present mechanical disease concepts reflect the superficiality of our pathophysiologic concepts. These tenets are easy to grasp, but fail to accurately segregate TMD patients from normal patients, and cannot explain adaptation differences between patients. The research on inflammatory mediators and their effect on tissue types appears to possess greater pathophysiologic promise.

The two types of disk displacement include **disk displacement with reduction (DDWR)** and **disk displacement without reduction (DDNR)**, which are collectively referred to as **Internal Derangement**. These two disease entities are illustrated in Figures 9-6 and 7. Figure 9-5 shows the normal disk-condyle relationship during jaw opening. With teeth together, the disk is positioned anterior-superiorly to the condyle. The disk translates with the condyle on opening and simultaneously rotates posteriorly, placing the disk superior to the condylar head with maximal opening. Figure 9-6 illustrates disk displacement with reduction, in which the disk is anterior (and medial) to the condylar head in the closed mouth position. At some point during the opening, the disk is recaptured producing a popping or clicking sound that is usually palpable or audible on clinical examination. The point in the opening at which the disk is recaptured reflects the degree of disk displacement, whereby, the later the pop, the greater the degree of disk displacement. On closing, the disk remains recaptured and often displaces at the very end of closing when the teeth are nearly together. Therefore, a closing pop is frequently undetectable. When present, the closing pop usually occurs with the mouth more closed than with the opening pop. It is important to understand that in DDWR, the patient is functioning on the retrodiskal tissue prior to the opening pop and after the closing pop occurs. Locking, either open or closed, may accompany DDWR. Because locking is a dysfunctional symptom, some authors segregate DDWR with and without locking, which will also be a part of this classification scheme. The practitioner should keep in mind that DDWR with locking may represent a transitional stage between DDWR and DDNR, and as such, the presence of locking may signal an unstable DDWR with the potential to degenerate. The incidence of Internal Derangement, either DDWR or DDNR is reported to be 30% of all TMD patients.

The singular difference between DDWR and DDNR is that the disk is not recaptured with DDNR. As such, DDNR is, in essence, a closed lock. Figure 9-7 shows that the disk is anteriorly displaced in the closed mouth position and that the disk remains displaced with maximal opening. The inability to reduce the disk results from the severity of the disk displacement and, perhaps, from hypertrophy of the posterior band or the presence of adhesions. Acutely, DDNR is manifested by trismus, ipsilateral deviation and pain; in contrast, chronically, the disk attachments are stretched or torn with continued function, affording an improvement in all signs and symptoms. Chronic DDNR is perhaps the most difficult TMD diagnosis since the trismus and deviation are often mild and difficult to perceive. The associated pain is typically preauricular and elicited only by hard function or extended mandibular movement. As such, historical information and imaging are more important for the accurate diagnosis of chronic DDNR than with any other TM Disorder. In DDNR the patient is constantly functioning on the retrodiskal tissue rather than on the disk.

Degenerative joint disease (DJD) refers to intra-articular osteoarthritis that most commonly results from chronic joint loading. The occurrence of DJD is uncommon, accounting for 20% of all TMD clinic cases. Chronic bruxism is the most likely contributor, however, severe or repeated external joint trauma can be important in a smaller percentage of cases. Patients are generally older (> 40 years old) and the problem tends to be unilateral (or joint specific). The degenerative changes include soft tissue alterations in the disk such as a change in collagen type, calcifications and perforations (Figure 9-8). Associated hard tissue changes in the eminence and condyle can include erosion, sclerosis, and osteophyte formation. Adaptive remodeling of the joint is not pathologic and must be distinguished from these maladaptive, degenerative changes. Also, evidence of DJD is expected with aging, therefore, the diagnosis of degenerative joint disease is reserved for degenerative changes that are uncharacteristic for the age of the patient. For example, radiographic evidence of mild degenerative changes would only be significant on a young patient. DJD is closely associated with DDNR because DJD rarely occurs in the absence of DDNR. Thus, it can be accurately assumed that patients manifesting clinical signs and symptoms of DJD will have DDNR. Clinical manifestations of DJD include crepitus, (usually) episodic trismus, ipsilateral deviation and intra-articular pain. As with arthritic conditions elsewhere in the body, TMJ DJD is associated with episodic flare-ups in which patients experience pain and dysfunction. A positive history of osteoarthritis is important in the diagnosis of these patients.

In contrast to DJD, erosive forms of arthritis, of which rheumatoid arthritis (RA) is the most common, may also occur in the TMJs. However, this form of arthritis is very uncommon compared to DJD. Rheumatoid arthritis is a systemic, inflammatory form of arthritis that is associated with erosive hard tissue lesions. Joint sounds and the hard and soft tissue lesions previously described for DJD, also characterize RA. Clinically, this disease is more common in younger patients, is more frequently bilateral and tends to affect multiple joints. A significant clinical finding is the tendency for occlusal changes with RA. Erosion of the condylar head shortens the height of the condyle and ramus, allowing the teeth on the affected side to contact prior to the teeth on the opposing arch. Therefore, a unilateral erosive lesion will produce an occlusion that has a posterior premature tooth contact ipsilaterally, and an open bite elsewhere. Bilateral erosive lesions, which are more common with erosive forms of arthritis, result in an anterior open bite with bilateral posterior premature tooth contacts. One clue that the observed occlusal changes are acquired and not congenital or developmental is wear patterns on teeth that no longer occlude. Typically, these patients have not experienced movement of their teeth and the open bite is solely the result of the rheumatologic disease. Dental models taken on such patients can be articulated to closely replicate the original occlusion. This finding is also true of patients whose occlusal changes are secondary to intra-articular tumors, but is uncommon in patients whose occlusal changes result from iatrogenic splint wear. The latter have typically suffered tooth movement in addition to musculoskeletal changes and, therefore, their dental models cannot be accurately articulated. Practitioners should be aware of these occlusal findings in patients diagnosed with rheumatoid arthritis and when evaluating patients with open bites, especially when the open bite appears to be changing or progressing. Some classification schemes divide the DJD patients into symptomatic and asymptomatic subgroups; however, for the purpose of this text, we will consider all DJD patients encountered in the acute care setting as symptomatic.

Central to the pathophysiologic concept of TMD for both intra-articular and extra-articular disorders is inflammation. The presence of myositis has been supported by thermographic and spectrographic findings in humans, and by palpation tenderness noted on clinical examination. However, all of the aforementioned evidence is indirect and there is no direct evidence of inflammation being the cause of myalgia. Therefore, although the role of inflammation appears likely, there has been no confirmation of the relationship between inflammation and myalgia. Consequently, the extra-articular disorder is termed myalgia, recognizing the lack of understanding regarding the underlying pathophysiology.

Intra-articularly, inflammation, disk displacement, adhesions and alterations in cellular mediators have all been promoted as agents in the pathophysiology of capsulitis, internal derangement and DJD. Unlike the extra-articular disorders, many of these changes have been substantiated in animal models and in humans, both directly via TMJ surgery and at autopsy, and indirectly by magnetic resonance imaging (MRI). Inflammation and disk displacement were once considered the mediators of intra-articular disease until the development of arthroscopy. Subsequently, the pathophysiologic focus shifted to adhesions. Pathophysiologic thoughts prior to this time had been mechanical, focusing on disk position to explain the presence of disease. However, the incidence of displaced disks in asymptomatic populations and in TMD patients following successful treatments has questioned this simplistic concept of disease. Although adhesions appear to play a role in the pathophysiology of some TMD patients, the inconsistency with which adhesions are identified questions their role in the disease process of most TMD patients. Presently, significant attention is being paid to the role of inflammatory mediators on disease development and progression. Preliminary findings suggest that this line of investigation may lead to a more consistent explanation of intra-articular diseases.

For many TMD patients the disease is cyclical, marked by recurrences and remissions over one's lifetime. However, regarding disease progression, it appears that TMD is a self-limiting disorder for most patients, subject to spontaneous remissions and uncommonly associated with progressive degeneration. Therefore, assumptions that joint clicking in the absence of pain or dysfunction will progress to a painful joint, or that disk displacement with reduction will progress to disk displacement without reduction, or that disk displacement without reduction will progress to degenerative joint disease are unsupported. It does appear, however, that a small percentage of patients with DDWR do progress to DDNR and that a small percentage of DDNR patients develop DJD. Unfortunately, we are presently unable to segregate those patients who adapt from

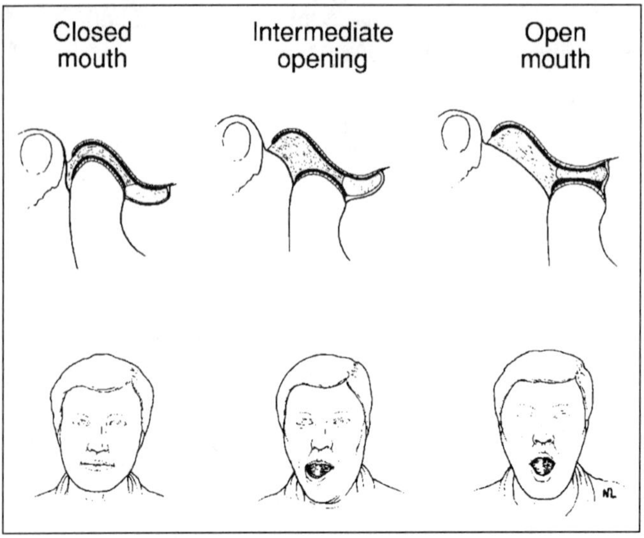

Figure 9-6: Disk Displacement With Reduction (DDWR). Closed Mouth - disk is displaced anterior to the condyle. Intermediate Opening - disk remains anterior causing ipsilateral deviation until clicking occurs. Open Mouth - disk has been recaptured following click and no deviation is observed.

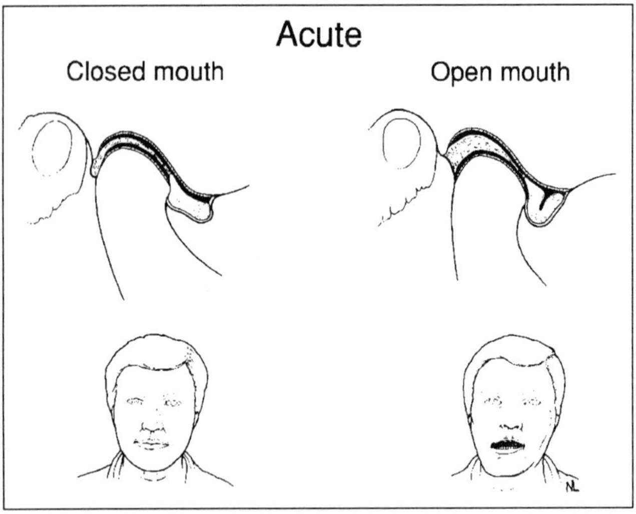

Figure 9-7a: Disk Displacement Without Reduction - Acute Injury. Closed Mouth - disk is displaced anterior to the condyle and shows some morphologic changes (thickened posterior band). Open Mouth - disk remains anteriorly displaced causing marked ipsilateral deviation and trismus.

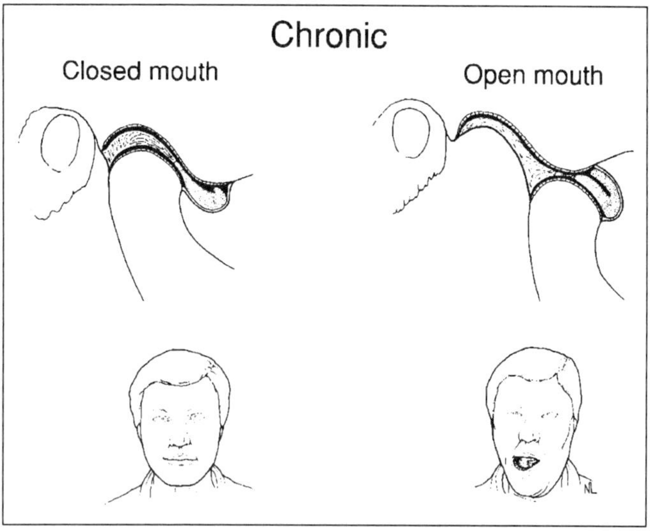

Figure 9-7b: Disk Displacement Without Reduction - Chronic Injury. Closed Mouth - disk is displaced anterior to the condyle and shows some morphologic changes (thinning posterior band). Open Mouth - disk remains anteriorly displaced, associated with subtle trismus and ipsilateral deviation.

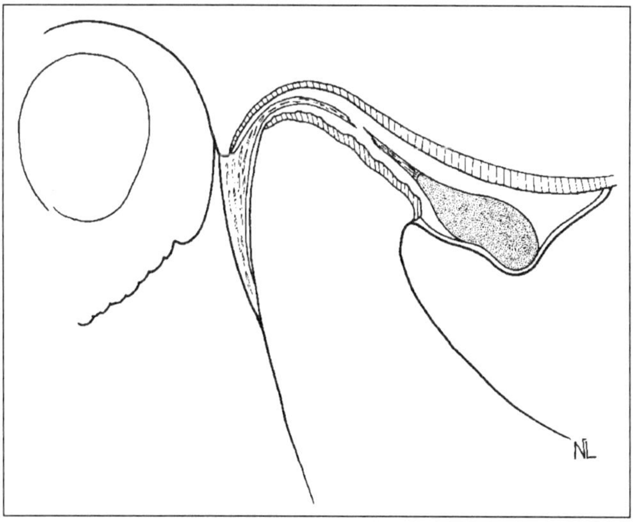

Figure 9-8: Degenerative Joint Disease (DJD). The degenerative changes illustrated include a thickening of the cortical bone on the condyle and articular eminence (eburnation or sclerosis), erosion of the condylar head with anterior beaking, flattening of the articular eminence, morphologic distortion of the disk and perforation of the retrodiskal tissue.

those prone to disease progression. Similarly, it is not possible to accurately predict the occurrence of TMD or to identify patients at risk for disease development. Therefore, efforts aimed at disease prevention cannot be endorsed at this time.

A final point to be contemplated concerns the role of **host adaptation** in disease development and progression. As is true of many diseases, there is an obvious discrepancy between objective findings and symptoms in TMD. In addition, discrepancies exist between etiologic factors and the presence of disease. Some patients have multiple etiologic factors or behaviors and yet are free of disease. An example is the asymptomatic patient with severe bruxism and numerous stressors. In contrast, symptomatic patients with minimal etiologic factors and objective findings offer a second discrepancy. A third example is the asymptomatic patient with radiographic evidence of severe DJD and trismus. Certainly, some of these disparities can be attributed to current misconceptions regarding signs of disease, pathophysiology and etiologic factors. However, some part of the discrepancy is the result of differences in host adaptation or susceptibility. A patient who is less susceptible or more adaptive, may possess a higher pain reaction threshold, better joint remodeling capacity, improved muscle fatigability (secondary to variances in muscle fiber make-up) and be more capable of balancing occlusal loads. Although all of these suggestions are theoretical, some of these factors may account for the obvious discrepancies between signs and symptoms, etiologic factors and disease occurrence.

A final intra-articular disease that is not considered a TM disorder, but should be contemplated, are **tumors** within the TMJ. Such tumors are uncommon and are generally benign. The most common examples of benign TMJ tumors include chondromas, osteomas and osteochondromas involving either the condylar head or the mandibular fossa. Rarely, malignant tumors have been reported of which osteosarcomas are the most common. Intra-articular tumors should be investigated whenever patients report progressive changes in their bites. The presence of occlusal changes such as open bites, arch-long crossbites as well as discrepancies between dental and facial midlines should heighten this suspicion. Unilateral tumors are associated with an ipsilateral open bite, contralateral shifting of the mandibular midline, a contralateral crossbite and an ipsilateral scissors bite. Contralateral deviation of the jaw can also be noted on gross head and neck examination. The presence of open bites and crossbites are observed with rapidly growing tumors, while tooth movement may compensate in slower growing lesions, thereby, masking these findings. However, even with slow growing tumors, the contralateral deviation should be visible. Confirmation will require TMJ imaging that can begin with simple plane films (e.g., panoramic, transcranial, lateral cephalograms, tomography and lateral obliques) in the acute care setting, followed by more detailed images (e.g., linear tomography, computerized tomography and magnetic resonance) after patient referral.

IV. ETIOLOGIES

Trauma, malocclusion, stress and bruxism are the most commonly proposed causes for TMD. **Malocclusion**, or the malalignment of the teeth, has been intensely scrutinized as a cause of TMD over the past fifty years. However, to date, neither the presence of various malocclusions nor their combination has been able to accurately distinguish patients from non-patients. These malocclusions or combinations of malocclusions exist in similar frequencies in both populations (TMD and non-TMD). Also, malocclusion as an etiology has never been able to show a cause and effect relationship to bruxism or been compatible with the cyclic, dynamic nature of the disorder. Because of these paramount discrepancies, malocclusion is not presently considered a primary etiologic factor in the development of TMD. As was suggested in the previous section, occlusion may play a role in defining the host's adaptive capabilities to bruxism, and thus be a secondary factor. However, even this suggestion is presumptive given the lack of scientific support. The aforementioned explanation excludes the role of iatrogenic dentistry as a cause of TMD or facial pain. It is accepted that acute, unbalanced occlusal changes from dental restorations (e.g., high fillings or crowns) can result in odontogenic pain and at times, TMD complaints. This problem is discussed in Chapter 1 and accounts for a small portion of TMD patients.

Another proposed etiology for TMD is **external trauma** secondary to events that place sudden or prolonged pressure on the mandible. Examples include a MVA, fisticuffs, extended dental appointments, mandibular tooth extractions and endotracheal intubation. The research to support this proposed etiology is based on retrospective case reports that generally fail to require any temporal relationship between the proposed traumatic event and the ensuing TMD complaints. As such, this body of literature assumes that a history of facial or head and neck trauma, irrespective of its relationship to the onset of TMD signs and symptoms, is etiologic. This line of thinking is without merit and provides whimsical support for trauma-related litigation. It is reasonable to assume that etiologically-related trauma would produce TMD signs and symptoms immediately, rather than weeks to months later, as this close relationship characterizes trauma-related musculoskeletal injuries in general. At present there is no creditable, pathophysiologic explanation for delayed manifestations. A recent study by Heise et al. examined a large group of MVA (whiplash) subjects and followed them one year post head and neck trauma. The authors found that TMJ pain or joint sounds occurred in less than 15% of the subjects and this prevalence decreased over a one year follow-up period. The presence of radiographic evidence of cervical-skeletal injury did not increase the likelihood of TMD. Therefore, the study showed that the chance of TMD developing following a whiplash-type injury was extremely low and that the resultant TMD signs and symptoms improved over time in most subjects. Epidemiologic studies have also found that head and neck trauma histories are not significantly different between TMD and normal patients. Furthermore, most TMD complaints do not follow physically traumatic events, as the majority of patients are unable to determine a cause for their problem on clinical examination. Therefore, it appears that external trauma is an uncommon and overstated cause of TMD. However, recognizing that external trauma is a possible cause of TMD, special attention should be paid to recording TMJ signs and symptoms and to performing a head and neck examination on patientsinvolved in MVAs or who have suffered direct head and neck trauma. For example, signs and symptoms of TMJ capsulitis would be expected following a blow to the mandible. These signs and symptoms often resemble those of a subcondylar fracture and distinguishing the two is essential for an accurate diagnosis. Because TMJ trauma, especially of the "whiplash variety", is frequently associated with litigation, it is equally important to record the absence of TMD signs and symptoms by signifying "TMD negative". This recommendation also applies to complaints of back and neck pain in patients who suffer head and neck trauma, which represents a more ubiquitous source of litigation. These entries can assist in determining the veracity of a patient's allegations at a later date.

A final proposed cause for TMD is the clenching or grinding of one's teeth, termed **bruxism**. Bruxism is a parafunctional behavior that is usually unconscious and most commonly occurs nocturnally, however, diurnal activity is also observed. This behavior appears to be mediated by the central nervous system, although the pathophysiologic pathways have not been determined. A relationship between nocturnal bruxism and sleep behavior has also been reported. Initially, bruxism was thought to occur during REM sleep, however, more recent research suggests that this motor outburst occurs during the lightening of sleep. These findings define bruxism as part of an "arousal reaction" that occurs when patients go from a deeper to a lighter sleep stage. This lightening of sleep is accompanied by an increase in heart rate, vasoconstriction and increased EMG activity. Clinical research has shown that stress/anxiety can initiate or exacerbate bruxism activity. This relationship, coupled with the psychological profile of TMD patients, the cyclic nature of the disorder and the success of diverse therapeutic approaches, support the role of stress-related bruxism in the disorder's etiology. Of all the potential etiologic factors previously discussed, bruxism/ stress is the most compelling because it can explain the disease process

Table 9-3: Diagnosing TMD

Screening Examination- conduct on all patients

History - ask questions to determine the presence of TMD pain and dysfunction such as:
- Do you experience pain or difficulty opening your mouth?
- Does your jaw ever get stuck?
- Do you have difficulty or pain with eating, talking or yawning?
- Do your jaws feel stiff or sore?
- Have you noticed a recent change in your bite?
- Have you been previously diagnosed or treated for a TMD problem?

Head and Neck Exam:

Observation - look for asymmetries, signs of tension/stress

Palpation Exam - bilaterally palpate head and neck muscles and TMJs; muscles to palpate include the anterior and posterior temporalis, masseters, medial pterygoids, suprahyoids, cervical neck muscles, sternocleidomastoids and trapezius

Joint Sounds - palpate the TMJs during opening and closing both preauricularly and endaurally; use a stethoscope if sounds are faint or light crepitus is suspected

Range of Motion - measure vertical opening

Screening Radiographs:
panoramic or transcranial radiograph if warranted by signs and symptoms

Diagnosis: TMD - negative
TMD - positive; pre-existing or new onset

Comprehensive Examination
-conduct on patients with positive findings on the screening exam; can be performed by the referral general dentist

History:

Chief Complaint (CC)

Past Medical History (PMH) - look for other sources of facial pain (e.g. neuralgias and vascular headaches), other musculoskeletal illnesses (e.g. arthritis and fibromyalgia) and stress related illness (e.g. gastritis, back pain, oral ulcers)

Past Dental History (PDH) - look for odontogenic sources of pain and occlusal changes

History of Present Illness (HPI) - examine each sign and symptom for onset, duration, frequency, timing, quality; look for relationships between the complaints and associated manifestations; inquire about potential etiologic factors regarding onset and exacerbations and record the efficacy of past treatments

Psychiatric History (PH) - explore past treatments for anxiety/stress or psychiatric illnesses; specifically question the patient about life stressors such as job, marriage, relationships, school, deaths, illnesses, children and finances; signs and symptoms of depression should be noted; adjunctive tests such as the TMJ Scale, Impath or the SCL 90 may be helpful

Bruxism - inquire about jaw stiffness and soreness or pain on wakening, sleep disruption, awareness of sleep partner, daytime awareness

Locking - distinguish open from closed; note onset, frequency and initiation

Trismus - does opening seem diminished and when did patient first notice this

Sleep Disruption - explore difficulty getting to or staying asleep; what awakens patient; onset and frequency

Systemic Signs and Symptoms - systemic myalgia and arthralgia suggesting a systemic rheumatologic disorder

Dietary Changes - question about ability to chew hard and chewy foods and foods requiring wide opening; diet should be modified with a significant problem

Treatment Expectations - note the realism of the patient's desires

Clinical Examination:

Observation - look for asymmetries, signs of tension/stress

Palpation Exam - bilaterally palpate head and neck muscles and TMJs; muscles to palpate included the anterior and posterior temporalis, masseters, medial pterygoids, suprahyoids, cervical neck muscles, sternocleidomastoids and trapezius

Joint Sounds - palpate the TMJs during opening and closing both preauricularly and endaurally; use a stethoscope if sounds are faint or light crepitus is suspected

Range of Motion - measure vertical opening and lateral movements; note if accompanied by pain, deviation or deflection

Occlusion - look for gross occlusal changes such as open bites, skeletal distortions and attrition

Screening Radiographs:

Panoramic or transcranial radiograph if warranted by signs and symptoms in most patients with the least incongruities. However, recognizing that bruxism/stress may explain the disease in the largest population of patients, TMD is presently considered to have a multifactorial etiology, which includes trauma and occlusion (as a secondary factor). Some authors consider the cause of TMD to be idiopathic, a reflection of the theoretical and imprecise nature of our present understanding. From a scientific standpoint, this is an appropriate conclusion.

V. DIAGNOSIS

TMD is essentially defined by patient self-report, as there are no signs that define the presence of this disorder in the absence of pain and/dysfunction (Dysfunction is defined as any activity limitations that involve mandibular movement, such as eating, kissing and yawning). For example, if a patient presents with crepitus and slight trismus, but has no pain or functional limitations, the patient is not suffering from TMD. The argument can be made that this patient has TMD that is minimally symptomatic, however, the diagnosis of TMD based solely on objective findings promotes overdiagnosis and treatment. Because our present level of understanding is primitive, the suggested demeanor more accurately reflects our lack of sophistication and, thereby, protects the patient. Certainly, this approach will need to be modified as the sophistication of our knowledge improves.

Diagnosis is comprised of a history, a clinical examination and, at times, imaging. The history is considered the most essential component because of the need to rely on subjective data to determine the presence of TMD and its classification. Following a thorough history, the clinical examination confirms the historical findings. An abbreviated **screening examination** is recommended to determine the presence of a TM disorder when initially evaluating a patient (Table 9-3). If positive findings exist, a thorough comprehensive examination is indicated (Table 9-3). In the screening examination, the history should consist of a few simple questions that assess the presence of pain and dysfunction. For a positive diagnosis, the investigation should determine whether the pain is located on the sides of the head (i.e., temporal, pre-auricular and/or masseteric regions). This pain should increase with mandibular movement or with functions such as eating, talking and wide opening. The presence of trismus, joint sounds and locking are also key symptoms to be investigated. Caution is advised if the only positive findings are joint sounds. Although the incidence of joint sounds is significantly higher in the TMD population compared to normal patients, the correlation of joint sounds with disease is weaker than with other symptoms. This is because joint sounds appear to be compatible with health, existing without other signs and symptoms in 15-30% of the normal population. Therefore, the presence of joint sounds should be in combination with other symptoms to support a positive diagnosis.

The screening history should be followed by a brief clinical examination that is comprised of a palpation examination for muscle/joint tenderness and joint sounds, a range of motion examination, and when indicated, a screening radiograph. Muscle and joint palpation should be conducted bimanually with the practitioner standing in front of the patient. Two to four pounds of pressure is recommended to determine the presence of pain or discomfort. Muscles to be palpated include the temporalis (anterior and posterior bellies), the masseters, the medial pterygoids, the sternocleidomastoids, the suprahyoids (floor of the mouth), the cervical neck muscles (splenius capitus and semispinalis capitus) and the trapezius muscles. The temporomandibular joints should be palpated preauricularly and endaurally against the anterior wall of the external auditory meatus. The presence of joint sounds should be evaluated by preauricular and endaural palpation, while having the patient open and close through a full range of vertical opening. Practitioners should ensure that patients are opening maximally and closing with their teeth opposed, as patients may limit their range of motion to avoid pain or joint sounds. The type of joint sound (clicking or crepitus) should be noted, as well as when the sound occurs during the opening and closing movement. The presence of clicking should be determined by palpation alone and the practitioner is discouraged from over-interpretation of sounds. For example, using a stethoscope to detect clicking will result in a twofold increase in the incidence rates and it is unclear whether these additional joint sounds represent pathological or incidental findings. The amplification of joint sounds is appropriate when degenerative changes are suspected and no joint sounds are audible. In such cases, a stethoscope can be used to elicit the presence of light grating. The range of motion examination should record the vertical opening (maximal opening) in millimeters between the incisal edges of the front teeth. Generally, a vertical opening less than 35-40 millimeters can be considered trismus. This objective finding can be combined with the patient's subjective perception in order to diagnose the presence of trismus.

A screening TMJ image is intended to provide visualization of the intra-articular hard tissues. As such, screening radiographs are recommended only when ruling out an intra-articular tumor, TMJ fracture, severe degenerative disease or idiopathic intra-articular disease. The need for imaging is determined by the presence of suggestive clinical findings, such as progressive lateral skeletal deviations and open bites, severe crepitation and trismus. Preferred screening radiographs include panoramic, transcranial/ transpharyngeal, and lateral oblique radiographs. Although, it is recognized that these images are distorted, cortical outlines of the hard tissues are clearly identifiable. Linear and computerized tomography as well as magnetic resonance imaging can provide more precise hard tissue analysis and allow visualization of disk tissue (CT and MRI only). However, the cost of these images prohibits their use as screening films.

On a **comprehensive examination**, the **history** is comprised of a chief complaint, a past medical history, a past dental history, a history of present illness and a brief psychological history. The chief complaint provides incite into the patient's most bothersome symptom, which can be important in selecting and monitoring a treatment modality. The importance of the past medical history is its incite into underlying illnesses that can directly or indirectly affect a TMD problem. Examples include musculoskeletal illnesses such as arthritis, fibromyalgia and low back pain, and stress-related illness such as gastritis, vascular headaches and oral ulcerations. The past dental history principally identifies potential, although uncommon etiologic factors such as long dental appointments and third molar extractions. The past dental history is also important in evaluating odontogenic and occlusal factors in disease onset and exacerbations. The history of present illness should evaluate the development of the disorder, the effectiveness of previous treatments and the characteristics of each sign and symptom. Information concerning disease development should include the onset, relief and exacerbation of signs and symptoms. Potential etiologic factors (external trauma, stress and bruxism) should be analyzed for their relationship to disease onset and episodes of relief or exacerbation. Queries concerning external trauma should include motor vehicle accidents, falls, blows to the face, long dental appointments, mandibular extractions and general anesthetic intubations. The analysis of stress should include major life stressors such as job, school, marriage, personal relationships, family, children, finances and family deaths. It is important to conduct the examination in a private environment with minimal distractions because of the personal nature of these questions. Symptoms of depression such as aberrant sleep behavior, changes in dietary habits, significant weight fluctuations and malaise should be recognized. Various psychological instruments such as the TMJ Scale, Impath, or the SCL 90 may be used to augment and intensify the psychological examination.

Nocturnal bruxism can be evaluated by asking about sleep partner corroboration of tooth grinding, sleep disruption because of facial pain and tenseness/soreness of facial muscles upon wakening (or increased pain in the morning). The diagnosis of diurnal bruxism depends on patient awareness and more grossly on the presence of diurnal pain patterns. The relative history of signs and symptoms should be explored to determine their relatedness and to reveal unrecognized diagnostic constellations or patterns. For example, it is especially important to determine the relationship of joint sounds or neck pain to facial pain since these symptoms are commonly unrelated. Temporally distinct and distant onsets or disjointed fluctuations suggests that these complaints represent independent problems. Past treatments should be evaluated for their efficacy, which can provide guidance in choosing a combination of therapeutic modalities. This information can also assist the practitioner in identifying chronic pain patients and in determining if you can help the patient. Each symptom should be characterized by anatomic location, onset, intensity, frequency, duration and associated manifestations. Headaches, facial pain, ear pain, neck and shoulder pain, locking and trismus are symptoms to be evaluated in this manner. This information not only assists in the diagnosis, but also provides a benchmark for future comparisons over time to assess patient progress. When investigating headaches, questions concerning signs and symptoms specific to vascular headaches and neuralgias should be posed to ascertain the presence of other types of headaches. Similarly, questions concerning pain with neck movement can reveal a coexisting cervical disorder. Dysfunctional signs and symptoms (i.e., trismus, locking and restrictions in mandibular movement and diet) deserve special attention because of their importance in defining TMD and their impact on treatment. The presence of systemic musculoskeletal signs and symptoms should be evaluated to uncover undiagnosed arthritis and fibromyalgia. Finally, it is important to determine the patient's treatment expectations to ensure that these desires are therapeutically attainable.

The **clinical examination** is comprised of observation, a muscle and joint palpation exam, a range of motion examination and an occlusal examination. Observation involves visual inspection of the head and neck for asymmetries and signs of stress/tension. An asymmetrical appearance (i.e., deviation of the mandible to one side) can be the initial clue to either a developmental or traumatic disturbance of condylar growth (condylar hyperplasia or hypoplasia) or to an intra-articular tumor. Signs of stress to recognize include anxious behaviors such as a furrowed brow, hand wringing, muscle rigidity and a depressed or fatigued appearance.

Muscle and joint palpation was previously described under the screening examination. The range of motion examination can include lateral movements in addition to vertical opening measurements. Lateral movement is evaluated by having the patient move their mandible as far laterally as possible and measuring the distance between maxillary and mandibular dental midlines. This measurement should be corrected for midline discrepancies when the teeth are maximally occluded. Normal lateral movement is 6-12 mm. The occlusal examination should note the number of missing teeth, the presence of dental disease and attrition. Dental disease may represent an additional source of facial pain, while attrition is consistent with past or present tooth grinding activity.

Imaging can consist of the screening films previously suggested on the screening examination, panoramic and transcranial radiographs (Figure 9-9). Although these films are recommended, screening radiographs are not cost-effective because of the rare occurrence of intra-articular tumors and the gross nature of the information provided. Therefore, these images are only recommended when a significant intra-articular disorder involving the hard tissue is suspected, such as degenerative joint disease or intra-articular tumors. This suspicion can arise from evidence of skeletal asymmetries or occlusal changes such as new or progressive open bites and/or crossbites. When more detailed hard tissue images are needed, linear or computerized tomograms are appropriate. When intra-articular soft tissue images are

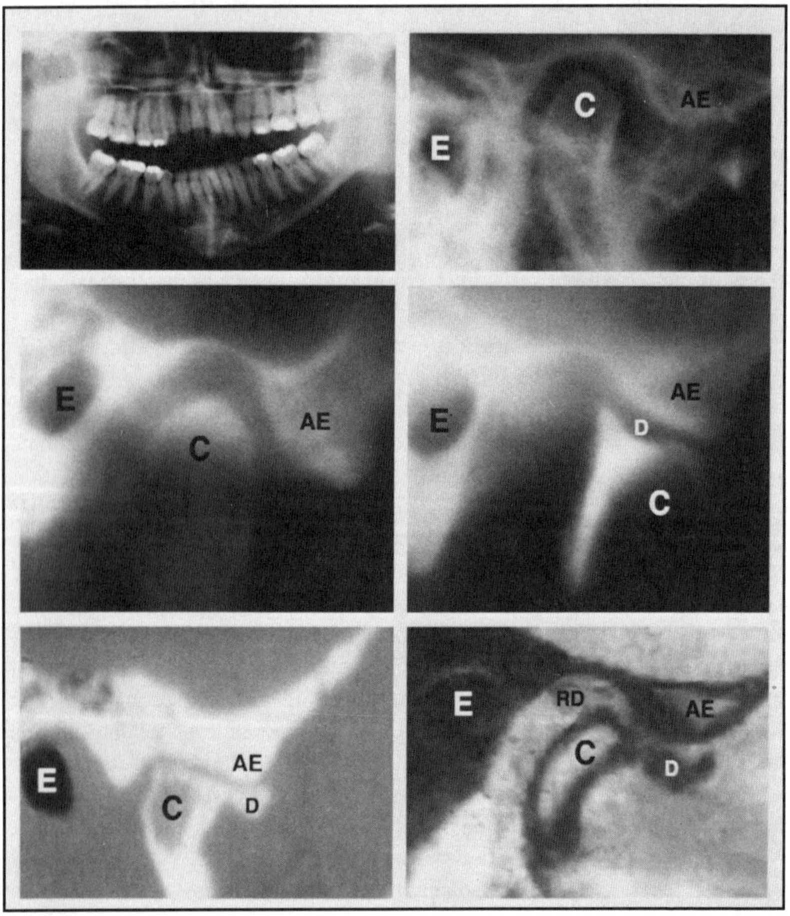

Figure 9-9: TMJ Imaging. Upper left - panoramic radiograph, Upper right - transcranial radiograph, Middle left - tomogram, Middle right - arthrogram, Bottom left - computerized tomogram, Bottom right - magnetic resonance image. AE - Articular eminence. C - condyle. D - disk. E - ear. RD - retrodiskal tissue.

desired (i.e., with disk displacement or degenerative joint disease), magnetic resonance imaging, arthrograms or computerized tomography can be used. These images are usually reserved to confirm the presence of the aforementioned intra-articular problems following the failure of nonsurgical therapies and prior to performing TMJ surgery. MRIs accurately depict soft tissues, but are less sensitive to hard tissue disease. Although MRIs are expensive, their accuracy and minimal invasiveness make them a preferred method of TMJ imaging for disk displacements. Computerized tomography affords an accurate hard tissue assessment and a less detailed soft tissue analysis. As such, they are indicated for disk displacements and degenerative disease. Arthrography is an invasive method of intra-articular imaging that requires the injection of radio-opaque iodine into the joint space (usually the superior joint space) followed by linear tomography. Arthrograms are the only form of TMJ imaging that will accurately depict perforations of the disk or retrodiskal tissues. The dye reveals the outline of the soft tissues, but the disk itself is not visible. The position of the disk is inferred by the indentations on the dye material during opening. The tomography also affords an accurate hard tissue evaluation. Although this technique is the least expensive, the invasiveness has limited its use since the advent of MRIs and CTs.

In summary, the diagnosis is based on the culmination of historical, clinical and imaging results. Sophisticated diagnostic adjuncts such as electromyography, sonography and kinesiography are not presently recommended. This advice is based on the inability of these diagnostic tests to accurately distinguish TMD patients from normal patients, and the inability of these tests to improve the diagnostic accuracy of the standard history and clinical examination. Because of this, the validity of these diagnostic adjuncts is unsupported scientifically.

In the acute care setting, all patients who complain of head and/or neck pain, or who suffer direct or indirect head and neck trauma, should receive a screening TMD examination (Indirect trauma refers to jolting body forces that do not involve direct impact to the head and neck region). Positive findings should be noted, palliative treatment rendered (discussed in next section) and the patient referred to a general dentist who has expertise in the management of TMD. At a minimum, recognizing the presence of a TM Disorder is essential for health care providers in this setting. If the expertise and time exists, a comprehensive examination and more definitive therapy is encouraged in the acute care environment.

VI. TREATMENT

TMD therapy can be divided into nonsurgical and surgical methods. Recognizing the behavioral component (bruxism and stress) of T-M Disorders and the possibility of disease recurrence, TMD therapy should attempt to educate patients regarding the nature of the disease and should provide patients with an effective method of self-treatment. In the acute care setting, only nonsurgical therapy is indicated (Table 9-4). These treatments can include patient education, pharmacotherapy, physical therapy, orthotic therapy and behavioral therapy.

Table 9-4: TMD Treatments

Treatment	Indications
Nonsurgical	
Patient Education	-all patients; is the foundation for all treatments
Pharmacotherapy	
-NSAIDS	-all patients; especially with intra-articular inflammation, DJD and diurnal pain patterns
-Muscle Relaxants	-nocturnal bruxism, sleep disruption
-TCAs	-nocturnal bruxism, sleep disruption
Orthotic	
-Flat Plane	-bruxism; most patients
-Anterior Repositioning	-not recommended
Physical Therapy	-trismus; acute DDNR; following TMJ surgery
Behavioral Therapy	
-Stress Management	-significant stressors or anxiety; many patients and most chronic pain patients
-Psychotherapy	-psychopathology beyond stress/anxiety
Surgical	
Arthrocentesis	-acute DDNR
Arthroscopy or Open Joint Surgery	-failure of nonsurgical therapies -intractable residual pain -major source of pain is intra-articular -intra-articular disorder confirmed by imaging -refractory bruxism and stress have been addressed

Patient education is essential to the success of all other forms of therapy, underscoring the importance of patient understanding to therapeutic outcome. Patient education should include an overview of the disease with special reference to the tissues affected (musculoskeletal disease), potential etiologic factors (stress, bruxism and trauma) and their affect on disease onset and recurrence. Patients should also understand the dynamic nature of the disease, treatment options (with special emphasis on self-treatment) and prognosis.

Pharmacotherapy generally consists of anti-inflammatory drugs, muscle relaxants and agents intended to improve sleep quality. Pharmacologic agents are commonly used only in the acute period; however, at times chronic dosing is necessary. Nonsteroidal anti-inflammatory drugs (NSAIDs) are indicated for the treatment of inflammatory musculoskeletal disorders and, therefore, are administered to most TMD patients. These drugs inhibit the conversion of arachadonic acid to prostaglandin by blocking the essential enzyme, cyclooxygenase. NSAIDs have both analgesic and anti-inflammatory actions. The analgesic activities are seen with a single dose, while the anti-inflammatory actions require approximately one week of dosing to achieve therapeutic blood levels. Although these agents have proven efficacy in the treatment of systemic musculoskeletal disorders (i.e., arthritidies, SLE and fibromyalgia), recent research findings have questioned the efficacy of these agents in the treatment of TMD. The studies show little to no benefit over placebo, suggesting a dissimilar pathophysiology between TMD and other musculoskeletal disorders. This finding supports the pathophysiologic process proposed by the recent TMJ cellular mediator research.

Over-the-counter agents such as aspirin and ibuprofen are recommended when patient's finances are limited. Otherwise, agents capable of single and twice a day dosing are preferred to improve patient compliance. Such agents include piroxicam, diflunisal, nabumetone, diclofenac, and anaprox DS, among others (Table 9-5). Because gastrointestinal disturbance

Table 9-5: Drugs Used in the Treatment of TMD

Drugs	Max. Recc. Dose	Cost/Day
Simple NSAIDs and Analgesics		
Acetominophen (Tylenol)	1 gm q6h	.10
Naproxen (Anaprox DS)	550 mg bid	2.00
Aspirin	325-650 mg q6h	.10
Diclofenac (Voltaren)	75 mg bid	2.00
Diflunisal (Dolobid)	500 mg bid	2.00
Fluorbiprophen (Ansaid)	50-100 mg tid	3.00
Ibuprofen (Motrin)	800 mg q 6 h	.20
Ketoprofen (Orudis)	150-300 tid	2.00
Nabumetone (Relafin)	500 mg bid	1.50
Piroxicam (Feldene)	20 q d or 10 mg bid	2.00
Ketorolac (Toradol)	60 mg IM or 10 mg q6h PO	7.00 or 4.00
Muscle Relaxants and Antianxiety Agents		
Alprazolam (Xanax)	.25-1 mg HS	.40
Diazepam (Valium)	5-10 mg HS	.54
Buspirone (BuSpar)	5 mg TID	2.40
Cyclobenzaprine (Flexeril)	10 mg HS	.68
Clonazapam (Klonopin)	.50-1 mg HS	.68
Baclofen (Lioresal)	10-20 mg HS	.34
Tricyclic Antidepressants (TCAs)		
Amitriptyline (Elavil)	10-50 mg HS	.10
Desipramine (Norpramin)	25-50 mg HS	.61

is the predominant side-effect, NSAIDs should be avoided in patients with gastrointestinal disorders (i.e., gastritis, gastric ulcers, Crone's Disease etc.) and in patients who have manifested sensitivity reactions. Nabumetone and ibuprofen are thought to produce the least G.I. side-effects. Although narcotic analgesics can be effective in the relief of pain, these drugs are not recommended in the treatment of TMD because of the possibility of dependency in a potentially chronic disorder.

Muscle relaxants and/or antianxiety agents are intended to reduce muscle tension and provide overall relaxation effects. None of these agents are direct skeletal muscle relaxants, causing muscle relaxation indirectly from central nervous system depression. Because the major side-effect is drowsiness, it is recommended that these agents only be used at bedtime to improve sleep and decrease nocturnal EMG activity. Patients should be alerted to the possibility of drowsiness upon wakening. Because of this the weekend is often the best time to initially evaluate the agent. It is also recommended to begin with half the maximum dose at bedtime and have the patient double the dose if no effect is noted. This can avoid a negative experience which may preclude the subsequent use of these agents. Scientific studies have shown these agents to be effective in decreasing TMD signs and symptoms and in decreasing EMG activity in approximately 50% or 80% of patients. The main difference between these agents is their duration and site of action. Notable distinctions include alprazolam's short duration of action, clonazepam's effectiveness in decreasing motor output and buspirone's lack of drowsiness. Buspirone's unique quality makes it a preferred agent when diurnal dosing is desired.

In low doses, the tricyclic antidepressants (TCAs) possess analgesic and sleep stabilizing qualities via their inhibitory effects on serotonin and norepinephrine. The recommended doses (10 to 50 mg) are well below the daily antidepressant doses (150 to 200 mg), therefore, depression is not usually affected. TCA's effect on sleep include limiting the number of awakenings, increasing the time spent in deep sleep stages and decreasing the time in REM sleep. Recent research has shown that among TCAs, amitriptyline was the most effective analgesic in the treatment of chronic pain. Scientific support for the use of these agents in the management of TMD patients is minimal, although empirical clinical experience has been positive. These agents are indicated for the long-term management of refractory nocturnal bruxism because TCAs do not possess the addictive side-effect of most muscle relaxants.

Orthotic or splint therapy involves the use of interocclusal appliances to relax masticatory muscles, protect the occlusal tooth surfaces from attrition (bruxism) and/or recapture a displaced disk. Orthotics can be classified as either flat plane or anterior repositioning. **Flat plane splints (FPS)** attempt to relieve the signs and symptoms of bruxism and to protect the teeth from excessive wear (Figure 9-10a). These orthotics

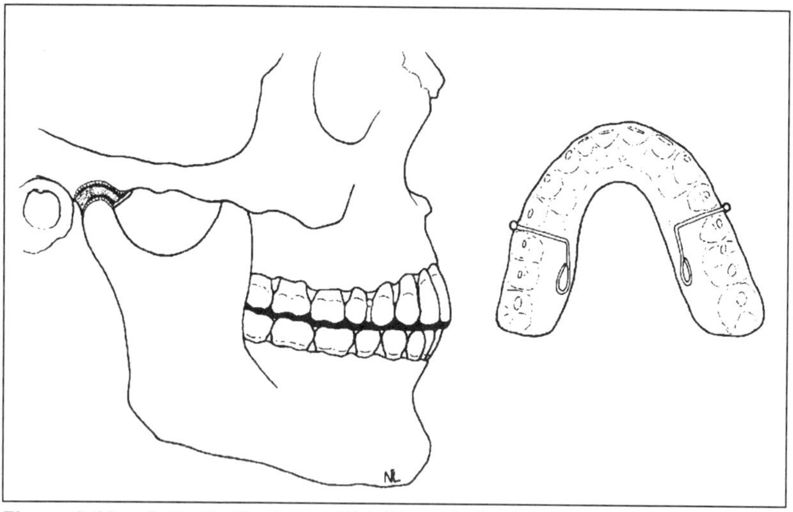

Figure 9-10a: Orthotic Designs. Flat Plane Orthotic. The flat plane orthotic is designed to minimize signs and symptoms from bruxism. The appliance is made of clear acrylic with minimal indentations of opposing teeth in the occlusal surface. Ball clasps are used for retention.

are the most commonly used and are not intended to recapture a displaced disk. The splints can be fabricated over the maxillary or mandibular teeth, and research findings suggest that therapeutic success does not depend on which arch is utilized. Also, the scientific data suggests that the type of occlusal design is not important to the efficacy of the orthotic. For example, partial coverage splints and splints without canine guidance appear to work as well as full coverage splints and splints with canine guidance. Similarly, splints fabricated in centric occlusion are as successful as splints made in centric relation. This data is consistent with the lack of data supporting occlusion as an etiologic factor in TMD. Therefore, it appears that potential mechanisms of orthotic therapy success may be behavioral and/or neuromuscular in nature. It is theorized that splints may remind patients not to clench or grind their teeth during waking hours and that orthotics may alter neuromuscular feedback from the periodontal ligaments during sleep and, thereby, decrease masticatory muscle output. Important aspects of orthotic design include the preference of full coverage, rigid appliances. Clinical findings have shown that partial coverage splints are more likely to result in irreversible tooth movement with chronic, continual wear. Hence, if a patient is not followed regularly or is lost to follow-up, these undesirable consequences may result. Also, research data suggests that partial coverage splints and splints fabricated from soft materials are less effective in improving signs and symptoms than are full coverage splints made of a rigid material.

Initially, flat plane splints are usually worn constantly, except when eating, for patients with nocturnal and diurnal pain patterns. In patients who appear to have either nocturnal or diurnal pain, the pattern of splint wear can be limited to these times. However, because most patients are unaware of bruxism and typically have nocturnal and diurnal pain patterns, constant splint wear is appropriate for most patients as a starting point. The duration of flat plane splint therapy is dependent on patient response and the achievement of therapeutic goals. Therefore, the treatment can be as short as a week or as long as 6 months. Long-term, continuous orthotic therapy is discouraged because the benefits of splint wear appear to wane with chronic use. For example, when patients' residual signs and symptoms fail to show further improvement with orthotic wear, additional splint therapy is not likely to be of benefit. Flat plane splint therapy appears to improve signs and symptoms in approximately 70-90% of all TMD patients, although recent studies suggest that FPS are no more effective than placebo splints. Research has also shown that these splints will reduce the electromyographic activity of masseter and temporalis muscles in approximately 60% of TMD subjects; however, the magnitude of this effect is variable.

Anterior repositioning splint therapy (ARS) is a therapy that can have two distinct intentions. The first is to advance or protrude the mandible and, thereby, allow the condyle to recapture an anteriorly displaced disk. This therapy is only indicated for cases of DDWR, because the disk must be displaced and reducible for recapture to occur. Hence, patients with DDNR are not candidates for this treatment. The therapy involves the placement of an orthotic that is fabricated to hold the mandible in a protruded position, just enough to allow disk recapture. This position is determined by having the patient open and close along the anterior border path (in the most protruded position), followed by retrusion of the mandible until the closing click is noted. The mandible must be maintained anterior to this point (the click) in order to recapture the disk. It is not recommended to protrude the mandible more than 2 to 4 mm beyond intercuspal position, because of the subsequent difficulties encountered with permanent disk retention. The orthotic can be placed on the maxilla or the mandible, and is fabricated with deep indentations and a ramp in order to both guide and retain the mandible in the desired position (Figure 9-10b). Because the intent of the treatment is to permanently recapture the disk, the orthotic must be worn constantly, even during eating. When compared to FPS therapy, the ARS orthotic is also more likely to impair phonation, therefore, this treatment places greater demands on host compliance. The orthotic treatment tends to be prolonged, lasting for 4 to 9 months and must be followed by some type of permanent dental alteration to retain the mandible in the anterior position. In a few cases with minimal disk displacement,

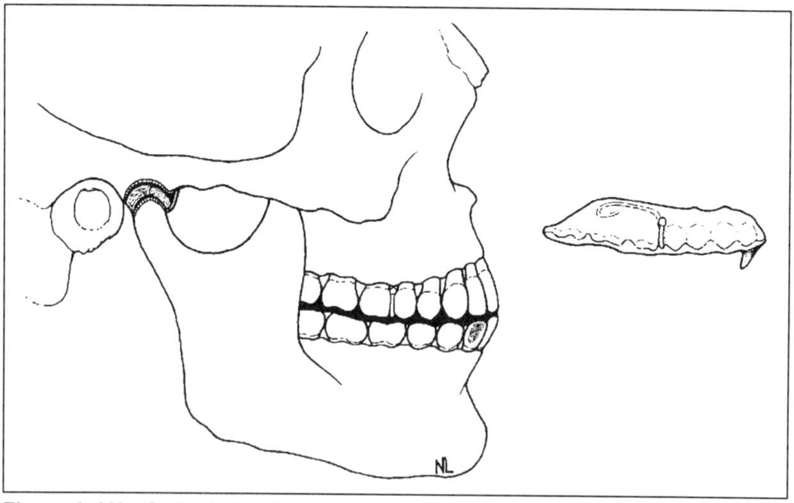

Figure 9-10b: Orthotic Designs. Anterior Repositioning Orthotic. The anterior repositioning splint is designed to recapture a displaced disk in DDWR. The appliance is distinguished by the ramp and the deep indentations of the opposing teeth in the occlusal surface which attempt to maintain the mandible in a protruded position.

this treatment can be an occlusal adjustment; however, most cases require more invasive therapies such as orthodontics or full-mouth prosthetic dentistry to permanently maintain the position. The research literature has produced equivocal support for the long-term success (disk recapture and the elimination of pain and dysfunction) of this treatment approach. Most authors suggest that the treatment is most successful in minimally displaced disks and that the success diminishes as disk displacement increases. Some authors purport a 70% success rate, however, most report less predictable results. In addition, this treatment approach is questioned because the occlusion is permanently altered as a method of disk recapture, even though the occlusion is not problematic. Therefore, why disk displacement is not managed by surgical repositioning of the disk when this is believed to be pathologic, rather than permanently altering mandibular position to accommodate a displaced disk, is puzzling. This therapy is further questioned by other treatment outcome results which show that disk repositioning is not needed to eliminate pain and dysfunction. As such, this treatment approach is not recommended at this time.

A second and distinct objective of anterior repositioning splint therapy is to temporarily take the condyle off the retrodiskal tissues for a period of time in order to promote healing and adaptation of the tissue. This treatment approach does not intend to recapture the disk, since the condyle is allowed to return to the retrodiskal tissue after a period of time (i.e., 2-6 weeks). The orthotic is fabricated in a similar manner, but its use and objectives differ. This treatment approach is consistent with our present understanding of the importance of host adaptation in successful outcomes, as opposed to disk repositioning.

Orthotics are generally fabricated from either processed acrylic, a light-cured composite material, or rigid vacuform materials. The splint occlusion can be determined indirectly by mounting casts on an articulator before fabricating the splint, or directly by relining the occlusal surface at chair-side with cold cure acrylic or a light-cured composite material. Retention on the orthotics can be acquired by using wrought wire clasps or by applying the splint material to undercuts on the teeth surfaces. The former method is preferred because it allows easy adjustment of the retentive properties and obviates the need to cover the buccal tooth surfaces, allowing the splint to be more esthetic. The issue of esthetics is important to diurnal wear because of its impact on patient compliance.

Potential advantages to orthotic therapy include the ease of patient self-treatment, the cost and the minimum number of treatment visits required. Disadvantages can include negative effects on speech and appearance and the potential for irreversible occlusal changes with chronic, continual wear.

Physical therapy involves the use of thermal applications (heat and cold), exercises (range of motion and isometric), ultrasound, laser therapy, and electrical therapies (TENS and electrical stimulation) to improve joint range of motion and decrease pain. Research has shown that physical therapy improves patient recovery following TMJ surgery, and it is a routine therapy for most musculoskeletal problems. However, research is lacking to support the routine use of physical therapy in the management of TMD. Empirically, physical therapy appears more effective in improving range of motion with TMD, than with reducing pain. Commonly, patients report improvement in their pain while undergoing physical therapy, however, the improvement abates when the sessions are concluded. Therefore, the use of physical therapy is recommended when range of motion is restricted (i.e., acute DDWR and exacerbations of DJD), especially in young patients who appear to possess improved adaptation capabilities. This youthful advantage in host response may be secondary to differences in the retrodiskal tissues, such as a higher concentration of elastic connective tissue, improved vascularity and less degenerative changes. A second indication for physical therapy is following TMJ surgery, when postsurgical joint mobility is limited by intra-articular edema, which increases the risk of adhesion formation. Although this therapeutic modality has the potential of allowing self-treatment, the self-treatment is usually less intense than that which is professionally delivered and, hence, is probably less effective. Typically the physical therapy is delivered on an alternating daily schedule for a

2 to 4 week period. Extended administration of this therapy is not recommended because of the lack of scientific evidence supporting efficacy.

Behavioral therapy is indicated for TMD patients whose problem involves stress/anxiety or psychopathology as etiologic or perpetuating factors. Patients may be aware of their stress and its relationship to the TM Disorder, or they may be oblivious to both. Once identified by history or psychological testing, some form of stress management or counseling is indicated. Stress management is intended for patients whose anxiety has not resulted in psychopathology (i.e., significant neurosis or psychosis). Appropriate stress management techniques can include biofeedback, hypnosis, relaxation tapes and progressive relaxation. These therapies can be delivered by either a psychologist or a psychiatrist. When psychotherapy is indicated, a psychiatrist may be preferred because of their ability to utilize additional therapies such as pharmacotherapy. Research has shown behavioral therapy to be as successful as orthotic therapy. Additional therapeutic advantages include the ability to transfer knowledge to the patient, which promotes self-treatment following professional care and the potential curative role of this modality. The latter advantage refers to the potential etiologic relationship of stress to the initiations or exacerbations of many patients' problem. Behavioral therapy is the only therapeutic modality that can be both palliative and curative (address the cause). Disadvantages include the number of visits required (usually a minimum of 12), the cost and the intense reliance upon patient motivation for success.

The duration of nonsurgical therapies is generally 6 weeks to 6 months. Typically, the length of time required is determined by patient response. For many patients as little as 2 weeks of therapy is required to control their symptoms. Multiple therapies are common and can consist of any combination of pharmacotherapy, orthotic therapy, physical therapy and behavioral therapy. The desired therapeutic combination is determined by the patient's disease history and signs and symptoms. For example, a patient with a positive stress history, sleep disruption and nocturnal bruxism would be a candidate for stress management, pharmacotherapy (muscle relaxant or tricyclic antidepressant) and nocturnal orthotic wear. Similarly, a patient with trismus and a diurnal, intra-articular pain pattern may be treated with physical therapy, diurnal splint wear and anti-inflammatory agents. Therapeutic success is more likely if the treatments are initially comprehensive followed by gradual weaning, rather than relying on single therapies, to which other treatments are added following failure. In the latter technique, patients lose confidence in the value of the treatments and in the practitioner, which undermines future success. Therefore, a comprehensive approach is recommended initially, followed by selective weaning of therapies once treatment objectives are accomplished. The desired therapeutic goals should be explained to the patient prior to initiating any therapy. Patients should clearly understand which signs and symptoms can be reduced, and which are unlikely to be affected by treatment. For example, joint sounds are refractory to therapy in most patients. Similarly, signs and symptoms from separate disorders, such as migraine headaches and cervical dysfunction, or idiopathic complaints, such as hearing loss, tinnitus, dysequilibrium, fatigue and changes in taste, should not be therapeutic goals. Finally, relieving all TMD-related symptomatology is not possible for every patient, therefore, a realistic goal of successful nonsurgical therapy would be the improvement of signs, symptoms and associated dysfunction to a tolerable level. With the exception of patient education and pharmacotherapy, the remaining therapies (orthotic therapy, behavioral therapy and physical therapy) should be left to the discretion of the general dentist to whom the patient is referred from the acute care provider.

When nonsurgical therapies are successful, the treatments are selectively weaned beginning with medications. Medications are weaned first, secondary to the potential side-effects associated with chronic use of muscle relaxants and NSAIDs. In contrast, the chronic administration of antidepressants poses less concern, since long-term administration is well tolerated. Patients are asked to cut their dosing regimen in half for the first week, followed by complete cessation or ad lib dosing by the second week. Some rebound insomnia may occur when reducing the use of muscle relaxants and antidepressants. When decreasing orthotic wear, the time period during which orthotic wear is least necessary for most patients is in the morning, between waking and noon. Therefore, this is a prime target time for weaning splint wear in patients who appear to constantly need the orthotic. For most patients, however, their history and/or treatment response will clearly define the best weaning pattern. Nocturnal bruxers, for example, can begin with decreasing their diurnal wear, while diurnal bruxers can follow the reverse pattern. Remember that patients can provide invaluable assistance in making these decisions. Patients are usually aware of the relative worth of the various treatments and have some idea of when the treatments are most needed.

When nonsurgical therapies are unsuccessful, practitioners are advised to closely re-evaluate the case to insure that the diagnosis and treatment were appropriate. Close attention should be paid to the potential role of stress, psychopathology and bruxism in the perpetuation of signs and symptoms. Such patients are now candidates for invasive therapies and these treatments are also prone to fail if the reason for failure is uncontrolled stress, bruxism activity, or unrecognized psychopathology. In patients diagnosed with a significant intra-articular problem, the failure of nonsurgical therapy may have been expected and some form of invasive management is appropriate. Such invasive therapies can include intra-articular corticosteroid injections and TMJ surgery. **Intra-articular corticosteroid**

injections involve the injection of a local anesthetic and a corticosteroid into the superior joint space. The intent of this therapy is to relieve pain and decrease intra-articular inflammation. Suitable patients include those who have failed conservative therapies and who have intractable intra-articular pain. The injected solution typically contains a 50:50 mixture of a local anesthetic without a vasoconstrictor (e.g., bupivicaine or lidocaine) and a potent corticosteroid (e.g., 4-8 mg dexamethasone or 3 mg betamethasone). The total volume of the injected solution is 1-2 cc and a 27 guage, 1 1/2 inch needle is suggested. The injection technique involves having the patient open and close while palpating the joint to locate the condylar head and glenoid fossa (Figure 9-11). Once oriented,

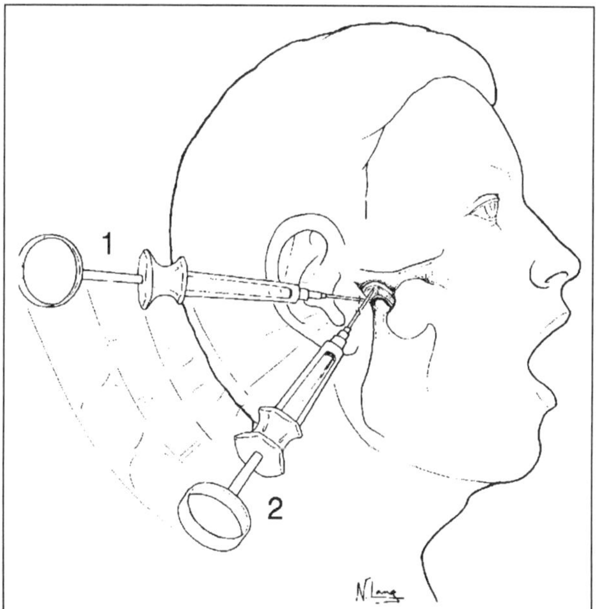

Figure 9-11: Intra-articular Injections. Position 1 - With the patient in maximal opening, the needle is inserted between the ear and the translated condyle, until contact is felt with the posterior aspect of the condylar head. Position 2 - The needle is slightly retracted and advanced in an anterior-superior direction over the condylar head and into the superior joint space. Upon contact with the fossa, the needle is slightly retracted and the solution injected.

the preauricular skin should be prepared with a disinfectant such as iodine. The patient should be prepared psychologically and asked to open maximally. The operator should keep one hand on the condylar head for orientation, while the other hand directs the needle. The skin should be punctured between the external auditory meatus and the condylar head and the needle should be directed anteriorly, superiorly and medially towards the posterior aspect of the condylar head. Upon boney contact, the needle should be slightly withdrawn and advanced in a more superior direction, to slide over the condylar head. After entering the superior joint space the needle will contact the glenoid fossa. At this point, the needle should be slightly withdrawn and the solution injected following aspiration. The operator will have difficulty advancing the needle when in contact with the capsular ligament (when entering the joint space) and should notice significant opposing pressure during the injection when the needle is correctly positioned within the joint space. In the absence of this last sensation, the operator is likely outside the joint. After removing the needle, the patient will encounter difficulty moving their jaws for the next few days. This therapy can be used in conjunction with physical therapy to improve range of motion during a period of comfort.

The most notable, potential side-effect of this treatment is condylar head resorption, which has been reported with repeated injections. This caution is based on animal studies and is presently in question concerning the extrapolation of these results to humans. Nonetheless, the present recommendation is not to exceed three injections per joint separated by two week rest periods. The research literature supports the use of intra-articular corticosteroid injections as both a short-term and a long-term treatment measure. Seventy percent of patients' pain improves, both acutely and chronically, without significant side-effects. Acutely, patients' range of motion is also significantly improved. The use of corticosteroids has been compared with a more biocompatible agent, hyaluronate, showing no significant differences in outcome. This naturally occurring connective tissue enzyme is not associated with the potential boney degeneration side-effect and, therefore, may be the preferred agent for intra-articular injections. Irrespective of outcome success, this therapy has been used sparingly in the United States, which may reflect the ill-ease of both patients and operators with facial injection and the fear of boney degeneration.

TMJ Surgery is reserved for patients who satisfy the following five basic criteria: 1) failure of a thorough attempt at nonsurgical therapy 2) refractory pain that is intolerable to the patient 3) the pain source is intra-articular 4) intra-articular pathology is documented by imaging 5) attempts have been made to control bruxism and psychopathology when present. TMJ surgery can be divided into categories of open joint surgeries, arthroscopy and arthrocentesis. Open joint surgery entails a myriad of soft and hard tissue manipulations following surgical exposure of the joint. For example, the disk can be repositioned (plication), recontoured or replaced with autogenous (dermis, fascia, muscle or cartilage) or alloplastic materials (silastic). Similarly, the condyle and eminence can be recontoured (alveoloplasty) or replaced with autogenous (ribs) or alloplastic materials (titanium-teflon condyle, fossa and total joint prostheses). Because of the invasive nature of these therapies, open joint therapy is typically reserved for patients who fail less aggressive surgical approaches. In addition, minimal surgical manipulation is preferred to aggressive surgical approaches, and autogenous grafts are preferred over alloplastic materials. Arthroscopy involves the placement of an arthroscope (metal cannula with a camera on one end) inside the superior joint space. This allows the surgeon to visualize the disk, retrodiskal tissues and the synovium for pathologic changes (fibrillation, perforations, adhesions). Blunt dissection can be used to break up adhesions and the joint is mobilized, flushed out with saline and a corticosteroid deposited. The aforementioned steps represent the standard surgery, although some surgeons also use specialized instruments to recontour hard and soft tissues.

Arthrocentesis involves all of the procedures associated with arthroscopy except the arthroscope. In this new procedure, the joint is flushed out, mobilized and steroids are injected without visualization of the joint or blunt dissection. Arthrocentesis had shown promise with acute locks, although the available research literature is scant.

Usually, all forms of TMJ surgery are accompanied by postsurgical physical therapy, intended to prevent permanent limitations in range of motion associated with intra-articular edema and pain during surgical recovery. Continuous passive motion (CPM) is a new physical therapy technique that involves involuntary movement of patients' mandibles via a mechanical device. The success of this technique is presently ill-defined.

Outcome comparisons between arthroscopy and open joint surgery have shown very little differences. Both techniques improve pain and dysfunction in 70-90% of the patients, but leave some level of residual pain and dietary limitations in 40-60%. With arthroscopic surgery, patients tend to improve more rapidly and have less residual trismus. Arthroscopic surgery is also associated with a smaller surgical incision and shorter surgical time. For these reasons, arthroscopy is typically performed as an out-patient surgical procedure, while open joint surgery requires a hospital stay of 1 to 3 days. Finally, the success of repeat surgeries is poor, therefore, it is essential that patients are carefully selected for surgery and that failing patients are closely scrutinized for occult or unrecognized psychopathology and/or uncontrolled stress/bruxism before a second surgery is attempted.

In the acute care setting, patient education, moist heat, dietary restrictions and nonsteroidal anti-inflammatory agents are recommended for patients suffering from myositis and capsulitis. This will represent most of the TMD patients encountered, but is also applicable to other intra-articular disorders (internal derangements and degenerative joint disease).

Table 9-6: Reduction of Closed and Open Locks

Open Locks

1 - Discuss the problem with the patient and explain what you plan to do and what the patient will likely experience. Discomfort is minimal.

2 - Standing in front of the patient, place your thumbs on the external oblique ridges of the mandible, bilaterally, with your fingers grasping the inferior border. Avoid placing your fingers on the occlusal surfaces to prevent being bitten.

3 - Place pressure on the mandible in an inferior-posterior direction, attempting to distract the condyle from the articular eminence and allow the mandible to slide back into the fossa. Typically, the condyles will reduce rapidly and sequentially. Thus the practitioner should attempt to distract the condyles and then to lightly guide them into the fossas. Sedation or, less commonly, general anesthesia may be employed on anxious patients to assist in muscle relaxation and patient cooperation.

4 - Following successful reduction, the patient should be advised to refrain from wide opening (i.e. with yawning and eating), placed on a soft diet, provided with simple analgesics if pain control is indicated and referred for a definitive TMD evaluation.

Closed Locks

1 - Discuss the problem with the patient and explain what you plan to do and what the patient will likely experience. Discomfort in the form of pressure or pain is common.

2 - Standing in front of the patient, place your thumbs on the occlusal surfaces of the mandibular posterior teeth, bilaterally, with your fingers grasping the inferior borders.

3 - Ask the patient to relax and the practitioner can begin to move the mandible in small circles getting the patient use to movement and allowing time for the patient to demonstrate relaxation. When the patient seems relaxed, place superior pressure on the unaffected side, attempting to stabilize the unlocked condyle. Simultaneously, place pressure on the locked condyle, to bring it inferiorly, medially and anteriorly. Remember that the disk is most frequently displaced in an anterior-medial direction because of the pull of the superior head of the lateral pterygoid muscle. Numerous attempts may be necessary to successfully reduce the disk, although the likelihood of reduction cannot be predicted. Successful reduction can be confirmed by a popping sensation and the immediate improvement in vertical opening with the mandible protruded. Sedation or, less commonly, general anesthesia, may be employed on anxious patients to assist in muscle relaxation and patient cooperation.

4 - Following successful reduction, the patient must maintain their mandible in a protruded position to ensure the reduction. An orthotic that holds the mandible anteriorly (i.e an anterior repositioning orthotic) is commonly used for this purpose. This orthotic must be worn constantly, even during eating. Should the patient allow their mandible to slide back, the patient will return to a closed lock position. Because of the technical difficulty of fabricating the orthotic and the problems created with permanently maintaining this position, this therapy is questionable in the acute care setting.

5 - Irrespective on one's success in reducing the displaced disk, the patient should be placed on a soft diet, encouraged to place moist heat on the TMJ and muscles of mastication at least 4 times a day, provided with simple analgesics and referred for a definitive TMD evaluation.

Patient education is essential and has been previously described. Moist heat should be applied to the painful areas four times a day using a warm wet wash cloth, a wet heating pad or a hot water bottle. Patients should limit

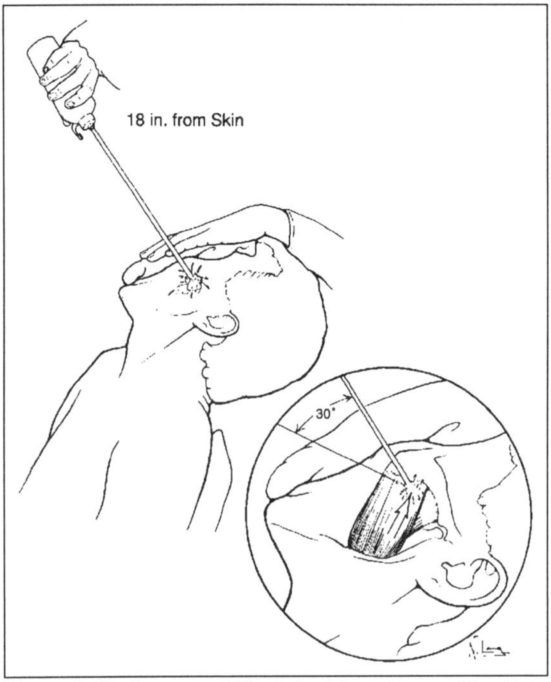

Figure 9-12: Spray and Stretch. A towel is used to shield the patient's face, while a vapor coolant spray (i.e., ethyl chloride or Fluori-Methane) is directed along the orientation of the muscle fibers. The coolant is held 18 inches from the skin and at a 30 degree angle to the muscle. Two to three sweeps are performed followed by passive stretching.

chewy foods (e.g., pizza and candies) and tough foods (e.g., meats, chips and uncooked vegetables) from their diets. A normal diet can be reintroduced with symptomatic improvement. For patients in moderate to severe discomfort, intramuscular ketorolac should be considered. This agent has been exceptional in the relief of postsurgical pain, has a long duration of action and avoids the undesirable side-effects associated with narcotic administration. The outstanding efficacy of this agent appears to be secondary to the route of administration (IM) which avoids the gastrointestinal tract and, thereby, allows delivery of a much higher drug dose. For patients with painful muscle trismus, an intraoffice physical therapy technique that can be used in the acute care setting is "spray and stretch". This involves spraying the tender muscles with a vapor coolant material such as fluoromethane. A towel is used to keep the aerosol out of the patient's face and the material is applied in thin layers along the muscle's fiber orientation (Figure 9-12). Three applications are suggested and the patient's mandible should be passively stretched between each application.

Acute disk and condylar displacements generally require manual reductions to expediently afford these patients a normal range of motion. This is best exemplified in open locking, when patient's jaws are locked in an open position secondary to condylar hypermobility and perhaps, spasm of the temporalis and masseter muscles. This problem can be easily corrected with manipulation of the jaw and minimized by having patients restrict their diets and their vertical opening (especially during yawning, talking and eating). In contrast, reducing closed locks is less likely to be successful and once reduced, they are extremely difficult to maintain without fixing and maintaining the mandible in a protrusive position. Following successful reduction, closed lock patients must maintain their mandible in a protruded position to avoid relapse. Fabrication of an anterior repositioning splint would be required which is technically difficult, although possible, on an emergency basis. The protocols for reducing both open and closed locks is presented in Table 9-6 and Figures 9-13 and 14.

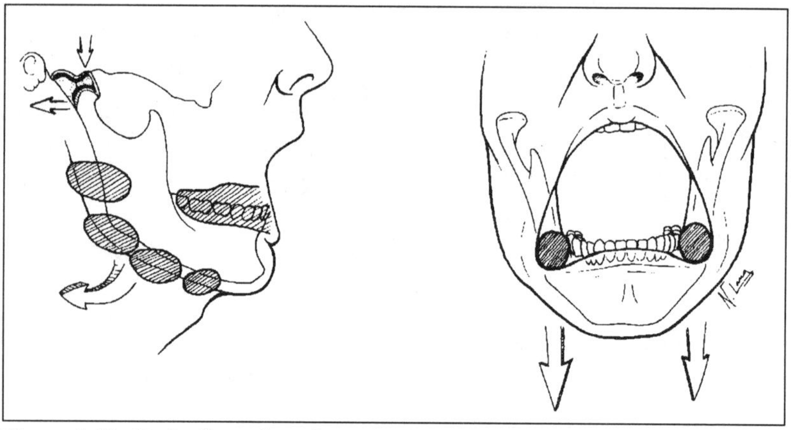

Figure 9-13: Reduction of an Open Lock. Thumbs are placed on the external oblique ridges with the fingers grasping the inferior border of the mandible. Pressure is applied in downward (inferior) and back (dorsal or posterior) directions.

The most critical aspect of managing the TMD patient in the acute care setting is diagnosis, especially distinguishing a TMD problem, such as capsulitis, from more serious problems (i.e., condyle, fossa and mandible fractures, intra-articular tumors and odontogenic infections). Generally, the signs and symptoms of capsulitis resemble those of fractures, especially when patients have generalized facial pain from trauma. In such circumstances, when a fracture cannot be visualized radiographically and the patient does not have clinical signs of a fracture (Chapter 8), then a capsulitis

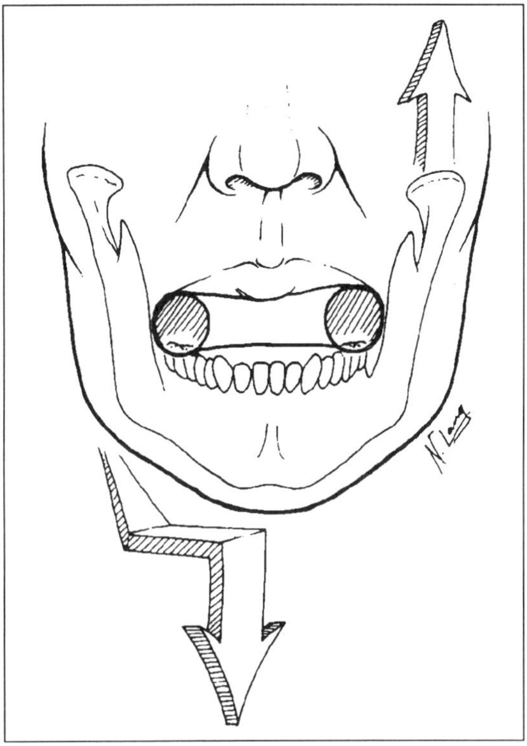

Figure 9-14: Reduction of a Closed Lock. Thumbs are placed on occlusal surfaces of the teeth with the fingers grasping the inferior border of the mandible. The unlocked joint is stabilized with superior pressure, while downward (inferior), medial and forward (ventral or anterior) pressure is applied to the locked joint.

is the likely diagnosis. The reader is reminded that although patients with capsulitis may be unable or unwilling to occlude their teeth, there is no true occlusal discrepancy. The presence of fever, lymphadenopathy and/or odontogenic pathology must be recognized in order to distinguish odontogenic infections from capsulitis, keeping in mind that trismus may be common to both problems. The vascular and neurogenic sources of facial pain can be distinguished by differences in pain character, but most importantly by the exacerbation of pain with mandibular movement that is unique to TMD. All of these differential diagnoses are covered in more detail elsewhere in this text and the reader is referred to the appropriate chapters for further insight. Finally, it is imperative to always remember that patients can have more than one problem and that it is the confluence of multiple problems that present the greatest challenge to diagnosis and treatment.

VII. PROGNOSIS

The majority of TM disorders are mild and self-limiting, therefore, the prognosis for most patients is good. Host adaptation appears capable of alleviating the problems for most patients and the treatments serve to accelerate this recovery or perhaps, only to minimize signs and symptoms during the recovery period. A small percentage of TMD problems tend to be chronic or progressive in nature, however, we are presently unable to prospectively identify these patients. Psychopathologic factors are associated with chronic pain, although the etiologic relationship of the pain to these factors appears bidirectional. Eighty to ninety percent of all TMD patients improve with nonsurgical therapies. An additional eighty to ninety percent of the patients who are refractory to the nonsurgical treatments improve with surgical therapies. Thus, the percentage of patients who fail to respond to some form of TMD therapy is exceptionally small. The key to successful patient treatment is devoting the time and effort required for accurate diagnosis, and apportioning treatments according to patient need, rather than following a cookbook approach of escalating therapies. In addition, the goal of treatment is to have the patient reach a tolerable level of pain/dysfunction with the expectation that the problem may recur or require periodic maintenance. Curing patients as a treatment objective fails to recognize the behavioral nature of TMD and, thus, is prone to overtreatment and disappointment by both the practitioner and patient. These factors promote the development of chronic pain scenarios in which overtreated patients who have been told that a cure is possible, desperately seek a permanently asymptomatic state.

VIII. PATIENT REFERRAL

After providing initial care to TMD patients, referral is suggested to a general dentist with expertise in treating the disorder. General dentists are recommended because their expertise is primary care, their treatment capabilities are broad and because of their commitment to a variety of conservative treatment methods. Referral is required when a patient's problem fails to show signs of improvement, shows a pattern of relapse or is desired by a concerned patient. In addition, TMD problems with a chronic history and those involving a significant intra-articular disorder are candidates for referral. The need for patient referral can be determined on a one week follow-up visit to the acute care provider.

References

Aufdemorte T.B., Van Sickels J.E., Dolwick M.F., Sheridan P.J., Holt G.R., Aragon S.B., Gates G.A., "Estrogen receptors in the temporomandibular joint of the baboon (Papio cynocephalus): An autoradiographic study." *Oral Surg, Oral Med, Oral Pathol* 61 (1986): 307-314.

American Academy of Orofacial Pain., ed. McNeill C., *Temporomandibular Disorders Guidelines for Classification, Assessment, and Management.* Chicago: Quintessence, 1993.

Bean L.R., Thomas C.A., "Significance of condylar positions in patients with temporomandibular disorders." *J Am Dent Assoc.* 114 (1987): 76-77.

Bezuur N.J., "The effect of therapeutic laser treatment in patients with craniomandibular disorders." *J Craniomandib Disord.* 2 (1988): 83-86.

Boero R.P., "The physiology of splint therapy: a literature review." *Angle Orthodontist.* 59 (1989): 165-180.

Braun B.L., "The effect of physical therapy intervention on incisal opening after temporomandibular joint surgery." *Oral Surg Oral Med Oral Pathol.* 64 (1987): 544-548.

Burgess J.A., Dworkin S.F., "Litigation and post-traumatic TMD: How patients report treatment outcome." *J Am Dent Assoc.* 124 (1993): 105-110.

Christiansen L.V., "Effect of ibuprofen on isometric contractions and associated pain of the human masseter muscle." *Am J Orthod Dentofacial Orthop.* 92 (1987): 144-150.

Clark G.T., "A critical evaluation of orthopedic interocclusal appliance therapy: design, theory, and overall effectiveness." *J Am Dent Assoc.* 108 (1984): 359-363.

Clark G.T., "A critical evaluation of orthopedic interocclusal appliance therapy: effectiveness for specific symptoms." *J Am Dent Assoc.* 108 (1984): 364-368.

Clark G.T., Siligman D.A., Solberg W.K., Pullinger A.G., "Guidelines for the treatment of temporomandibular disorders." *J Craniomandib Disord Facial Oral Pain.* 4 (1990): 80-88.

Clark G.T., Adachi N.Y., Doran M.R., "Physical medicine procedures affect temporomandibular disorders: a review." *J Am Dent Assoc.* 121 (1990): 151-161.

De Laat A., Van Steenberghe D., Lesaffre E., "Occlusal relationships and temporomandibular joint dysfunction. Part II: Correlations between occlusal and articular parameters and symptoms of TMJ dysfunction by means of stepwise logistic regression." *J Prosthet Dent.* 55 (1986): 116-121.

Dixon C.D., Graham C.S., Mayhew R.B., Oesterle L.J., Simms D., Peirson W.P., "The validity of transcranial radiography in diagnosing TMJ anterior disk displacement." *J Am Dent Assoc.* 108 (1984): 615-618.

Dworkin S.F., Huggins K.H., LeResche L., Korff M.V., Howard J., Truelove E., Sommers E., "Epidemiology of signs and symptoms in temporomandibular disorders: clinical signs in cases and controls." *J Am Dent Assoc.* 120 (1990): 273-281.

Dworkin S.F., Burgess J.A., "Orofacial pain of psychogenic origin: Current concepts and classification." *J Am Dent Assoc.* 115 (1987): 565-572.

Gale E.N., "Behavioral approaches to temporomandibular disorders." *Ann Behav Med.* 8 (1986): 11-16.

Gordon S.M., Montgomery M.T., Jones D.L., "Comparative efficacy of Prioxicam, Acetominophen and placebo for temporomandibular pain." *J Dent Res.* 70 (1991): 329.

Greene C.S., Olson R.E., Laskin D.M., "Psychological factors in the etiology, progression and treatment of MPD syndrome." *J Am Dent Assoc.* 105 (1982): 443-448.

Greene C.S., "Managing TMD patients: Initial therapy is the key." *J Am Dent Assoc.* 123 (1992):43-45.

Harkins S., Linford J., Cohen J., Kramer T., Cueva L., "Administration of clonazepam in the treatment of TMD and associated myofascial pain: A double-blind pilot study." *J Craniomandib Disord Oral Facial Pain.* 5 (1991): 179-186.

Heise A.P., Laskin D.M., Gervin A.S., "Incidence of temporomandibular joint symptoms following whiplash injury." *J Oral Maxillofac Surg.* 50 (1992): 825-828.

Kaplan P.A., Helms C.A., "Current status of temporomandibular joint imaging for the diagnosis of internal derangements." *Am J Radiol.* 152 (1989): 697-705.

Kinney R.K., Gatchel R.J., Ellis E., Holt C., "Major psychological disorders in chronic TMD patients: Implications for successful management." J Am Dent Assoc. 123 (1992): 49-54.

Kirk W.S., Calabrese D.K., "Clinical evaluation of physical therapy in the managment of internal derangement of the temporomandibular joint." *J Oral Maxillofac Surg.* 47 (1989): 113-119.

Kopp S., Wenneberg B., Haraldson T., Carlsson G.E., "Short-term effects of intra-articular injections of sodium hyaluronate and corticosteroid on temporomandibular joint and dysfunction." *J Oral Maxillofac Surg.* 43 (1985): 429-435.

Kopp S., Carlsson G.E., Haraldson T., Wenneberg B., "Longitidinal effect of intra-articular injections of sodium hyaluronate and corticosteroid on temporomandibular joint arthritis." *J Oral Maxillofac Surg.* 45 (1987): 929-935.

Kopp S., Akerman S., Nilner M., "Short-term effects of intra-articular sodium hyaluronate, glucocorticoid, and saline injections on rheumatoid arthritis of the temporomandibular joint." *J Craniomandib Disord Facial Oral Pain.* 5 (1991): 231-238.

Kriesberg M.K., "Tricyclic antidepressants: Analgesic effect and indications in orofacial pain." *J Craniomandib Disord Facial Oral Pain.* 2 (1988): 171-177.

McNeill C., Mohl N.D., Rugh J.D., Tanaka T.T., "Temporomandibular disorders: diagnosis, management, education, and research." *J Am Dent Assoc.* 120 (1990): 253-262.

Milam S.B., Klebe R.J., Triplett R.G., Herbert D., "Characterization of the extracellular matrix of the primate temporomandibular joint." *J Oral Maxillofac Surg.* 49 (1991): 381-391.

Mohl N.D., Ohrbach R., "The dilemma of scientific knowledge versus clinical management of temporomandibular disorders." *J Prosthet Dent.* 67 (1992): 113-120.

Mohl N.D., McCall W.D., Lund J.P., Plesh O., "Devices for the diagnosis and treatment of temporomandibular disorders. Part I: Introduction, scientific evidence, and jaw tracking." *J Prosthet Dent.* 63 (1990): 198-201.

Mohl N.D., Lund J.P., Widmer C.G., McCall W.D., "Devices for the diagnosis and treatment of temporomandibular disorders. Part II: Electromyography and sonography." *J Prosthet Dent.* 63 (1990): 332-336.

Mohl N.D., Orbach R.K., Crow H.C., Gross A.J., "Devices for the diagnosis and treatment of temporomandibular disorders. Part III: Thermography, ultrasound, electrical stimulation, and electromyographic biofeedback." *J Prosthet Dent.* 63 (1990): 472-477.

Montgomery M.T., Gordon S.M., Van Sickels J.E., Harms S.E., "Changes in signs and symptoms following temporomandibular joint disc repositioning surgery." *J Oral Maxillofac Surg.* 50 (1992): 320-328.

Montgomery M.T., Van Sickels J.E., Harms S.E., Thrash W.J., "Arthroscopic TMJ Surgery: Effects on signs, symptoms and meniscal position." *J Oral Maxillofac Surg.* 47 (1989): 1263-1271.

Montgomery M.T., Van Sickels J.E., Harms S.E., "The success of TMJ arthroscopy in meniscal subluxation and meniscal dislocation." *Oral Surg Oral Med Oral Pathol.* 71 (1991): 651-659.

Nitzan D.W., Dolwick M.F., Martinez G.A., "Temporomandibular joint arthrocentesis: A simplified treatment for severe, limited mouth opening." *J Oral Maxillofac Surg*. 49 (1991): 1168-1170.

Obeid G., Zhang X., Wang X., "Effect of ibuprofen on the healing and remodeling of bone and articular cartilage in the rabbit temporomandibular joint." *J Oral Maxillofac Surg*. 50 (1992): 843-849.

President's conference on the examination, diagnosis and management of temporomandibular disorders. ed. Laskin D., Greenfield W., Gale E., Rugh J., Neff P., Alling C., Ayer W.A., Chicago, *American Dental Association*, 1-184, 1983.

Pullinger A.G., Seligman D.A., Gornbein J.A., "A multiple logistic regression analysis of the risk and relative odds of temporomandibular disorders as a function of occlusal features." *J Dent Res*. 72 (1993): 968-979.

Report of the president's conference on the examination, diagnosis and management of temporomandibular disorders. ed. Griffiths R.H., *J Am Dent Assoc*. 106 (1983): 75-77.

Research diagnostic criteria for temporomandibular disorders: Review, criteria, examinations and specifications critique. ed. Dworkin S.F., LeResche L., *J Craniomandib Disord Facial Oral Pain*. 6 (1992): 302-355.

Reynders R.M., "Orthodontics and temporomandibular disorders: A review of the literature (1966-1988)." *Am J Orthod Dentofac Orthop*. 97 (1990): 463-471.

Roberts C.A., Tallents R.H., Katzberg R.W., Sanchez-Woodworth R.E., Manzione J.V., Espeland M.A., Handelman S.L., "Clinical and arthrographic evaluation of temporomandibular joint sounds." *Oral Surg Oral Med Oral Pathol*. 62 (1986): 373-376.

Roberts C.A., Katzberg R.W., Tallents R.H., Espeland M.A., Handelman S.L., "Correlations of clinical parameters to the arthrographic depiction of temporomandibular joint internal derangements." *Oral Surg Oral Med Oral Pathol*. 66 (1988): 32-36.

Rugh J.D., Harlan J., "Nocturnal bruxism and temporomandibular disorders." *Adv in Neurol*. 49 (1988): 329-341.

Rugh J.D., Solberg W.K., "Oral health status in the United States: Temporomandibular disorders." *J Dent Educ*. 49 (1985): 398-405.

Satoh T., Harada Y., "Electrophysiologic study on tooth-grinding during sleep." *Electroenceph Clin Neurophysiol*. 35 (1973): 267-275.

Schiffman E.L., Fricton J.R., Haley D.P., Shapiro B.L., "The prevalence and treatment needs of subjects with temporomandibular disorders." *J Am Dent Assoc*. 120 (1990): 295-303.

Schumann S.D., Nohr A.P., Hagen J.D., Jones D.L., Montgomery M.T., "Comparative efficacy of maxillary and mandibular splints for TMD pain." *J Dent Res*. 70 (1991): 441.

Seligman D.A., Pullinger A.G., Solberg W.K., "Temporomandibular disorders. Part III: Occlusal and articular factors associated with muscle tenderness." *J Prosthet Dent*. 59 (1988): 483-489.

Solberg W.K., "Temporomandibular disorders: data collection and examination." *Br Dent J*. 160 (1986): 317-322.

Solberg W.K., "Temporomandibular disorders: masticatory myalgia and its management." *Br Den J*. 160 (1986): 351-356.

Solberg W.K., "Temporomandibular disorders: management of internal derangement." *Br Den J*. 160 (1986): 379-385.

Solberg W.K., "Temporomandibular disorders: management of problems associated with inflammation, chronic hypomobility, and deformity." *Br Den J*. 160 (1986): 421-428.

Solberg W.K., "Temporomandibular disorders: physical tests in diagnosis." *Br Dent J*. 160 (1986): 273-277.

Speculand B., Goss A.N., "Psychological factors in temporomandibular joint dysfunction pain: A review." *Int J Oral Surg.* 14 (1985): 131-137,.

Truelove E.L., Sommers E.E., LeResche L., Dworkin S.F., Von Korff M., "Clinical diagnostic criteria for TMD: New classification permits multiple diagnoses." *J Am Dent Assoc.* 123 (1992): 47-54.

Van den Berg L.I., de Boever J.A., Schautteet H., "Double-blind clinical study of Piroxicam as adjuvant in the treatment of the pain and dysfunction of the temporomandibular joints." *Cranio.* 4 (1986): 351-356.

Wenneberg B., Kopp S., "Short term effect of intra-articular injections of corticosteroid on temporomandibular pain and dysfunction." *Swed Dent J.* 2 (1987): 189-196.

Wenneberg B., Kopp S., Grondahl H-G., "Long term effect of intra-articular injections of a glucocoticosteroid into the TMJ: A clinical and radiographic 8-year follow-up." *J Cranio Craniomandib Disord Facial Oral Pain.* 5 (1991): 11-18.

Yemm R., "A neurophysiological approach to the pathology and aetiology of temporomandibular dysfunction." *J Oral Rhabilit.* 12 (1985): 343-353.

Zamburlini I., Austin D., "Long-term results of appliance therapies in anterior disk displacement with reduction: A review of the literature." J Craniomandib Prac. 9 (1991): 361-368.

10 Extraoral Sources of Facial Pain

Mary K. Hagemeier, D.D.S.

Gary J. Nishioka, D.M.D., M.D.

INTRODUCTION

Craniofacial pain is a common chief complaint and can be among the most challenging and frustrating diagnostic and treatment problems encountered by primary care dentists and physicians. The numerous organs that lie within the face and skull, their rich innervation and the variety of ailments to which they are susceptible, account for the multitudinous and complicated array of pains found in the craniofacial region. To illustrate this intricacy, pain may arise from intraoral sources such as the teeth, periodontium and jaws; and from extraoral sites including ligaments and muscles of the head, neck and face; the nasal cavity and paranasal sinuses; the temporomandibular joints; eyes and ears; blood vessels of the scalp and face (including the venous sinuses and their tributaries); dural and intracerebral arteries; and, finally, from cranial and cervical nerves.

Furthermore, another complexity arises in that these pains may be referred from their site of origin to many distant locations (referred pain). Finally, there are a limitless number of ways in which people perceive and react to pain which serves to further complicate the formidable task of identifying causes and providing adequate treatment. The pathophysiology responsible for most of the facial pain entities is ill-defined, requiring that most treatment approaches be palliative rather than disease specific. In addition, the debilitating nature of many conditions may give rise to numerous aggressive therapies with potentially devastating side-effects. This scenario of idiopathic etiologies and symptomatic therapies is typical of chronic pain in general. For example, indomethacin is the treatment of choice for many of the more obscure facial pains, even though the proposed pathophysiologic mechanisms are dissimilar. Therapies can also include intracranial surgeries and chemotherapeutic agents with potentially serious morbidities. In addition, many of the facial pain entities manifest similar signs and symptoms, which further questions the present scheme of classification. Finally, many of the signs and symptoms are vague and vary significantly between patients, which complicates a diagnosis that is essentially based on signs and symptoms.

The goal of this chapter is to assist primary care providers in the development of a differential diagnosis, the delivery of any needed emergency treatment and the appropriate referral of patients who present with craniofacial pain from nonodontogenic sources (i.e., neuralgias, headaches, sinusitis, etc.). A diagnostic workup format appropriate for the emergency setting is presented, along with descriptions and treatment (both emergency and definitive) of some of the more common craniofacial pain entities. Temporomandibular disorders are discussed as a single entity in Chapter 10. A synopsis of the more common causes of facial pain can be found in Table 10-5.

I. DIAGNOSIS

The most important tool in developing a differential diagnosis is a thorough medical and dental history. A detailed history will usually differentiate odontogenic from nonodontogenic pain, even when the pains occur simultaneously. Such a history should elicit the information contained in Table 10-1 and requires careful attention to detail. The nature of the condition must be explored with respect to the onset and nature of pain and associated symptoms. A useful mnemonic when gathering information about pain is "PQRST." ***P*** represents provoking and palliating factors including movement, thermal changes, medications, swallowing, talking, etc. ***Q*** indicates pain quality which can be segregated into three types: 1) sharp, cutting, lightning-like or stabbing; 2) burning, stinging or hot; 3) deep aching, boring, gnawing or throbbing. The first two types of pain are usually more superficial, better localized and more commonly associated with paresthesia, itching or hyperalgesia. In contrast, the third type of pain is more deeply perceived, diffuse, and tends to persist for a longer period of time. To differentiate these pains, clinicians must insure that patients are specific when describing their pain. Oftentimes this requires persistent questioning from multiple perspectives to accurately distinguish the pain type. ***R*** refers to the anatomic distribution of the pain, including the points of origin and referral patterns, and the presence and location of trigger points. ***S*** describes subjective pain severity and patients are commonly asked to compare this pain to other pains previously experienced and rate the pain on a 1 to 10 scale. Finally, ***T*** indicates the timing of the pain including initial onset, duration, frequency, remissions and exacerbations, seasonal and daily (nocturnal/diurnal) variations, the association of the pain with other symptoms during an attack (i.e., nausea, flushing, changes in sensory perception) and the relationship of the pain to stress, illness or injury.

Desired physical examination data is also listed in Table 10-1 and includes a thorough intraoral examination to rule out odontogenic causes, tumors, etc., and a physical evaluation comprised of vital signs, assessment of cranial nerve function, detailed descriptions of areas of paresthesia, dysesthesia, anesthesia (especially of the face, lips and hands), and trigger point regions. Additional neurologic evaluation should be performed to determine the presence of arm or leg weakness, aphasia, dizziness, altered gait, changes in sensory perception (especially visual disturbances such as flashing points or lines, scintillations), and changes in mental status (confusion, lethargy, altered speech). Other symptoms to assess include the presence of nausea/vomiting and nuchal rigidity.

TABLE 10-1: Steps in the Diagnosis of Facial Pain

A. HISTORY
   I. General information
      a. name, race, age, and sex
      b. address and occupation
      c. name and address of family physician
   II. Chief complaint
   III. Medical and dental histories
      a. previous dental treatment and problems
      b. previous illnesses and injuries
      c. previous medical and surgical treatments
      d. results of prior examinations
      e. medication history
      f. family history
   IV. Social history
      a. birthplace and former residences
      b. occupational and educational history
      c. habits - former and/or current use of tobacco, alcohol, illicit drugs
      d. marital history
      e. pertinent stress-related matters (recent loss of job, death in the family, etc)
   V. Review of systems
   VI. History of present illness
      P - provocative/palliative
      Q - quality
      R - region
      S - severity
      T - temporal character
B. PHYSICAL EVALUATIONS
   I. Vital signs
   II. Neurologic examination and assessment of cranial nerve function
   III. Head and neck palpation
   IV. Intraoral exam

II. TYPES OF PAIN

A. Cranial neuralgias

Neuralgias are a group of clinical entities affecting one or more nerves which supply sensation and motor function to the head and neck. As such, health care providers must have at least a rudimentary understanding of head and neck neuroanatomy. The face and mouth are supplied by cranial nerves and nerves of the cervical plexus, as illustrated in Figure 10-1. Cutaneous sensation of the face, head and neck is supplied by the cervical plexus and trigeminal nerve (CN V). The first division of the trigeminal nerve, the ophthalmic branch or V1, innervates the forehead and nose. The second division, the maxillary or V2, supplies the upper jaw and a portion of the temporal region. The third division, the mandibular or V3, supplies the majority of the lower jaw and temporal region. The cervical plexus innervates the neck and a small portion of the lower jaw at the mandibular angle. The glossopharyngeal nerve (CN IX) supplies the major portion of the pharynx, the posterior third of the tongue and the epiglottis, while the larynx is supplied by the vagus nerve (CN X).

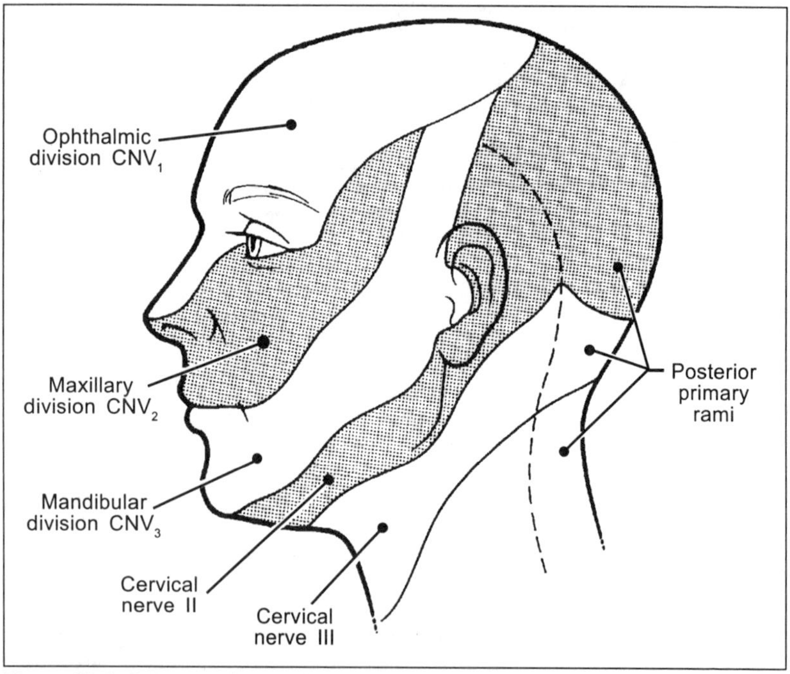

Figure 10-1: Cutaneous Innervation of the Head and Neck.

Trigeminal neuralgia (TGN)

TGN is a disorder characterized by recurrent episodes of high-intensity, lightning-like pain restricted to the distribution of the trigeminal nerve. This condition is also called tic doloreaux ("painful tic") because of the twitching that can accompany the affected area during an episode. The pain has been described as an "electric shock," "lightning," "stabbing," and is always "excruciating" and "sharp." The onset and termination of episodes are usually paroxysmal and patients are generally free of pain between attacks. The attacks occur while patients are awake and are rarely, if ever, reported during sleep. Episodes are of short duration lasting seconds to minutes, and it is common for patients to experience a number of closely-spaced attacks over several hours. Ninety-five percent of the cases involve the second and/or third divisions of CN V, and in the vast majority of patients the pain is unilateral. Only 4 to 8% of the patients experience bilateral symptoms, and in these patients, a given attack occurs on just one side of the face. No preference for the right or left side of the face has been demonstrated for TGN.

Many TGN patients report the presence of a "trigger zone," a discrete area within the trigeminal distribution which when stimulated can precipitate an attack. Potential stimuli can include talking, eating, touching, washing, shaving or slight movement of the trigger zone. The trigger zone is almost always ipsilateral to the affected side, but can reside in either the same or a different trigeminal division. Trigger zones have been reported to migrate, though most are located in the nasolabial fold, upper and lower lips. At times, an "aura" of altered sensation (i.e., paresthesia, an abnormal sensation; dysesthesia, a partial loss of sensation; or anesthesia, a total loss of sensation) within the trigger zone will precede and signal the onset of an attack. However, the aura occurs in only a small percentage of TGN patients.

The overall age and sex-adjusted incidence of TGN in the U.S. is about 5 per 100,000 patients per year. Females are favored 2:1, and incidence rates increase sharply in older (over 60) populations. Patients with multiple sclerosis are somewhat predisposed to TGN, and estimates of TGN in MS patients range from 1-8%. In addition, there appears to be a hereditary distribution to the disease.

For most TGN patients, the etiology of the disease is idiopathic. Some cases, however, appear to be caused by compression of the sensory root of the trigeminal nerve, as the nerve leaves the pons and crosses the apex of the petrous bone (Figure 10-2). This compression is generally attributed to the distribution of blood vessels in the region, and much less commonly to A-V malformations, aneurysms and tumors. Demyelination has also been implicated in the etiology of TGN, an idea which is supported by

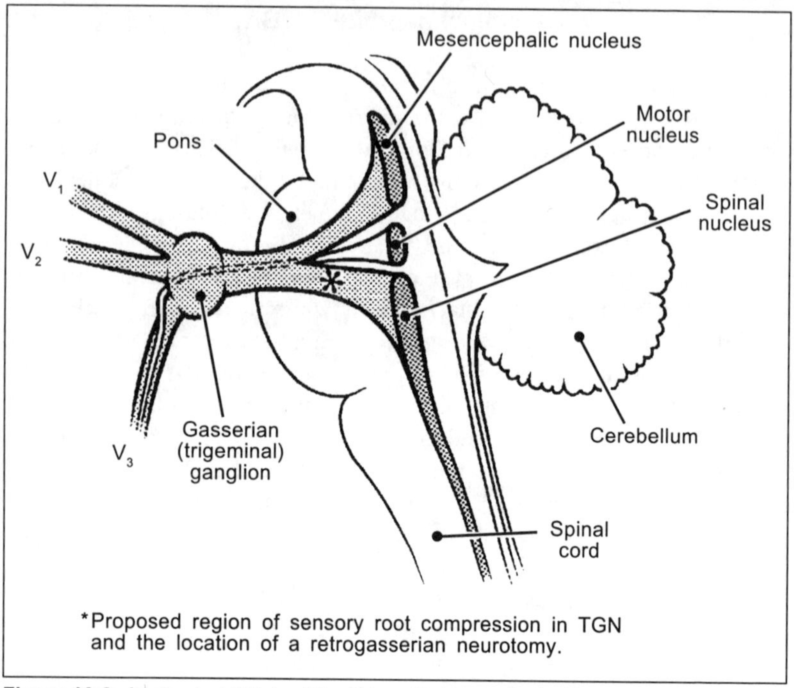

Figure 10-2: Anatomical Origin of the Trigeminal Nerve in the Brainstem.

the increased incidence of TGN in MS patients. Finally, TGN has been associated with virally-mediated diseases such as recurrent herpes zoster episodes.

The initial onset of TGN in a previously unaffected patient, especially in one experiencing multiple, closely-spaced attacks, prompts many patients to seek emergency care. Most TGN cases are easily diagnosed by history, signs and symptoms. Once TGN is suspected, emergent treatment consists of explanation, reassurance and referral to a neurologist for definitive evaluation and therapy. Carbamazepine, 100 mg twice daily may be prescribed for one to two days until the patient is evaluated by a neurologist, and parenteral analgesics (i.e., meperidine 50-100 mg IM or IV) may be given in the emergency setting for patients suffering considerable pain and anxiety.

Most patients require definitive treatment for the signs and symptoms of TGN, and a variety of medical and surgical therapies is available. Initial management is usually pharmacologic, consisting of either carbamazepine, phenytoin or baclofen. 200 to 1600 mg of carbamazepine in 3 to 4 daily oral doses provides complete or acceptable partial relief for two-thirds of the patients. The drug must be used on a long-term basis, however, and this pattern of use can lead to the insidious development of mental and physical sluggishness. One-quarter of the patients benefit from phenytoin (300 to 500 mg in 3 daily doses), and a smaller percentage respond to baclofen (50 to 60 mg per day in 6 divided doses). In addition, these agents may be used in combination to achieve therapeutic efficacy when necessary.

Surgery is generally considered when medical management fails to provide adequate relief. Surgical success is claimed with complete or acceptable partial relief of symptoms in the absence of intolerable side-effects such as severe dysesthesia. Gangliolysis involves the insertion of a needle into the trigeminal rootlets behind the trigeminal ganglion, through which radiofrequency, heat or glycerol is applied. Five-year success rates of 60% are claimed, however, 5% of the patients develop severe dysesthesias in the denervated areas following the procedure. A second surgical approach, termed microvascular decompression, involves coagulation or repositioning of the vessels impinging upon the trigeminal rootlets. The long-term success rate is reported to be 75%, while operative mortality is approximately 1%. If compression is not discovered during this surgery, a retrogasserian neurotomy may be performed, in which the trigeminal root is sectioned between the pons and the ganglion (Figure 10-2). Dysesthesias and anesthesia dolorosa (painful anesthesia) are occasional complications, with corneal and facial anesthesia occurring more frequently. As a last resort, a surgery may be performed in which the trigeminal tract is sectioned in the medulla, thereby eliminating pain and, unfortunately, temperature sensation in the ipsilateral pharynx and face.

Glossopharyngeal Neuralgia

This condition is similar to TGN regarding the character of the pain, temporal occurrence patterns, the presence of trigger zones and the lack of neurologic deficits. However, the entity is 10 to 100 times less common than TGN, and the glossopharyngeal nerve (CN IX), rather than the trigeminal nerve, is affected. The glossopharyngeal nerve supplies the lateral pharyngeal wall, tonsillar pillar and base of the tongue, and as such, during the attack the resulting pain may radiate ipsilaterally to the ear, upper areas of the neck or to the angle of the jaw. Triggers commonly include swallowing, eating, yawning, clearing the throat, talking and temperature changes.

Treatment is similar to that for TGN, including carbamazepine and phenytoin as potential medical therapies and a glossopharyngeal tractotomy as the surgical option. Suspected patients should be referred to a neurologist for definitive diagnosis and treatment.

Superior Laryngeal Neuralgia

As with glossopharyngeal neuralgia, the character of the pain associated with superior laryngeal neuralgia mimics that of TGN. However, the condition is much less common than TGN and the anatomic distribution of the pain follows the branch of the vagus nerve, which innervates the undersurface of the epiglottis and the larynx. Distinctive of this disorder is syncope during an attack that can result from bradycardia or even asystole. Long-term management is similar to that for TGN and should be directed by a neurologist.

Occipital Neuralgia

Occipital neuralgia is characterized by neurogenic pain over the entire distribution of the greater occipital nerve in a manner similar to that in TGN with several unique features. Paresthesia can be intermittent or continuous and is not always painful. Also, there is a decrease in abnormalities of sensation both during and between episodes of paresthesia. The problem can arise spontaneously or result from trauma to the dorsal ramus of C II or its extension, the greater occipital nerve. Other symptoms of occipital neuralgia can include the presence of a trigger point along the nuchal ridge, which may be stimulated by pressure. Tenderness of the occipital nerve to palpation and vertigo are also reported. Treatment success has been purported with the use of analgesics, cervical collars, and injections of local anesthetic and corticosteroids along the occipital nerve distribution.

Alcoholic Facial Neuralgia

In this uncommon condition, chronic alcohol consumption is associated with an atypical neuralgia involving the second and third divisions of the trigeminal nerve. Patients complain of recurrent bilateral, dull, aching pain in one or both jaws that is sometimes lancinating. Pathophysiologic mechanisms are poorly understood and abstinence from alcohol usually provides complete relief within two to three days.

Postherpetic Neuralgia

Postherpetic neuralgia is associated with the reactivation of a Varicella zoster infection in the trigeminal ganglion. Patients usually have a history of shingles and experience an intense pain that is often associated with hyperesthesia and paresthesia. These symptoms can last weeks to months and can cause patients to suffer sleep disruption and depression. Like TGN, the pain location is defined by the distribution of CN V; however, with postherpetic neuralgia the ophthalmic division is most often affected.

Regarding treatment, the usual drug regimens for TGN are sometimes effective, however, for many patients pharmacologic therapy is unsuccessful. Antiviral agents such as acyclovir and gancyclovir may hold some promise, although information on therapeutic efficacy is presently unknown.

Geniculate Neuralgia (Ramsey-Hunt syndrome)

Geniculate neuralgia is also caused by Varicella zoster reactivation; however, in these cases the geniculate ganglion is the source of viral replication. Patients usually experience a deep facial pain in the retro-orbital, inner ear or posterior nasal cavity regions. Cutaneous vesicular lesions in the outer ear, facial paralysis and the loss of taste in the anterior two-thirds of the tongue are characteristic signs and symptoms. In addition, some patients report a bitter taste, increased salivation, vertigo and tinnitus during an attack.

Potential therapies are identical to those discussed with postherpetic neuralgia and are characterized by the same ineffectiveness. New antiviral agents may also possess therapeutic benefit.

Idiopathic Cranial Polyneuropathy

This condition involves the motor portions of cranial nerves II through XII in any combination. Patients experience a constant, deep aching pain in the temporal and frontal areas with occasional lightning-like, stabbing pains that radiate to the nose, scalp, cheek, neck or earlobe. Additional signs and symptoms can include ptosis, conjunctivitis, eyelid edema, nystagmus, tinnitus and temporary decreases in hearing, taste and visual acuity. The symptoms usually last from several days to over six months before spontaneous resolution occurs. These neuropathies have been associated with many entities, including herpes zoster, herpes simplex, and mycoplasma infections, Guillain-Barre syndrome, giant-cell tumors, epidermoid tumors and lymphomas.

Management consists of corticosteroid therapy which will usually decrease pain and ophthalmologic symptoms within a few days.

B. Eagle's Syndrome

This syndrome is associated with an elongation of the styloid process and/or ossification of the stylohyoid ligament. The resulting constellation of symptoms include dysphagia, sore throat, headache, ear pain, vague orofacial pain and sometimes dizziness upon turning the head to one or both sides. The latter symptom is believed secondary to constriction of the carotid artery by the styloid process with rotation of the head. Of the aforementioned signs and symptoms, pharyngeal pain is the most common complaint and most patients are over 40 years of age. It is estimated that radiographic evidence of stylohyoid ossification exists in 4 to 40% of the population, though most people are asymptomatic. This discrepancy in the incidence of signs and symptoms questions the significance of stylohyoid ossification as an etiologic factor. A rapidly-progressing form of Eagle's syndrome has occasionally been described following cervicopharyngeal trauma, such as a tonsillectomy.

Patients able to tolerate their symptoms may be managed conservatively with local corticosteroid injections. Surgical excision of the offending stylohyoid ligament and/or the styloid process can be performed should nonsurgical therapy fail.

C. Intracranial Tumor Pain

Intracranial tumors can produce a large and confusing array of symptoms creating a formidable diagnostic challenge. Also, the incidence of such tumors is low (10 per 100,000); therefore, a high index of suspicion is necessary for an early diagnosis. Many cases present with facial pain of an aching or stabbing nature, with or without facial numbness. The manifestation of neurological deficits is not always obvious and can precede the localizing signs of the tumor for years. Some of these deficits include: numbness or tingling of the hands, lips, or face; weakness of the extremities, altered motor function of one or more cranial nerves; aphasia, gait disturbances; visual defects such as flashes or lines of light; dizziness, and altered consciousness such as drowsiness and confusion. A number of patients present with pain similar to atypical facial pain or TGN which responds to standard TGN medication. This can further confuse and delay the diagnosis, hence, such treatments are not diagnostically significant in determining the underlying pathology when intracranial tumors are suspected.

Although sensory disturbances occur commonly with migraine headaches and occasionally with TGN, paresthesias should be regarded suspiciously. Areas of facial anesthesia can be an ominous sign, and neoplasia should be high on the differential diagnosis. Altered motor function of cranial nerves should also alert the clinician to the possibility of a neoplastic process and headache is a common symptom of intracranial tumors. The reader is referred to the "Headache" section of this chapter for further discussion. Prompt evaluation of such symptoms by a neurologist is essential for early diagnosis and treatment.

D. Trotter's Syndrome

This condition is caused by malignant tumors in the lateral pharyngeal recess and presents as a triad of symptoms including neuralgia within the trigeminal distribution, unilateral deafness and defective mobility of the soft palate. Infiltration of the tumor into the eustachian tube, tensor and levator palatini muscles, and mandibular branch of the trigeminal nerve is responsible for the symptomatic triad. Such patients should receive careful examination of the lateral pharyngeal recesses and be referred to an otolaryngologist for definitive diagnosis and treatment.

E. Ictal Facial Pain

Ictal facial pain is an unusual presentation of sensory epilepsy presumed to be caused by episodic discharges from the reticular formation. The pain attacks produce facial numbness or tingling that results in a burning pain deep in the facial tissues. Symptoms wax and wane over 15 to 20 minutes, followed by a numb or cold sensation in the affected areas, lasting several hours. The condition is commonly manifested in adulthood, and patients often relate a significant family history of seizures. Anticonvulsant medications are the treatment of choice and patients should be referred to a neurologist for management.

F. Atypical Facial Pain

Atypical facial pain (ATP) is characterized by unilateral or bilateral constant, burning pain that crosses neuroanatomic boundaries of the trigeminal, glossopharyngeal, second and third cervical nerves. The pain can persist without disruption for weeks to years, and there are no identifiable trigger points. Accompanying symptoms can include slight paresthesia, dysesthesia or hypoesthesia. Stress may exacerbate the symptoms, and women of all ages are afflicted more commonly than men. Although the majority of cases are idiopathic, ATP has been associated with a number of pathologic

Table 10-2: Potential Causes of Headache

1. Muscle contraction (tension)
2. Vascular
    A. Migraine
    B. Nonmigranous vascular causes
        1. Cluster headache
        2. Physical activity
        3. Hypertension/hypotension
        4. Cerebrovascular disease
        5. Post-seizure
        6. Hypoglycemia
        7. Toxic vascular (fever, infections, alcohol, hypoxia, high altitude, hypercapnia, foods [nitrates, tyramine, MSG], and drugs/toxins [theophylline, caffeine, dextroamphetamines, histamine, disulfiram and alcohol, carbon monoxide, insecticides, and nitroglycerin])
3. Intracranial causes
    A. Post-traumatic
    B. Tumors
    C. A-V malformations
    D. Aneurysm
    E. Subdural hematoma
    F. Encephalitis
    G. Cranial inflammation
        1. Meningeal irritation/infection
        2. Vasculitis (i.e., temporal arteritis)
4. Extracranial causes secondary to trauma/inflammation
    A. Ears (otitis media, otitis externa)
    B. Eyes (glaucoma, optic neuritis)
    C. Sinuses (acute and chronic sinusitis)
    D. Teeth (pulpitis and periodontitis)
    E. TMJs (capsulitis)
    F. Cervical spine ligaments and muscles (spondylitis, arthritis)
5. Psychogenic
    A. Hypochondriasis
    B. Anxiety states

processes including infections of the sinuses or jaws, malignancies which invade the cranial foramina, benign tumors, traumatic sectioning of trigeminal branches and vascular compression. Treatment of the underlying cause in these cases should resolve the facial pain. In many of the idiopathic cases, the symptoms are believed to be of psychogenic origin, resembling Munchausen syndrome. These patients often relate a history of chronic sickness, failure of extensive treatments to alleviate the pain, the tendency to seek care from numerous providers, the aggressive pursuit of invasive therapies, and a detailed recollection of all events connected with the condition. However, the suggestion of a psychogenic etiology and subsequent referral to a psychiatrist should be deferred until other potential causes have been ruled out. Pharmacotherapy including tricyclic antidepressants and phenothiazines have been successful in providing symptomatic relief.

G. Headaches

According to the National Ambulatory Care Medical Survey, headaches are the eighth and thirteenth most common problem encountered by family practitioners and internists, respectively. Surveys report that 73 to 85% of the general adult population suffers from recurrent headaches, which can be severe and disabling. To underscore this point, headache is the leading cause of lost workdays among adults employed full-time. Headaches, however, are a symptom rather than a specific disorder, and can signify anything from a physiologic response to an emotional insult, to intracranial or extracranial diseases. Fortunately, less than 1% of patients with acute headaches suffer from an underlying disorder that is life-threatening. The more common causes of headaches are listed in Table 10-2.

In the ***emergency assessment of headache***, the history is the most important and useful diagnostic tool. This is because pain's subjectivity hinders accurate quantification and because most headaches are usually not accompanied by physical findings. Patient evaluation should consist of a detailed history and physical examination as outlined in the "Diagnosis" section of this chapter, accompanied by a fundoscopic exam and limited laboratory tests in certain cases. A thorough evaluation coupled with explanation and reassurrance should play a large role in emergency management, as many patients are concerned that the headache is a manifestation of a severe underlying disease. This approach is oftentimes necessary for patients' physical and psychological well-being. Three types of headache patients are typically seen on an emergency basis and include those with a severe, first headache; chronic headache sufferers whose current headache is different from previous ones (i.e., change in character, increase in intensity); and previously-evaluated chronic sufferers seeking pain control for their typical headache. The risk of serious disease is greatest with the first group and least in the third.

When headaches are secondary to a serious underlying disease, most patients present with one or more positive neurologic findings or other abnormalities listed in Table 10-3. Some of the more serious causes of

Table 10-3: Indications of a Serious Headache

- When initial onset is severe ("worst headache ever")
- In a chronic sufferer with a significantly worse headache
- In a febrile patient or in one who looks ill.
- In a confused or drowsy patient.
- When accompanied by focal neurologic signs.
- When accompanied by neck stiffness
- When accompanied by papilledema

headache include subarachnoid hemorrhage, vasculopathies (i.e., temporal arteritis), meningitis and intracranial tumors. Patients presenting with such symptoms should receive immediate neurologic consultation for a more detailed evaluation that commonly includes CT or MRI scanning. The neurologist should also suggest treatment to control the headache pain and other symptoms as needed. Fortunately, over 99% of all headaches are benign, and 90% are of migraine or muscle contraction origin. Examples of benign headaches include muscle contraction (tension) and vascular headaches. Once a working diagnosis of an innocuous headache is established, emergency management consists of explanation, reassurrance, appropriate referral (i.e., to a neurologist or family physician) and control of pain and any associated symptoms. Oral or injectable analgesics, sedatives and antiemetics are examples of medications commonly administered for headaches in the emergency setting. Once the symptoms are controlled, patients should be discharged to the care of a responsible adult and referred for definitive evaluation and treatment. The management of specific headaches will be discussed under the respective sections which follow.

Tension Headache

Tension headaches are usually bilateral with a diffuse distribution over the top of the head in the manner of a "hatband" or "cap." However, the headaches can occur with an occipito-nuchal, frontal or temporal predominance. The pain has been characterized as a non-throbbing, dull ache that is frequently accompanied by tightness or pressure.

The prevalence of tension headache approximates that of migraine, affecting 3 to 30% of the population, and the two types of headaches commonly occur together. Like migraines, tension headaches are more common in women than in men, but unlike migraines, tension headaches are more likely to occur in middle age and are associated with anxiety and depression (Approximately one-third of patients with tension headaches exhibit symptoms of depression). Tension headaches have a more gradual onset than do migraine headaches, and also unlike migraine headaches, may persist unremittingly for weeks to years. In fact, this is the only headache that can persist without relief for extended periods. Though sleep is usually not disturbed, the headache is commonly present on waking or develops soon afterward. Simple analgesic medications are effective in minimizing the pain unless the pain is uncharacteristically intense. Tension headaches are a frequent sequel to head trauma, representing the most common type of chronic post-traumatic headache. Past theories regarding the etiology of tension headaches have included excessive muscle contraction and constriction of scalp arteries. However, secondary to a lack of scientific support, these theories are in question and today the etiology of tension headaches remains obscure.

The diagnosis of tension headaches is based on clinical signs and symptoms as there are no relevant objective clinical tests. Because many patients are fearful of an underlying, life-threatening illness, treatment should always begin with explanation and reassurrance. Psychiatric referral is appropriate if the headache is of psychogenic origin, as some form of stress management or psychotropic medication, such as tricyclic antidepressants and benzodiazepines may be beneficial. In cases such as post-traumatic headache, nonsteroidal anti-inflammatory agents are appropriate in the emergency setting, along with a referral to a family physician or neurologist for definitive management.

Vascular Headaches

Vascular headaches represent a heterogeneous group of disorders which are classified into three main types based on clinical and pathophysiologic features (Table 10-4).

Table 10-4: Classification of Vascular Headaches

1. Migraine
    - Classic
    - Common
    - Complicated
        - Ophthalmoplegic
        - Hemiplegic
        - Basilar artery migraine
2. Cluster
    - Episodic
    - Chronic
3. Chronic paroxysmal hemicrania
4. Miscellaneous
    - Carotidynia
    - Ice-pick headache
    - Exertional headache
    - Cough headache
    - Orgasmic headache
    - Toxic vascular headache

H. Migraine Headache

Migraine headaches account for 90% of all vascular headaches and are characterized by recurrent attacks that vary widely in intensity, frequency and duration. The headaches tend to be unilateral and are often associated with anorexia, nausea and vomiting. Some forms are preceded by neurologic and/or mood disturbances. Symptoms may vary with each episode, and some patients experience tension headaches between occurrences. Migraine headaches may begin at any age, but commonly start in childhood or early adulthood. Prevalence estimates range from 1 to 20% in males and 3 to 30% in females, and over 70% of migraine patients relate a positive family history. For some female patients, symptoms may be exacerbated or resolved during pregnancy, although pre-pregnancy patterns usually return after parturition. Up to 75% of female sufferers experience relief following menopause.

Based on proposed pathophysiologic events, migraine attacks can be divided into three phases: prodrome, headache and post-headache phases. Although these events concern vasomotor dysfunction, scientific support is equivocal, and the cause of the vasomotor disturbance is unknown. Nonetheless, in the prodromal phase, reduced blood flow from vasoconstriction of intracranial and extracranial arteries leads to local tissue hypoxia. This is followed by the headache phase, heralded by vasodilation of the extracranial arteries. Finally in the post-headache phase, vessel lumens return to the normal size, although edema and inflammation persist in the extravascular tissues. Though this pathophysiologic mechanism is conceptually tidy, the timing of the clinical features correlates poorly with these vascular changes. In addition, the two pathophysiologic stages of vasoconstriction and vasodilation are not always sharply defined. For example, the vasodilation is not consistently associated with the headache, and it is proposed that the headache pain may be secondary to other factors. One alternative mechanism for the headache pain is that affected arteries become hyperpermeable, resulting in a local sterile inflammatory reaction. Platelets and certain vasoactive substances are believed to play a role in this process. In some patients the headaches may be provoked by air pollution, perfumes, oversleeping, fatigue, hypoglycemia, drugs such as vasodilators and some ingested substances (e.g., chocolate, cheese, alcohol, MSG). Whatever the case, migraine headaches should be considered idiopathic in origin until further scientific insight is available.

Classic Migraine

The classic type comprises 15 to 20% of migraines and is characterized by a sharply-defined prodrome of neurological symptoms occurring contralateral to the side of the headache. The most commonly reported prodromal symptoms are visual disturbances such as photophobia, diplopia, scotoma, zig-zag lines or flashing lights. Arm or leg weakness, mild aphasia, confusion, as well as numbness and tingling of the lips, face or hands can also occur. Any one of these symptoms or a combination thereof can affect a given patient, and the same prodromal symptoms usually occur with each headache episode. These prodromal manifestations build gradually over 5 to 30 minutes, usually last 15 to 60 minutes, and fade slowly. Nausea and vomiting are common occurrences at the peak of the headache phase, which generally lasts 6 to 12 hours. The reader should be aware that the manifestations of vascular headaches and certainly migraine headaches are recalled by the distinctive signs and symptoms of classic migraines, when in fact, this type of migraine is uncommon and, hence, is unrepresentative of most migraines.

Common Migraine

Common migraines account for over 80% of all migraine headaches and differ from the classic variety in that there are no sharply defined neurologic symptoms. The prodromal symptoms vary greatly, ranging from psychic disturbances such as depression and irritability, to gastrointestinal symptoms or heightened energy. These manifestations may precede the headache by hours to days. The headache tends to escalate over a period of hours and persists for hours to days. The pain is usually unilateral and throbbing in nature, but can be bilateral. Nausea, vomiting, irritability, photophobia and tenderness of the superficial vessels in the area of the pain normally accompany the headache.

The term "complicated migraine" refers to those varieties in which the prodromal symptoms persist throughout or beyond the headache phase. Permanent neurological deficits may result with repeated attacks, and this type of migraine includes ophthalmoplegic, hemiplegic and basilar artery migraine.

Ophthalmoplegic Migraine

This unusual form occurs most often in children and young adults, especially in those with a history of common migraine. The third cranial nerve is affected in most cases and the pain is moderate in intensity and occurs on the same side as the ophthalmoplegia. The ophthalmoplegia typically includes dilation of the pupil, outward deviation of the eye, and ptosis. This ocular paresis usually begins as the headache subsides and persists for days to weeks. Permanent damage to the oculomotor nerve can follow repeated attacks and is thought to result from ischemic compression of the nerve secondary to vasodilation and resultant swelling of the posterior cerebellar arteries.

Hemiplegic Migraine

Hemiplegic migraine is an uncommon variant in which unilateral motor and sensory disturbances accompany and outlast the headache. Confusion, aphasia and visual symptoms can also occur. Total recovery from the paresis requires days to weeks, and permanent weakness occasionally results from multiple episodes. The majority of these patients have family histories of migraine, and 4 to 8% report a family history of hemiplegic migraine. Interestingly, the paresis always recurs on the same side in every affected family member, whereas in patients without a positive family history, the weakness can occur on either side. It is suggested that oral contraceptives may exacerbate the headaches.

Basilar Artery Migraine

The signs and symptoms of basilar artery migraine follow the distribution of the vertebrobasilar arterial system. Affected areas include the brainstem, thalamus, occipital lobe and cerebellum. Vertigo, disturbed consciousness, diplopia, tinnitus and ataxia can occur in various combinations and sequencing. Though the visual aberrations are similar to those seen in classic migraine, with basilar artery migraine, the disturbances can occur in both visual fields. Children and young women are most often affected.

The treatment of migraine headaches can be divided into the four categories of acute, general, abortive and prophylactic care. The ***acute treatment*** of emergency migraine patients depends on the severity of the attack and the associated symptoms. Patients with a history of migraine headaches will usually have attempted their normal therapies without success. These patients are typically in severe pain and are often considerably nauseated and dehydrated from vomiting and/or the inability to drink or eat. For patients who present during the neurologic phase or early headache phase, further pain can be aborted or greatly reduced in up to 75% of patients with the administration of ergotamine tartrate. The desired dose is 0.25 to 0.50 mg given subcutaneously or intramuscularly every 30 minutes or 2 mg uncoated tablets given sublingually every 30 minutes to a maximum dose of 8 mg. Once the pain becomes intense, ergotamine is of no abortive use, and potent analgesics are usually necessary for pain control. Parenteral narcotics (i.e., meperidine 50-100 mg or morphine

5-10 mg) may be used; however, because there is a potential for narcotic addiction with recurrent severe headaches, other medications such as the phenothiazines are commonly substituted (i.e., chlorpromazine 50-300 mg orally or intramuscularly). Dehydration may require intravenous fluid replacement, and nausea can be controlled with antiemetic drugs such as intravenous promethazine (25 mg) or metoclopromide (10 mg). The sedative properties of these medications may help allay anxiety, in addition to providing the needed analgesia. Emergency migraine headache patients should be referred to a neurologist for initial evaluation or re-evaluation of the problem. The ***general treatment*** for migraine headaches consists of avoiding known triggering factors, and maintaining regular times for sleeping and waking. ***Abortive therapy***, as the name implies, is employed to bring an end to an impending or on-going attack. Ergotamine tartrate is the mainstay of treatment, with individualized dosage regimens as previously described under "acute treatment". Other effective abortive agents for patients can include propranolol, naproxen and even aspirin in mild cases. ***Prophylactic treatment*** is prescribed for patients with frequent and disabling headaches and for patients who respond poorly to abortive therapy. Potential medications include beta-blockers such as atenolol, timolol, nadolol and metoprolol; calcium channel blockers such as verapamil, nifedipine and diltiazem; serotonin antagonists such as methysergide and cyproheptadine; naproxen; MAO inhibitors; and amitriptyline. Nonpharmacologic therapies such as biofeedback, behavioral counseling, and transcutaneous electrical nerve stimulation (TENS) have also been used with variable success. Combining medication and non-pharmacologic therapies is often more efficacious than either treatment alone.

I. Cluster Headaches

Also known as migrainous neuralgia, cluster headache is characterized by diurnal or, more commonly, nocturnal facial pain that is excruciating, unilateral and occurs for periods of several weeks to months. In ***acute cluster headache***, these episodes are separated by remissions lasting months to years. ***Chronic cluster headache*** is diagnosed when patients experience at least two attacks per week for more than two years. During an attack, the pain is present for 30 minutes to two hours, and commonly evokes a pacing behavior in patients. Associated with the headache are a group of ipsilateral autonomic symptoms that include rhinorrhea, nasal congestion, conjunctival infection and lacrimation. Ptosis and miosis are also present in about 20% of the patients and there are no identifiable provocative factors. The severity of the attacks can lead to severe depression and suicidal ideation, hence, these patients are candidates for acute psychiatric intervention. The prevalence of cluster headaches is estimated at 0.4 to 0.8% with a male to female ratio of 5:1. Most patients are between 20 and 40 years of age and there is no familial pattern. Many sufferers exhibit a "leonine" appearance, characterized by deep furrows in the forehead, and deep folds in the glabellar and nasolabial areas. The patients' skin tends to be thickened with large pores similar to that of an orange peel. Cluster headaches occur more often in smokers and in those who use alcohol, and the incidence of peptic ulcer disease is nearly four times greater in this population. However, the reasons for these relationships are unclear. Similarly, the etiology of cluster headache is obscure, but recent studies have implicated substance P, a vasoactive peptide and putative transmitter in the pathogenesis of both cluster and migraine headache. As with migraine headaches, the diagnosis is based solely on signs and symptoms.

The treatment of cluster headache can be divided into the treatment of an acute attack, prophylactic treatment and the treatment of a chronic headache resistant to medical management. The ***acute management*** of patients who present with cluster headache consists of reassurrance, pain control and appropriate referral. These patients are typically in excruciating pain and are often extremely anxious, being ignorant of the problem's benign nature. The pharmacologic management of pain and anxiety in the emergency setting is usually indicated and commonly administered drugs include parenteral narcotic analgesics (i.e., meperidine 50-150 mg IM or IV) and phenothiazines (i.e., chlorpromazine 50-300 mg IM). The inhalation of 100% oxygen and the instillation of 4% lidocaine nasally may also be useful in suppressing an acute attack. Once the symptoms are controlled, patients should be promptly referred to a neurologist for definitive evaluation and management. ***Prophylaxis*** is the preferred therapeutic approach because the headache's short duration makes acute management difficult. Medications that have been used with some success include methysergide, ergotamine tartrate, prednisone, lithium carbonate, propranolol, verapamil, and nifedipine. The ***treatment of chronic cluster headaches*** is usually surgical, because of the patient's unresponsiveness to medical therapy. Sectioning of the trigeminal root, avulsion of trigeminal nerve branches, and the injection of local anesthetic or glycerol into the trigeminal sensory root have all been attempted with variable success.

Chronic Paroxysmal Hemicrania

Chronic Paroxysmal Hemicrania is a rare condition first described in 1976. Like cluster headache, the pain is unilateral and excruciating, but differs in temporal character and response to indomethacin. Chronic paroxysmal hemicrania is characterized by numerous daily attacks of headache, which last approximately 15 to 20 minutes. The pain begins abruptly in the temporal region and may radiate to the ipsilateral orbit, maxilla, jaw, neck or shoulder. A partial unilateral Horner's syndrome (ptosis, miosis, anhidrosis and enophthalmosis) and rhinorrhea may accompany the headache. Unlike cluster headaches, there are no pain-free remissions, nor is there a nocturnal predominance. The etiology of chronic paroxysmal hemicrania is poorly understood; however, because virtually all patients respond dramatically to indomethacin and some to aspirin, prostaglandins are believed to play an important pathophysiologic role.

Carotidynia

Carotidynia is a vascular headache characterized by unilateral carotid bifurcation tenderness and anterior neck pain. This dull ache can be referred ipsilaterally to the face, ear, jaws and teeth. Also present is an exquisite tenderness in the floor of the mouth in the region of the facial artery and submandibular ganglion. This headache is commonly a symptom of intraluminal clots in the internal carotid artery, or of spontaneous arterial dissection. The clinical diagnosis of carotidynia is not difficult because of the uniqueness of the signs and symptoms; however, angiography is recommended after the first attack to rule out carotid artery dissection. Regarding treatment, patients appear to respond well to indomethacin.

Ice-pick Headache

These headaches are characterized by sudden, sharp stabbing pain or pricking sensations lasting seconds to minutes. The pain's location is variable, though the anatomical area involved is typically discrete and small. Although these headaches can occur as an isolated condition, they are common in migraine patients, especially in patients over 60 years old. The cause of the headaches is unclear, and patients respond to indomethacin therapy.

Exertional Headache

This condition usually affects men over 40 years of age and begins toward the end of sustained vigorous exertion (i.e., running) or shortly after cessation of the activity. Athletes and unconditioned persons alike are affected. The headache is usually severe, particularly in the frontal area and resembles migrainous pain. Unlike migraine, however, the pain is usually bilateral and takes minutes to hours to resolve. The symptoms mimic those seen with a leaking berry aneurysm, hence, a neurological workup is indicated when the headache first occurs. The etiology is idiopathic and the diagnosis is based on clinical signs and symptoms. Warmup exercises and indomethacin therapy are potentially beneficial treatments.

Cough Headache

This headache also commonly affects men over 40 years old and occurs with coughing and other forms of brief, intense activity such as weight-lifting. The pain is typically severe and diffuse and begins seconds after the triggering activity. The pain peaks rapidly and subsides over 30 seconds, although a residual ache can persist for hours. Because symptoms mimic those of intracranial neoplasms, a CT or MRI of the head is usually performed to rule out this possibility. The headache's etiology is unknown, and the diagnosis is based on signs and symptoms. Treatment consists of indomethacin therapy and the avoidance of conditions causing coughing.

Orgasmic Headache

This headache occurs during sexual activity and can be of two types. The first is a severe nucho-occipital or generalized headache that begins explosively at the time of climax and clears within minutes to hours. Because these headaches can be confused with leaking berry aneurysms or intracranial tumors, a CT or MRI of the head should be obtained to rule out these possibilities. The second type is a slowly building, dull occipital headache, thought to be caused by increasing muscle contraction or increasing blood pressure as sexual excitement builds. Once the diagnosis is made, ergotamine tartrate is a frequently effective treatment taken approximately 30 minutes before an expected sexual encounter.

Toxic Vascular Headache

This headache is precipitated by systemic vasodilation and is most commonly caused by fever. Additional precipitators include certain foods (MSG, tyramine, nitrites), hypoxia, infection, alcohol, carbon dioxide retention, high altitudes, and medications such as bronchodilators and various antihypertensives. The pain is bilateral, generalized, pulsatile, and moderate to severe in intensity. The duration is variable and depends on the etiology. Diagnosis is based on historical information, signs and symptoms, and treatment involves addressing the underlying cause. Emergency and short term management with mild analgesics such as acetominophen or aspirin with or without codeine is appropriate until the cause of the headache can be determined.

Cervical Spinal Disease Headache

This headache is associated with diseases of the cervical spine and essentially represents the radiation of pain to the head from the noxious stimulation of musculature and connective tissue in the cervical spine. The pain is most commonly referred to the back of the head, but can also occur in the eyes, temporal and maxillary regions. In the presence of cervical radiculopathy, the prevalence of headache is nearly 40%. However, radiographic findings of cervical arthropathies are common in the elderly, yet few of these patients complain of headache. As such, the relationship between headaches and cervical disease is poorly understood. Cervical collars, physical therapy and NSAIDs are commonly used therapies.

Temporal Arteritis

Temporal arteritis (TA) is an inflammatory disease characterized by headaches, temporal artery abnormalities, jaw claudication, weight loss, fever, fatigue, and ischemic symptoms such as visual deficits. Headache occurs in 90% of TA patients and is usually located in one or both temporal areas. The pain can be constant or episodic and is often described as sharp, burning, or throbbing. Scalp tenderness is common and can be so severe that sufferers cannot brush their hair or wear a hat. Jaw claudication occurs in up to 50% of TA patients, hence, patients often perceive the problem to be TMJ or odontogenic in origin. TA is thought to be caused by inflammation of a cranial artery, most commonly the temporal artery. Immune-mediated abnormalities have been demonstrated in a few studies to account for the inflammatory process; however, the etiology remains unknown. Depending on which cranial arteries are affected, a number of other symptoms can occur, of which blindness is the most serious. Up to one-third of untreated TA patients lose vision in one eye, and if treatment is not initiated, another third lose sight in the other eye within weeks of the initial visual symptoms (i.e., visual defects and hallucinations). Fortunately, blindness is rarely the first manifestation of TA, and systemic complaints usually precede eye symptoms by weeks to years. Forty to seventy percent of TA cases are associated with an arthritic condition called polymyalgia rheumatica, which is characterized by proximal limb pain without weakness, morning stiffness, fatigue, weight loss, low-grade fever, anemia, and elevated erythrocyte sedimentation rate. The typical TA patient is a Caucasian woman over 50 years of age, although the disease has also been reported in oriental and hispanic populations. Occasionally, familial clusters occur, and the prevalence ranges from 0.49 to 16.8 per 100,000 in Israel and Sweden, respectively.

Screening measures for TA can include history, an ophthalmologic evaluation, a physical examination of the temporal artery and cranial blood supply, and laboratory studies. An elevated ESR and mild normocytic or hypochromic anemia that is resistant to iron therapy are common findings. If TA is suspected, a temporal artery biopsy should be performed to confirm the diagnosis. Glucocorticosteroids are the mainstay of therapy because they usually lessen the symptoms and virtually eliminate the risk of blindness.

Some of the more serious causes of headache, which includes intracranial tumors, subarachnoid hemorrhage, and meningitis, are discussed in the following paragraphs.

Headaches Associated with Intracranial Tumors

Although the vast majority of headaches that are seen on an emergency basis are not caused by mass lesions, headache is a significant symptom in one-half to two-thirds of patients with intracranial tumors. The pain is typically deep-seated and can be described as "aching", "bursting" or "throbbing." Initially, the headaches tend to occur intermittently, lasting several minutes to hours and recur on a daily basis. As the tumor expands, the duration and intensity of the pain increase until the pain is severe and continuous. However, some patients experience only mild to moderate pain which is easily relieved with mild analgesics. This variability may relate to the tumor's location and rate of growth.

The pain is typically unilateral and usually overlies the tumor, although referred pain is common. Lesions above the tentorium refer pain anteriorly to the frontal region or vertex, whereas subtentorial masses refer pain posteriorly to the occipital region. A bilateral headache that occurs following a unilateral headache usually signifies an increase in intracranial pressure. Activity and frequent positional changes may intensify the headache, whereas rest diminishes the pain. Certain associated symptoms should arouse one's suspicion of an intracranial tumor, including nocturnal awakening secondary to headache pain, pain that is worse with the Valsalva maneuver or lowering the head, and a new or unfamiliar headache associated with nausea or vomiting. Of course, these characteristics can be associated with other causes of headache and, hence, are not pathognomonic of an intracranial mass. As previously mentioned, localizing neurological signs such as numbness or tingling of the face or hands, weakness of an extremity, altered motor function of one or more cranial nerves, visual defects (i.e., flashes or lines of light), dizziness and altered consciousness (i.e., lethargy, confusion) often do not present until months to years after the headache first appears. This fact, coupled with the low incidence of intracranial tumors (10 per 100,000 patients), necessitates a high index of suspicion and discrimination for early diagnosis.

When an intracranial tumor is suspected on the basis of signs and symptoms, emergency management should include immediate neurological consultation, coupled with a CT or MRI of the head. The headache pain can usually be managed with analgesics such as aspirin or acetominophen with or without codeine until definitive care is instituted.

Headaches Associated with a Subarachnoid Hemorrhage

The most common cause of subarachnoid hemorrhage is the rupture of an aneurysm in the Circle of Willis. These so-called "berry aneurysms" develop insidiously over years to reach sizes of 1 to 3 cm. This slow evolution accounts for the relative lack of ruptures prior to the age of 30. Typically, the aneurysms give no indication of their presence prior to the rupture and upon rupture, the ensuing symptoms are variable. Commonly, patients experience a relatively sudden severe headache, accompanied by an alteration of mental status, syncopy, and photophobia. Focal neurologic deficits are rare, and if present, intracerebral hemorrhage should be suspected. When a subarachnoid hemorrhage is suspected on the basis of signs and symptoms, neurological consultation and a CT or MRI of the head should be obtained immediately. The hemorrhagic lesion will be evident on the CT or MRI in the majority of cases, although a negative scan does not exclude the diagnosis. If the diagnosis remains unclear, a lumbar puncture can be performed, which will usually demonstrate a modest elevation of CSF pressure with blood in the spinal fluid for a positive diagnosis. During this procedure, it is important that the patients are kept calm and comfortable to avoid exacerbating the problem. As such, adequate local anesthesia for the puncture and careful use of analgesia and sedation, both during and after the procedure, are essential. Intravenous benzodiazepines and narcotics titrated to effect are frequently indicated. The patient's head should be elevated 20 to 30 degrees from the floor whenever possible. Most patients are admitted to the hospital for a period of stabilization (7 to 10 days), angiography and surgery.

Headaches Associated with Meningeal Irritation

The headache of meningitis resembles that of a toxic vascular headache, typically encompassing the entire head. The pain is usually acute in onset, severe, deep-seated, constant and often pulsatile. Unlike toxic vascular headache, however, most meningitis patients demonstrate significant stiffness of the neck upon bending the head forward (nuchal rigidity), a positive Kernig's sign (hamstring and paraspinal muscle pain on extension of the knee with the hips flexed), a positive Brudzinski's sign (flexion of the knees and hips when the neck is flexed), and retro-orbital pain exacerbated by eye movement. Photophobia, alteration of consciousness and fever greater than 101° degrees are common symptoms as well. Meningitis occurs more frequently in children, in lower socioeconomic groups and in the winter. Most cases of meningitis are bacterial or viral in origin, and hematogenous seeding from an existing infection is the predominant route of spread to the CNS. The disease is thought to result from the combination of a primary infection such as sinusitis, otitis, pneumonia and pharyngitis with a defect in the host's immunologic competency. Irrespective of the offending organism, signs and symptoms are similar; however, the manifestations are usually more severe with a bacterial etiology. In fact, few patients with viral meningitis require treatment beyond follow-up observation. Organisms commonly responsible for bacterial meningitis include *Haemophilus influenzae*, *Neisseria meningitidis*, and *Streptococcus pneumoniae*. Between the ages of 6 and 50, meningococci and pneumococci predominate, while in patients over 50 years old, gram negative bacilli and pneumococci are more common. Enterovirus and mumps virus are responsible for most cases of viral meningitis and *Cryptococcus neoformans* and *Candida albicans* account for uncommon fungal meningitis.

If bacterial meningitis is suspected on the basis of signs and symptoms, an immediate neurological consultation, blood cultures and a lumbar puncture should be performed. If focal neurologic deficits suggesting a mass lesion are observed, the lumbar puncture should be preceded by a CT or MRI of the head to rule out this possibility. In the presence of bacterial meningitis, the CSF pressure is elevated, the spinal fluid is often cloudy to frankly purulent and is infiltrated with neutrophils (up to 90,000 per cubic mm). Also, CSF protein content is increased, while sugar content is markedly reduced. The mortality rate with bacterial meningitis is greatest during the first 24 hours and patients with turbid CSF should begin receiving intravenous antibiotics in the emergency setting. Penicillin G (50,000 units/kg every 4 hours) is usually the drug of choice, while chloramphenicol (25mg/kg every 6 hours) is substituted for penicillin-allergic patients.

Table 10-5 is provided as a quick reference comparison of the more common headache and neuralgia entities.

Table 10-5: Extraoral Sources of Facial Pain

	TGN	Atypical Facial Pain	Migraine	Cluster HA	Temporal Arteritis	Tumors	Sinusitis	Tension HA	Meningeal Irritation
Site	2nd and/or 3rd div. of trigeminal nerve	face and upper neck	fronto-temporal, temporo-parietal	occulo-temporal, occulo-frontal	temporal	discrete or generalized	regions of paranasal sinuses	top of head, "hatband" or "cap"	bioccipital, bifrontal, or generalized
Type of Pain	severe. stabbing, electric	moderate to severe, burning, aching	moderate to severe, throbbing	excruciating, drilling (not throbbing)	moderate to severe, burning, throbbing, sharp	variable intensity, steady pain, deep-seated	moderate to severe, dull, aching	moderate to severe, dull aching, nonthrobbing	severe, steady, deep-seated
Side Affected	unilateral	unilateral or bilateral	unilateral or bilateral	unilateral	unilateral or bilateral	unilateral or bilateral	usually unilateral	usually bilateral	bilateral
Pattern of Occurrence	intermittent, with pain-free intervals	constant	intermittent	headaches for weeks to months; pain-free periods for months to years	intermittent, then continuous	abrupt onset, short duration, progresses to continuous	episodic or chronic	variable, post-traumatic	rapid onset in minutes to hours
Frequency	several per day	constant	1 - 8 per month	1 - 3 per day	intermittent, then continuous	continuous to many per day	variable, depends on drainage	usually constant	single episode
Duration	seconds to minutes	weeks to years	4 - 48 hours	½ - 2 hours	weeks to months	minutes to continuous	days to months	weeks to years	constant
Trigger Points	yes	no	no	no	no	no	no	no	no
Sensory Changes	minimal to none	frequent	visual aura	none	loss of visual acuity	usually none	none	none	none
Associated Features	usually triggered by touching face	stress, depression	photophobia, nausea, vomiting, somnolence	lacrimation, rhinorrhea, injected conjunctivum, pacing	polymyalgia rhuematica, fever, weight loss, elevated ESR	paresthesia, anesthesia, seizures, cranial nerve dysfunction	postnasal drip, fever, malaise, max. post. tooth pain	anxiety, depression	nuchal rigidity, Kernig's sign, Brudzinski's sign

J. Sinusitis

The paranasal sinuses include the maxillary, frontal, ethmoid and sphenoid sinuses, which are paired diverticula of the nasal cavity named according to the encasing bones (Figure 10-3). Each sinus is continuous with the nasal cavity through a small opening termed an ostium. Typically, infectious agents and other airborne matter entering the sinuses are trapped in the mucus layer overlying the epithelium and moved to the ostia via sweeping movements of the underlying cilia.

Impairment of this cleansing mechanism usually results in sinusitis, an infection of one or more of the paranasal sinuses, resulting from the opportunistic growth of relatively harmless bacteria normally found in the nose. However, the condition can also occur as a consequence of infectious diseases such as influenza or the common cold, and from traumatic injury to the sinuses (i.e., midface surgery or antral perforation during tooth extraction). Allergic rhinitis is a common cause of sinusitis in which edematous closure of the ostium produces sinus congestion and subsequent infection. Other predisposing factors include upper respiratory infections, deviated nasal septums, hypertrophied adenoids, swimming, smoking, tumors, immunodeficiency and cystic fibrosis. The maxillary sinus can also be infected by bacterial invasion from periapical odontogenic disease (i.e., dental abscess). The discomfort associated with sinusitis is believed to result from pressure changes and irritation of the pain-sensitive sinus walls. The pain usually waxes and wanes with the amount of drainage from the sinus. Sinusitis is possibly the most common cause of facial pain and occurs in both acute and chronic forms.

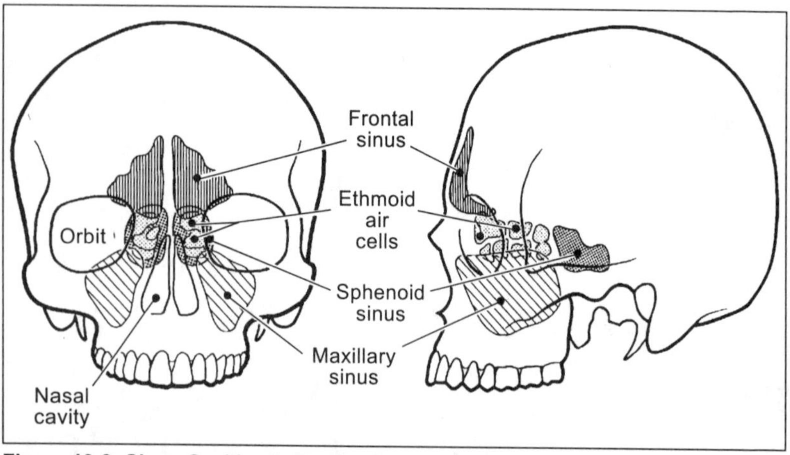

Figure 10-3: Sinus Cavities in the Head.

Acute Sinusitis

Patients with acute sinusitis usually complain of moderate to severe pain, accompanied by fullness and pressure in the region of the affected sinus(es). The pain can be referred to most areas of the face, including the ear and teeth, and the pain and pressure may increase when the head is lowered. Often, the area overlying the sinus is tender, and palpation can elicit significant discomfort. Patients may also complain of pharyngeal and external nasal drainage of pus or thick mucus, fever and malaise. Sinusitis most commonly affects the maxillary sinus, followed by the ethmoid, frontal and sphenoid sinuses. Typically, more than one sinus is involved. Pain from ethmoid and sphenoid sinusitis is perceived to be deep in the midline region behind the nose, while pain from frontal sinusitis occurs supra and retro-orbitally. Maxillary sinusitis produces pain in the maxillary region which can be referred to the ipsilateral eye and maxillary posterior teeth. As such, facial pain coupled with percussive sensitivity of several maxillary posterior teeth, strongly suggests maxillary sinusitis. Pain from frontal and ethmoid sinusitis is usually worse on waking and subsides during the day, presumably because the gravitational effects of postural change improves drainage. In contrast, with sphenoid and maxillary sinusitis, the reverse occurs. This phenomenon is attributed to the superior location of the ostia of these sinuses relative to the sinus floor, affording poorer drainage with the patient upright.

Regarding diagnosis, patients should be questioned about the historical presence of allergy, asthma and previous sinus infections. Teeth should be examined (pulp and percussion testing, observation, and/or periapical radiographs) for evidence of pathology that could account for tooth pain. Because cloudiness of the sinus is often evident radiographically with sinusitis, sinus imaging can assist in making the diagnosis. Waters and Caldwell views, along with lateral skull films are commonly used for this purpose. Once dental disease is ruled out, referring symptomatic patients to an Otolaryngologist is indicated.

Although the incidence of acute sinusitis complications has greatly decreased with the widespread use of antibiotics, complications still occur and are most likely to be present on an emergency visit. In descending frequency of occurrence, complications of acute sinusitis include orbital cellulitis, intracranial infection (epidural or subdural abscesses, and meningitis), chronic sinusitis and osteomyelitis. Symptoms of orbital cellulitis include edema of the eyelids and surrounding tissue, proptosis, restricted eye movements, visual disturbances, fever and malaise. Although uncommon, orbital abscess and cavernous sinus thrombosis can result from untreated orbital cellulitis and the latter is associated with an 80% mortality rate. Intracranial infection can produce subtle signs, such as periodic generalized headache, mental slowness, papilledema and confusion, which are commonly secondary to increased intracranial pressure. Nuchal rigidity will be present if meningitis occurs. Osteomyelitis is a very rare complication occurring most often in children. Radiographically, osteomyelitis can reveal boney erosions and loss of the intrasinus septa. If any of the aforementioned symptoms of acute sinusitis complications are present, immediate referral to an Otolaryngologist (and ophthalmologist for orbital symptoms) is essential. These complications usually require hospitalization and aggressive parenteral antibiotic therapy.

The treatment of uncomplicated acute sinusitis consists of oral antibiotic therapy, decongestants, antihistamines, nasal drops or spray and analgesics. For adults, 250 mg of penicillin or erythromycin administered four times daily for 2 to 4 weeks is appropriate. For children under 20 kg, amoxacillin 20 mg/kg/day in divided doses every 8 hours is suggested. Any combination of a long-acting decongestant/antihistamine should be taken for 10-20 days, along with nasal drops or spray. Oxymetazoline (Afrin) or phenylephrine (Neo-Synephrine) administered three times daily for 10 days are effective nasal sprays. Non-steroidal anti-inflammatory agents, with or without a narcotic such as codeine, may be needed for the first several days of treatment. If purulence in the nasal cavity is obvious, a specimen should be obtained for culture and sensitivity testing. Patients should be advised to avoid smoking, flying, swimming and physical exertion until the sinusitis has resolved. Patients can also apply moist heat over the affected sinus(es) to aid in comfort and possibly promote sinus drainage.

Chronic Sinusitis

Chronic sinusitis affects 31 million Americans and can result as a sequel to an acute episode or may develop without precedent. The disease is a common finding in asthma patients and can significantly exacerbate asthmatic symptoms. Whereas acute sinusitis produces a typical acute inflammatory infiltration with edema of the connective tissue, chronic sinusitis usually results in moderate to extreme thickening of the mucosa lining and sinus polyps. The mucosal and hyperplastic granulation tissue of the polyps usually exhibits lymphocytic infiltration typical of chronic inflammation.

Unlike acute sinusitis, symptoms of chronic sinusitis can be quite vague, and often the condition is an unexpected finding during a routine examination. Sometimes mild discomfort, pressure or stuffiness are present on the affected side. The discharge of small amounts of pus into the nose may also occur, and radiographs of the affected sinus are usually cloudy.

A number of surgical approaches are employed to treat this condition including intranasal antrostomy, Caldwell-Luc and sinus endoscopy. These treatments are intended to relieve the ostial obstruction and to remove the infected or inflammatory tissues, thereby creating a patent airway and avenue for drainage. An intranasal antrostomy involves creating a permanent opening between the maxillary sinus and the inferior meatus of the lateral nasal wall to restore drainage. An intranasal antrostomy is accomplished by removing diseased tissue through a sublabial opening. The Caldwell-Luc procedure is performed via a sublabial approach and provides excellent access to the entire antrum. A transantral ethmoidectomy, can also be performed through the same incision during a Caldwell-Luc operation, allowing entry into, and debridement of, the ethmoid air cells. Maxillary, frontal and ethmoid sinusitis can also be treated by endoscopic surgery, in which diseased tissue is removed from affected areas of the middle turbinate and meatus as well as the anterior ethmoid sinus.

Aerosinusitis

Also known as barosinusitis, aerosinusitis occurs when the ostium is obstructed, typically by boggy membranes during the resolution of a sinus infection. Air that is trapped in the sinus is absorbed by the sinus membrane, creating a negative pressure which is believed to be responsible for the discomfort. Activities such as descent in an aircraft or scuba diving have been implicated in the trapping of air and the creation of negative sinus pressures. The condition can produce severe pain, transudation of tissue fluids and hemorrhage into the affected sinus. Diagnosis is based on historical information and signs/symptoms. Treatment involving the restoration of sinus aeration generally relieves the discomfort.

References

Adams R.D., Victor M., *Principles of Neurology*. 4th ed., New York: McGraw-Hill Book Co, 1989.

Camarda A.J., et al., "Stylohyoid chain ossification: A discussion of etiology." *O Surg O Med O Path*. 67 (1989): 508.

Drinnan A.J., "Differential diagnosis of orofacial pain." *Dent Clin N Amer*. 31 (1987): 627.

Edmeads J., "The worst headache ever." *Postgrad Medicine*. 86 (1989): 93.

Ferguson B.J., et al., "Giant cell arteritis and polymyalgia rheumatica." *Ann Otol Rhinol Laryngol*. 96 (1987): 373.

Flynn T.R., Eisenberg E., "Computerized tomography and Trotter's syndrome in the diagnosis of maxillofacial pain." *O Surg O Med O Path*. 61 (1986): 440.

Hansotia P., "Evaluation and treatment of headache." *Postgrad Medicine*. 79 (1986): 75.

Harlin S.L., et al., "A clinical and pathologic study of chronic sinusitis: The role of the eosinophil." *J Allergy Clin Immunol.* 81 (1988): 867.
Kahn C.H., Warfield C.A., "Orofacial pain." *Hospital Practice*. Feb 15 (1989): 247.
Katusic S., et al., "Incidence and clinical features of trigeminal neuralgia, Rochester, Minnesota, 1945-1984." *Annals of Neurology*. 27 (1990): 89.
Kravis T.C., et al., *Emergency Medicine. A Comprehensive Review*. 2nd ed. Rockville: Aspen Publications, 1987.
Kumar K.L., Cooney T.G., "Vascular headaches." *J Gen Int Med.* 3 (1988): 384.
Lamey P.J., Lewis M.A.O., "Oral medicine in practice: orofacial pain." *Brit Dent J.* 167 (1989): 384.
Linet M.S., et al., "An epidemiological study of headache among adolescents and young adults." *JAMA*. 261 (1989): 2211.
Mastrocola R., et al., "Atypical facial pain of psychogenic origin." *Gen Dent*. May/June (1987): 207.
McKenna J.P., "Cluster headaches." *AFP*. 37 (1988): 173.
Mulry J.T., et al., "Alcoholic facial neuralgia: report of three cases." *JADA*. 112 (1986): 847.
Onofrio B.M., Campbell J.K., "Surgical treatment of chronic cluster headache." *Mayo Clin Proc.* 61 (1986): 537.
Robbins S.L., et al., *Pathologic Basis of Disease*. 3rd ed. Philadelphia: WB Saunders Co., 1984.
Rose F.C., *The Management of Headache*. New York: Raven Press, 1988.
Rovit R.L., et al., *Trigeminal Neuralgia*. Baltimore: Williams & Wilkins, 1990.
Schnetler J., Hopper C., "Intracranial tumors presenting with facial pain." *Brit Dent J.* 166 (1989): 80.
Shafer W.G., et al., *A Textbook of Oral Pathology*. 4th ed. Philadelphia: W.B. Saunders Co, 1983.
Slavin R.G., "Sinusitis in adults." *J Allergy Clin Immunol.* 81 (1988): 1028.
Stewart J.D., *Focal Peripheral Neuropathies*. New York: Elsevier, 1987.
Sweet W.H., "Treatment of trigeminal neuralgia (tic doloreaux)." *New England J Med*. 315 (1986): 174.
Warner J.J., "Headaches in older patients: Dx and Tx of common nonvascular causes." *Geriatrics*. 40 (1985): 69.
Wilkins E.W. Jr., *Emergency Medicine. Scientific Foundations and Current Practice*. 3rd ed. Baltimore: Williams & Wilkins, 1989.

11 Psychological and Behavioral Evaluations in the Acute Care Setting

Gerald W. Talcott, Ph.D.

John D. Rugh, Ph.D.

Robert R. Lemke, D.D.S., M.D.

INTRODUCTION

Approximately one-third of all emergency room visits are solely for mental health reasons (Yoder & Jones, 1982). Thus, psychological and behavioral abnormalities must be recognized and frequently managed in the acute care setting. In addition, psychological maladies frequently accompany other emergency complaints, such as those associated with physical abuse, personal injury, serious injury or death of a loved one. As such, during an examination of patients with acute illnesses and injuries, it is beneficial for health care providers to differentiate that part of a complaint related to purely organic pathology from secondary psychological and behavioral disorders such as anxiety disorders, alcohol abuse, drug abuse and physical abuse. Likewise, every practitioner should be capable of distinguishing between acute and chronic pain conditions and be capable of managing the assaultive or violent patient.

The purpose of this chapter is to provide the acute care practitioner with guidelines for the diagnosis and management of patients suffering from primary and secondary psychological and behavioral maladies. This chapter includes information on common presenting complaints (psychological and behavioral) and provides a brief outline to aid in the diagnosis of behavioral and psychosocial problems.

I. COMMON DISORDERS

Generally, psychological and behavioral disorders are categorized according to type, i.e., non-psychotic verses psychotic, or according to etiology, i.e., organic verses functional (Table 11-1). The term “somatoform” refers to a group of disorders with physical symptoms suggesting a physical disorder where there are no organic findings and where there is evidence that symptoms are linked to psychological factors (DSM III-R, 1987). Somatoform disorder can be associated with stress but is expressed as a preoccupation with having a physical disorder. Examples of Somatoform disorder include, Conversion disorder, Hypochondriasis, and Somatoform Pain disorder. Psychosis on the other hand is much more severe and represents a gross impairment in reality testing and the creation of a new reality (DSM III-R, 1987). These disorders are severe enough to interfere with a patient's capacity to meet ordinary life demands. The associated behavior is generally bizarre, irrational and delusional. Schizophrenia, Brief Reactive Psychosis, Organic Delusional Disorder, and Major Depression with psychotic features are several examples of psychotic disorders.

“Personality disorders” is a general term used to describe a group of behavioral disorders characterized by life-long, ingrained, maladaptive patterns of behavior. Subtypes include antisocial, passive aggressive, histrionic and borderline.

The term “mood disorder” refers to a disorder in which the patient's mood is the primary problem. A mood disorder is characterized by a "pervasive and sustained emotion that in the extreme, markedly colors the persons perceptions of the world," (DSM-III-R, 1987). This condition can be psychotic or non-psychotic. Examples of mood disorders include, Bipolar disorder, Major Depression and Dysthymia. Depression is characterized by depressed mood, and loss of interest in almost all activities of daily living. A major concern for patients who suffer from depressive mood is the presence of suicidal ideation or intent. “Dementia” refers to a deterioration of intellect that produces behavioral and psychological changes. Fourteen percent of elderly Americans (greater than age 65) are affected, and the disease is generally chronic and progressive. The most common form of dementia (55%) results from diffuse degenerative diseases such as Alzheimer’s, senile dementia, and Huntington’s Chorea. Drugs represent the second most common cause accounting for 10% of all patients with dementia. “Delirium” describes a condition of extreme mental and motor excitement, marked by a rapid succession of confused and unconnected ideas. Delirious behavior is generally acute in onset, transient in duration and is often accompanied by illusions and hallucinations. Patients appear intense and agitated with frenzied excitement and creations of imagination. The onset of delirium is hailed by an inability to concentrate, restless irritability, tremulousness, insomnia and a poor appetite.

Table 11-1: DSM-III-R Classification Axis I and II Categories

1 - DEVELOPMENTAL DISORDERS
- Mental Retardation
- Pervasive Developmental Disorders
- Specific Developmental Disorders
- Disruptive Behavior Disorders
- Anxiety Disorders of Childhood or Adolescence

2 - ORGANIC MENTAL DISORDERS
- Dementias Arising in the Senium and Presenium
- Psychoactive Substance-Induced Organic Mental Disorders

3 - PSYCHOACTIVE SUBSTANCE USE DISORDERS

4 - SCHIZOPHRENIA

5 - DELUSIONAL (PARANOID) DISORDER

6 - MOOD DISORDERS
- Bipolar Disorder
- Depressive Disorder

7 - ANXIETY DISORDERS
- Panic Disorder
- Agoraphobia
- Social Phobia
- Simple Phobia
- Obsessive Compulsive Disorder
- Post-traumatic Stress Disorder
- Generalized Anxiety Disorder
- Anxiety Disorder NOS

8 - SOMATOFORM DISORDERS
- Body Dysmorphic Disorder
- Conversion Disorder
- Hypochondriasis
- Somatization Disorder
- Somatoform Pain Disorder
- Undifferentiated Somatoform Disorder
- Somatoform Disorder NOS

9 - DISSOCIATIVE DISORDERS
- Multiple Personality Disorder
- Psychogenic Amnesia
- Depersonalization Disorder
- Dissociative Disorder NOS

10 - SEXUAL DISORDERS
- Paraphilias
- Sexual Dysfunctions
- Other Sexual Disorders

11 - SLEEP DISORDERS

12 - FACTITIOUS DISORDERS

13 - IMPULSE CONTROL DISORDERS NOT ELSEWHERE CLASSIFIED

14 - ADJUSTMENT DISORDERS

15 - PSYCHOLOGICAL FACTORS AFFECTING PHYSICAL CONDITION

16 - PERSONALITY DISORDERS

17 - CONDITIONS NOT ATTRIBUTABLE TO A MENTAL DISORDER THAT ARE A FOCUS OF ATTENTION OR TREATMENT

In emergency rooms, the most commonly encountered primary psychiatric and behavioral disorders are affective disorders, substance abuse-related conditions and schizophrenia. Family and other interpersonal problems are the most frequent precipitating conditions. In adolescents (ages 13 to 17), the most common problems are adjustment disorders, substance abuse and affective disorders (Hillard et al., 1987), while the usual presenting complaints are substance abuse and suicidal ideation or attempts. There is escalating concern over the dramatic increase in adolescent substance abuse and suicide attempts observed over the last decade. Data from the Drug Abuse Warning Network (DAWN 1990) reported 119,263 cases of drug abuse in emergency rooms across the country in 1986. By 1989, this figure had increased 29% to 153,650 cases, and 37% of the drug abuse episodes in 1989 were in individuals 20-29 years old. Substance abuse is usually associated with anxiety or depression and is 5 to 6 times more common in males. The prevalence of alcohol dependence in the United States is 13.3% compared to 5.9% for other substances. Suicide accounts for 30,000 deaths per year in the United States and suicide attempts are estimated to be 8 to 10 times more common.

Implied by the aforementioned figures, acute care facilities are frequently the first entry into the health care system for adolescents and young adults. As such, it is critical that the examining practitioner be alert to drug abuse, suicide and other conditions common to this segment of the population (Hillard et al., 1987). The crisis which brings both adolescents and adults into the emergency room may also represent the initiation of a long-term health care relationship. Hence, it is important that the practitioner provides appropriate reinforcement and referrals to strengthen this momentum if indicated. When the need for further health care is deemed appropriate, a motivational discussion should be provided to the patient and significant family members. The discussion should entail an explanation of the diagnosis or problem discovered, the importance of obtaining care for this problem, the type of care needed and the desired referrals.

II. EVALUATING PATIENTS FOR PSYCHOSOCIAL CONDITIONS

When a patient displays unusual behavior or psychological symptoms, it is important to initially ***determine if the behavior is secondary to an acute pain or disease condition, or represents a primary psychological problem***. Acute psychotic conditions may be divided into the two broad categories of organic and functional disorders. The organic psychoses are associated with actual changes in brain tissue which can produce severe alterations in mental state. Causes can include epilepsy, encephalitis, trauma, drugs and intracranial tumors. Conversely, the functional psychoses are characterized by similarly severe mental and behavioral manifestations that are classified as schizophrenia, manic-depressive illness and psychotic depression. It is important that the reader recognize that behavioral and psychological symptoms are commonly observed with and may result from acute physical illnesses (Hall & Gardner, 1980).

A second essential determination is to ***assess whether the patient may be harmful to themselves or others***. When suicidal or homicidal tendencies are suspected, a psychiatric consultation is indicated. Although most successful suicides occur in males (3:1), females are 4 times more likely to attempt it. Suicide is also more likely in caucasions (2:1) and in patients with physical illnesses. The likelihood of suicide increases with advancing age and in patients with higher social status. The two most reliable indicators of suicidal ideation are a positive history of suicide attempts in the past, and the presence of mental illness. Psychiatric patients are 3 to 12 times more likely to attempt suicide and the overwhelming majority of these patients are depressed (80%). Schizophrenia accounts for 10% of all suicides in psychiatric patients, while only 5% of suicidal patients suffer from delirium.

Patients whose agitation prohibits proper evaluation and/or treatment (i.e., delirious) can be sedated with haloperidol (Haldol), an antipsychotic agent. 0.5 to 2 mg may be administered intramuscularly for mild agitation, 2 to 5 mg for moderate agitation, and 5 to 10 mg for severely agitated patients. Low dosing is advised for elderly patients, and doubling of the aforementioned intramuscular doses is suggested for oral administration. Following these initial assessments, taking a careful history is the next step. Besides the patient, sources of historical information can include the family, friends and old medical records. ***Because many organic causes of delirium can be life-threatening, these potentially serious etiologies should be evaluated initially***. The mnemonic "WHHHIMP" may assist in recalling organic causes of delirium as follows:

W = Wernicke's encephalopathy
H = Hypoxia
H = Hypoglycemia
H = Hypertensive encephalopathy
I = Intracranial bleed
M = Meningitis/encephalitis
P = Poisoning

Another important determination to make early in the examination is the time of onset of the psychosis because this information can help ***distinguish organic and functional psychoses***. An acute psychosis (i.e., occurring within hours), suggests a metabolic, infectious, vascular or epileptic cause; while a psychosis that develops over weeks suggests a functional etiology (i.e., schizophrenia or manic-depression). Also, a functional psychosis usually begins after puberty and prior to age 40, while organic psychoses generally occur after age 40. However, the practitioner should be aware that major depression can be an exception to these delineators. A patient's memory recall can also assist in evaluating a potential psychosis. An intact recent memory recall is associated with functional psychosis, while recent memory loss is indicative of either delirium or dementia. The "Mini-Mental State" examination by Folstein et al., (1975) is a simple and standardized test to assess mental status (Table 2). A score of 20 or less is generally found in patients with dementia, delirium, schizophrenia or affective disorders. Healthy elderly patients and patients with a primary diagnosis of either neurosis or a personality disorder should score above 20.

In patients suffering from depression, it is often difficult to obtain a thorough history. A mnemonic for the common symptoms of depression is "SIG: E CAPS". Endorsement of a number of these symptoms suggests the presence of a depressed mood.

S - Sleep: insomnia or hypersomnia
I - Interests: Loss of interest or pleasure in activities
G - Guilt: excessive guilt, worthlessness, hopelessness, helplessness
E - Energy: fatigue or loss of energy
C - Concentration: difficulty concentrating, indecisiveness
A - Appetite: decreased appetite, >5% weight loss or gain
P - Psychomotor: psychomotor retardation or agitation
S - Suicidal: suicidal ideation, plan or attempt

Another essential part of patient assessment is an ***evaluation of the medication history***. The medication history has added importance in this patient population because numerous medications can produce behavioral and emotional features such as depression, delirium, dementia, psychosis, confusion, hypomania and/or hallucinations as side-effects. Some commonly used medications of this nature include the following:

Alcohol	Amphetamines	Barbiturates
Cimetidine	Corticosteroids	Digitalis
Isoniazid	Reserpine	

Also, in cases where patients are unaware of the nature of their underlying psychological problems, the medication history can provide valuable incite.

As a final note, during the examination one should ***observe the patient's behavior and speech to differentiate acute physical problems***

Table 11-2 : "MINI-MENTAL STATE" *

Maximum Score	Points Awarded	
		ORIENTATION
5	( )	What is the (year) (season) (date) (day) (month)?
5	( )	Where are we: (state) (county) (town) (hospital) (floor). Award one point for each correct answer.
		REGISTRATION
3	( )	Name 3 objects: 1 second to say each. Then ask the patient all 3 after you have said them. Give 1 point for each correct answer. Then repeat them until the patient learns all three. Count trials and record.
		ATTENTION AND CALCULATION
5	( )	Serial 7's. 1 point for each correct answer and stop after 5 answers. Alternatively spell "world" backwards.
		RECALL
3	( )	Ask for the 3 objects repeated above. Give 1 point for each correct answer.
		LANGUAGE
9	( )	Name a pencil, and watch (2 points) Repeat the following "No ifs, ands or buts." (I point)
		FOLLOW A THREE STAGE COMMAND:
		"Take a paper in your right hand, fold it in half, and put it on the floor" (3 points)
		READ AND OBEY THE FOLLOWING:
		"Close your eyes" (I point)
		WRITE A SENTENCE (1 point)
		COPY A DESIGN (I point)

TOTAL ________

ASSESS level of consciousness along a continuum:

Alert	Drowsy	Stupor	Coma

*From Folstein et al., 1975.

from psychosocial disorders. Psychosocial disorders should be suspected with positive responses to inquiries concerning the following signs and symptoms (Hall & Gardner, 1980):

- substance abuse
- hallucinations
- past or current psychiatric treatment
- suicidal ideation or attempts
- family and occupational difficulties
- changes in memory and/or mood
- disorientation (time and place)
- recent head trauma

Patients who respond positively to any of these questions should be referred for psychological or psychiatric consultation and/or other indicated medical specialists.

III. ACUTE VS. CHRONIC PAIN

Pain is generally classified as acute or chronic and usually results from either an injury or organic disease. Typically acute pain has a sudden onset, is associated with physical injury, and produces an emotional response of anxiety. Anxiety is characterized by symptoms of varying severity, but generally includes some or all the following features: shortness of breath, dizziness, accelerated heart rate, sweating, flushed appearance and chest pain or other discomfort (Diagnostic & Statistical Manual of Mental Disorders, 1987). In contrast, chronic pain is defined as pain of greater than six months' duration that is often accompanied by depression. The depressive symptoms can vary widely in severity, but usually include combinations of the following: depressed mood, general apathy, significant weight loss or gain, insomnia or hypersomnia, fatigue or chronic loss of energy and feelings of worthlessness that can lead to suicidal ideations (Diagnostic & Statistical Manual of Mental Disorders, 1987). Because of the prolonged nature of chronic pain, patients are more susceptible to emotional problems such as depression, superstitious behaviors, secondary gain, conversion reactions, hypochondriasis and abuse of pharmacotherapeutic agents. The aforementioned emotional problems describe a "chronic pain syndrome" which is a somatoform pain disorder whereby the patient is preoccupied with pain in the absence of adequate physical findings to account for the pain's behavior or intensity.

In evaluating pain, a thorough history is the centerpiece of diagnosis and should elicit approximately 90% of the physical exam findings (Sparger et al., 1987). In addition, the history is important in determining the subjective complaints that need to be validated during the physical examination. When taking a history, practitioners should avoid labeling the patient as hysterical or hypochondriacal. This pitfall only interferes with the evaluation process and can negatively impact future care if unsupported assumptions become part of the medical record (Stern & Anderson, 1989).

The following questions are suggested to help the practitioner obtain specific information about the patient's condition (Sparger et al., 1987):

1. Where is your pain today? (location)
2. How long have you had this pain? (duration)
3. Describe the pain. (quality)
4. What kinds of things increase your pain? (aggravating factors)
5. What kinds of things take away your pain? (relieving factors)
6. When did the pain first occur? (onset)
7. Can you rate this pain on a scale of one to ten? (intensity)
8. How have you dealt with this pain in the past? (history)
9. Are you currently using any methods of pain relief and, if so, what are they? (medications, biofeedback, cutaneous stimulation, etc.)

When treating any pain complaint in the acute care setting, the current trend is to treat conservatively because the relationship between the practitioner and the patient is too immature to justify an aggressive approach (Sparger et al., 1987). As such, practitioners should be concerned with contributing to drug addictions and be wary of patient noncompliance. Non-narcotic analgesics and nonsteroidal anti-inflammatory drugs are generally recommended for the treatment of minor to moderate pain (Sparger et al., 1987). Narcotic analgesics should be reserved for severe pains and then only prescribed for short-term relief. Intramuscular ketorolac (nsaid) or demerol (narcotic) are suggested for abrupt termination of severe, acute pain.

IV. CHILD ABUSE

Child abuse is defined as "any act by a parent, guardian or other person responsible for the well-being of a child, that is physically or mentally injurious to the child" (Bartlett, 1987). Incidence estimates range from 200,000 to 4 million cases annually (Zigler & Hall, 1989). The National Committee for the Prevention of Child Abuse estimated that 2,000 to 5,000 abuse-related deaths occurred in 1983 (Cohn, 1983). Although it is the obligation of health professionals to report child abuse, there are various reasons why this is not done. Explanations for failing to report these transgressions include personal, legal and economic factors, in addition to a lack of familiarity with local procedures and the inability to make a diagnosis. Morris (1985), in a survey of physicians, found out that 86% agreed that a spanking which resulted in bruises was inappropriate, yet only 25% would consider reporting this event as child abuse. Strauss et al. (1988), surveyed 1,146 American couples, of whom 73% reported using violence in the lives of their 3 to 17 year old children that included such acts as slapping, striking with objects, kicking, biting. Although child abuse may leave no physical signs, a review of cases in one children's hospital demonstrated 39% to have evidence of skin trauma, and 13% to have signs of head trauma (Johnson, 1990). Signs and symptoms suggesting the presence of child abuse are as follows:

1. Implausible history: The history is inconsistent with the injury. For instance, a child who reportedly tripped and fell when the severity and/or extent of the injuries suggests a more violent etiology.
2. Alleged self-inflicted injury: Is the child's injury appropriate for the child's age? To answer this question, remember to determine the child's developmental potential for self-injury.
3. Unexplained injury: Most non-abusive parents know exactly when, where and how their child was hurt. In addition, non-abusive parents will be eager to discuss the accident in detail.
4. Accusatory history: When a child reports that a particular adult has injured him or her, the history is generally true. Likewise, when one parent accuses the other of hurting the child, the story is usually accurate.
5. Discrepant history: This involves inconsistencies between the child's and parents' histories. If possible, parents should be interviewed separately to allow for comparative analysis.
6. Delay in seeking medical care: Most parents seek help immediately for their injured children. Abusive parents often delay seeking medical help for 24 hours or more following the incident.
7. Physical examination: If the injury is suspicious, request permission to perform a physical examination on the child. If permission cannot be obtained from the parents, a court order can be pursued. When child abuse is suspected, practitioners should immediately notify the appropriate child protective agency in their area.

V. ADULT ABUSE

As with child abuse, adult abuse should be a standard differential diagnosis to be ruled out on all patients. The extent of adult abuse spans from spouse abuse (wife or husband) to abuse of the elderly. Reviews of medical records have demonstrated histories consistent with batterings in 25% of females who suffer physical injury (Stark et al., 1979). When interviewing a person whom you suspect may have been abused, it's important not to prejudge the patient or their spouse. Remember, the patient may be ambivalent about their relationship with their spouse; hence, assumptions by the practitioner may deter openness. Rather, it is important to encourage the patient for the positive action they took in seeking help. The abuse suffered by elderly patients may include physical, emotional, financial or even medication abuse (Ross, 1988). As with all types of abuse, the incidence is hard to quantify, although one estimate suggests that 60% of professionals report encountering elderly abuse on a weekly basis (Hickey & Doulass, 1981). Characteristics of adult abuse include the following (Ross, 1988):

1. The injuries are uncharacteristic and vary widely from acute injuries to vague psychosomatic complaints.
2. The injury related activities also cover a wide spectrum from fists and kicks, to various weapons and instruments.
3. The most common injuries include those to the face and head.
4. Direct questioning concerning the injury can be helpful to determine the presence of abuse.
5. It's common for a patient to admit being hit, but then try to minimize the incident.
6. Patients often report falling to be the cause of the injury instead of abuse related activities.
7. Many abused women often have complaints of anxiety and depression in addition to their physical injuries.
8. Patients often have a history of prior abuse or trauma related injuries.

If abuse is confirmed or strongly suspected, referrals to a crisis center, social worker or other mental health resource are appropriate (Stern & Anderson, 1989). Many women crisis centers have volunteers who are willing to come to the practitioner and provide support for a battered female victim.

Although women are generally the targets of battering, men are also victims of abuse. In contrast to female abuse, battered men will often present with injuries to their legs, backs, heads or shoulders. In addition, the injuries will generally be caused by hard or sharp objects, rather than blunt instruments (Warner, 1987). As such, male injuries typically involve lacerations, rather than the bruising seen with blunt trauma.

VI. ASSAULTIVE/VIOLENT PATIENT

When evaluating the potentially assaultive or violent patient, it is important to stabilize the situation so the patient is less likely to act out aggressively. Generally these patients are fearful that others are going to hurt them (Rund, 1988). The practitioner should speak calmly and inform the patient that violent behavior is inappropriate. It is also suggested to ask the patient if he or she wants to be restrained, should the patient feel unable to maintain control. When restraints are needed, the patient should be reassured that the measure is for his or her protection and to control his or her behavior (Rund, 1988).

If the patient is potentially violent, but does not require restraints, the following guidelines are suggested (Rund, 1988):

1. Have physical assistance nearby.
2. Maintain an open, easy exit for the practitioner and the patient.
3. Allow the patient to talk or ventilate.
4. Be the patient's ally or at least be non-judgmental.
5. Avoid direct eye contact. This can be misperceived as a personal challenge.
6. Maintain a submissive posture by remaining relaxed and turning slightly away from the patient.

Medication to sedate the patient may also be indicated; however, most oral sedatives act too slowly to be useful. In addition, assaultive or violent episodes commonly have sudden onsets and brief durations (3 to 10 minutes), rendering them less susceptible to pharmacologic management. Hence, nonpharmacologic behavior management is generally more appropriate.

References

Bartlett G.S., "Child Abuse." In *Emergency Medicine: A Comprehensive Review.* Edited by Kravis T.C.; Warner C.G.; Benson D.R.; Cales R.H.; and Pierog J.E., Rockville: Aspen Publishers, Inc., 1987.

Cohn A.H., "An approach to preventing child abuse." Chicago: National Committee for Prevention of Child Abuse, 1983.

Data From the Drug Abuse Warning Network (DAWN): Annual Data 1989. National Institute of Drug Abuse Statistical Series I: 9., Rockville, MD: National Institute on Drug Abuse, 1990.

Diagnostic and Statistical Manual of Mental Disorders. Washington, D.C.: American Psychiatric Association, 1987.

Folstein M.F., Folstein S.E., McHugh P.R., "Mini-mental state: a practical method for grading the cognitive state of patients for the clinician." *J Psychiat Res.* 12 (1975): 189-198.

Hall R., Gardner E., "Physical illness manifesting as psychiatric disease." *Arch Gen Psychiatry.* 37 (1980): 989-95.

Hickey T., Douglass R.L., "Mistreatment of the elderly in the domestic setting: an exploratory study." *Am J Public Health.* 71 (5) (1981): 500-507.

Hillard J.R., Slomowitz M., Levi L.S., "A retrospective study of adolescents' visits to a general hospital psychiatric emergency service." *Am J Psychiatry.* 144 (4) (1987): 433-436.

Johnson C.F., "Inflicted injury versus accidental injury." *Pediatr Clin North Am.* 37 (4) (1990): 791-814.

Morris J.L., Johnson C.F., Clasen M., "To report or not to report: Physicians' attitudes toward discipline and child abuse." *Am J Dis Child.* 139 (1985): 194-197.

Ross D.S., "Adult abuse" In *Emergency Medicine: Concepts and Clinical Practice.* Edited by Rosen P.; Baker F.J.; Darkin R.M.; Braen G.R.; Dailey R.H.; and Levy R.C., St. Louis: C. V. Mosby Company, pp. 1929-1947, 1988.

Rund D.A., "Approach to violence" In *Emergency Medicine: Concepts and Clinical Practice.* Edited by Rosen P.; Baker F.J.; Darkin R.M.; Braen G.R.; Dailey R.H.; and Levy R.C., St. Louis, MO: C. V. Mosby Company, pp. 1827-1834, 1988.

Sparger G., Hoyt K.S., Heidenhoffer R., "Pain management" In *Emergency Medicine: A Comprehensive Review.* Kravis T.C.; Warner C.G.; Benson D.R.; Cales R.H.; and Pierog J.E., Rockville, MD: Aspen Publishers, Inc., pp. 815-827, 1987.

Stark E., Flitcraft A., Frazier W., "Medicine and patriarchal violence: the social construction of a "private" event." *Int J Health Serv,* 9 (3) (1979): 461-493.

Stern T.A., Anderson W.H., "Psychiatric emergencies" In *Emergency Medicine: Scientific Foundations and Current Practice.* Edited by Wilkins Jr. E.W., Baltimore: Williams and Wilkins, pp. 423-443, 1989.

Strauss M.A., Gelles R.J., Steinmetz S.K., *Behind Closed Doors: Violence in Family.* Garden City, NY: Anchor Books, pp. 60-61, 1988.

Warner C.G., "Domestic violence" In *Emergency Medicine: A Comprehensive Review.* Edited by Kravis T.C.; Warner C.G.; Benson D.R.; Cales R.H.; Pierog J.E., Rockville, MD: Aspen Publishers, Inc., pp. 773-786, 1987.

Yoder L., Jones S.L., "The emergency room nurse and the psychiatric patient." *J Psychosoc Nurs Ment Health Serv.* 20 (1982): 22-28.

Zigler E., Hall N.W., "Child abuse in America" In *Child Maltreatment: Theory and Research on the Causes and Consequences of Child Abuse and Neglect.* Edited by Cicchetti D., Carlson V., New York: Cambridge University Press, pp. 38-75, 1989.

Appendix A

Appendix A: Intraoral & Extraoral Injection Techniques to Achieve Local Anesthesia

Type of Injection	Indications	Landmarks	Procedure	Area Anesthetized
Inferior alveolar block (branch of the 3rd division of the 5th cranial nerve) **See Figure A-1**	Lacerations of the mandibular gingiva anterior to the molars, and of the lower lip & chin, extraction of mandibular teeth and vestibular I & D's in the mandible.	Pterygomandibular triangle bordered laterally by the ramus of the mandible and medially by the pterygo-mandibular raphe.	Direct a 1 - 1.5 inch 25 or 27 ga needle from the opposite sided of the dental arch and penetrate the pterygomandibular triangle 1cm above the mandibular teeth. Insert the needle 2.5 - 3 cm deep, aspirate, and deposit 1.5 - 2.0 ml of anesthetic solution.	Body of the mandible mandibular teeth, lip, chin, & the mucous membrane anterior to the 1st molar.
Mental nerve block (anterior portion of the 3rd division of the 5th cranial nerve) **See Figure A-2**	Lacerations of the mandibular gingiva anterior to the 1st molar & the lip & chin, extraction of mandibular incisors, premolars & canines and vestibular I & D's.	Mental foramen approximately 3 - 4 cm below the occlusal surface of the 1st or 2nd premolar. It is usually on a line with the pupil of the eye and the infraorbital foramen.	Direct a 1 inch 25 or 27 ga needle vertically and anteriorly toward the root apex of the mandibular premolar. The tip should penetrate the buccal vestibule to a depth of 2.5 - 3 cm from the occlusal surface of the premolar. Deposit 1.5 - 2.0 ml of anesthetic solution.	Lower lip & mucous membrane anterior to the mental foramen. The premolar and canine teeth.
Lingual nerve block (branch of the 3rd division of the 5th cranial nerve) **See Figure A-3**	Lacerations of the anterior 2/3 of the tongue & lingual gingiva, and lingual vestibular I & D's in the mandible.	Pterygomandibular triangle bordered laterally by the ramus of the mandible and medially by the pterygo-mandibular raphe.	Direct a 1 - 1.5 inch 25 or 27 ga needle from the opposite side of the dental arch and penetrate the pterygomandibular triangle 1 cm above the mandibular teeth. Insert the needle 1 - 1.5 cm deep, aspirate, and deposit 0.5 - 1.0 ml of anesthetic solution.	Lingual gingiva and the anterior 2/3 of the tongue.
Long buccal nerve block (branch of the 3rd division of the 5th cranial nerve) **See Figure A-4**	Lacerations & I & D's of the mandibular buccal gingiva and soft tissue manipulation during posterior tooth extraction	Anterior border of the ramus of the mandible and the mucous membranes adjacent to the 2nd or 3rd mandibular molar.	Direct a 1 inch 25 or 27 ga needle from the ipsilateral side of the dental arch and penetrate the mucous membrane distal to the 2nd or 3rd molar near the ramus of the mandible. Insert the needle 0.5 cm, aspirate, and deposit 0.5 - 1.0 ml of anesthetic solution.	Mandibular mucosa buccal to the molars.

Appendix A: Intraoral & Extraoral Injection Techniques to Achieve Local Anesthesia

Type of Injection	Indications	Landmarks	Procedure	Area Anesthetized
Maxillary superior alveolar nerve infiltration (branch of the 2nd division of the 5th cranial nerve) **See Figure A-5**	Lacerations of the maxillary gingiva and upper lip, extraction of maxillary teeth & I & D's in the maxillary vestibule.	Mucobuccal fold adjacent to the maxillary teeth.	Direct a 1 - 1.5 inch 25 or 27 ga needle into the mucobuccal fold adjacent to the maxillary tooth. Insert the tip approximately 2 - 3 cm ending at the apex of the tooth. Aspirate, and deposit 1.5 - 2.0 ml of anesthetic solution.	Facial gingiva, maxillary teeth and the upper lip.
Nasopalatine injection (branch of the 2nd division of the 5th cranial nerve) **See Figure A-6**	Lacerations and repair of trauma to the anterior portion of the hard palate and I & D's in the anterior hard palate.	Maxillary incisive papilla located between the two central incisor teeth and the incisive foramen.	Direct a 1 inch 25 or 27 ga needle vertically into the incisive foramen through the incisive papilla in the midline posterior to the two maxillary central incisors. Aspirate and deposit 0.5 ml of anesthetic solution.	Mucoperiosteum of the anterior 1/3 of the hard palate.
Greater palatine injection (branch of the 2nd division of the 5th cranial nerve) **See Figure A-7**	Lacerations, I & D's and repair of trauma to the posterior portion of the hard palate.	Greater palatine foramen located medially to the crest of the gingiva adjacent to the second maxillary molar.	Direct a 1 inch 25 or 27 ga needle to a point approximately 1 - 1.5 cm from the distal of the crest of the gingiva of the maxillary 2nd molar on a perpendicular toward the midline. Insert the tip into the foramen, aspirate and deposit 0.5 ml of anesthetic solution.	Mucoperiosteum or the hard palate from the tuberosity to the canine area.
Gow-Gates technique for the inferior alveolar block (branch of the 3rd division of the 5th cranial nerve) **See Figure A-8**	Lacerations of the mandibular gingiva anterior to the molars, and of the lower lip & chin, extraction of mandibular teeth and vestibular I & D's in the mandible.	Mesiolingual cusp tip of the maxillary 2nd molar, the head of the mandibular condyle intraorally and the inferior border of the tragus extraorally.	Direct a 1.5 inch 25 or 27 ga needle across the arch toward the inferior border of the tragus of the ear, penetrating the oral mucosa at the height of the mesiolingual cusp tip of the maxillary 2nd molar. Insert the needle until the head of the the mandibular condyle is contacted, withdraw the needle 1 - 2 mm, aspirate and deposit 1.8 ml of anesthetic solution.	Body of the mandible, mandibular teeth, lip, chin, & the mucous membrane anterior to the 1st molar.

Appendix A: Intraoral & Extraoral Injection Techniques to Achieve Local Anesthesia

Type of Injection	Indications	Landmarks	Procedure	Area Anesthetized
Akinosi technique for the inferior alveolar block (branch of the 3rd division of the 5th cranial nerve) **See Figure A-9**	Lacerations of the mandibular gingiva anterior to the molars, and of the lower lip & chin, extraction of mandibular teeth and vestibular I & D's in the mandible. Very useful when there is limited opening of the mouth.	Mucogingival junction of maxillary 2nd or 3rd molar adjacent to the maxillary tuberosity and the anterior, medial border of the mandibular ramus.	Direct a 1.5 inch 25 or 27 ga needle posteriorly penetrating the oral mucosa at the height to the muco-gingival junction adjacent to the maxillary 2nd or 3rd molar on the ipsilateral side parallel to the ramus of the mandible. With the mouth closed, insert the needle 2.5 - 3.0 cm, aspirate and deposit 1.5 - 2.0 ml of of anesthetic solution.	Body of the mandible, mandibular teeth, lip, chin, & the mucous membrane anterior to the 1st molar.
Maxillary 2nd division nerve block (2nd division of the 5th cranial nerve) **See Figure A-10**	Lacerations of the maxillary gingiva upper lip, cheek, lower eyelid & side of the nose, extraction of maxillary teeth and I & D's in the maxillary vestibule and palate.	Greater palatine foramen located medially to the crest of the gingiva adjacent to the second maxillary molar.	Direct a 1.5 inch 25 or 27 ga needle to a point approximately 1 - 1.5 cm from the distal of the crest of the gingiva of the maxillary 2nd molar on a perpendicular toward the midline. Insert the needle into the foramen to a depth of 2.5 - 3.0 cm, aspirate and deposit 1.5 - 2.0 ml of anesthetic solution.	All maxillary teeth, all buccal & palatal soft tissue, maxillary lip & cheek, side of nose and the lower eyelid.
Maxillary 2nd division nerve block (2nd division of the 5th cranial nerve) **See Figure A-11**	Lacerations of the maxillary gingiva upper lip, cheek, lower eyelid & side of the nose, extraction of maxillary anterior teeth and I & D's in the maxillary vestibule and palate.	Buccal vestibule adjacent to the maxillary 2nd molar and the pterygopalatine fossa.	Direct a 1.5 inch 25 or 27 ga needle into the buccal vestibule above the distal aspect of the maxillary second molar with an angulation toward the midline. Insert the needle to a depth of 3 cm, aspirate and deposit 1.5 - 2.0 ml of anesthetic solution in the pterygopalatine fossa.	All maxillary teeth, all buccal & palatal soft tissue, maxillary lip & cheek, side of nose and the lower eyelid.

Appendix A: Intraoral & Extraoral Injection Techniques to Achieve Local Anesthesia

Type of Injection	Indications	Landmarks	Procedure	Area Anesthetized
Intraoral Infraorbital block (branch of 2nd division of the 5th cranial nerve) **See Figure A-12**	Lacerations of the maxillary anterior gingiva, cheek and upper lip, extraction of maxillary anterior teeth and I & D's in the maxillary vestibule.	Mucobuccal fold adjacent to the maxillary lateral tooth and apex of the maxillary canine tooth, the pupil of the eye and the infraorbital foramen & infraorbital notch.	Direct a 1.5 inch 25 or 27 ga needle into the mucobuccal fold adjacent to the canine tooth. Insert the needle approximately 2 - 3 cm on a line with the canine tooth, pupil of the eye & the infraorbital notch, aspirate, and deposit 1.5 - 2.0 ml of anesthetic solution.	Facial gingiva, maxillary central, lateral and canine teeth, the upper lip, mid-facial area including the lower eyelid and the tip of the nose.
Extraoral Infraorbital block (branch of 2nd division of the 5th cranial nerve) **See Figure A-13**	Lacerations of the maxillary anterior gingiva, cheek and upper lip and side of nose extraction of maxillary anterior teeth I & D's in the maxillary vestibule.	Pupil of the eye, infraorbital notch, infraorbital foramen and the canine tooth.	Direct a 1 inch 25 or 27 ga needle through the cleansed skin 1.5 cm inferior to the infraorbital foramen. Advance the needle toward the infraorbital foramen, aspirate, and deposit 1.5 - 2.0 ml of anesthetic solution.	Facial gingiva, maxillary central, lateral and canine teeth, the upper lip, mid-facial area including the lower eyelid and the tip of the nose.

Appendix A
Figures

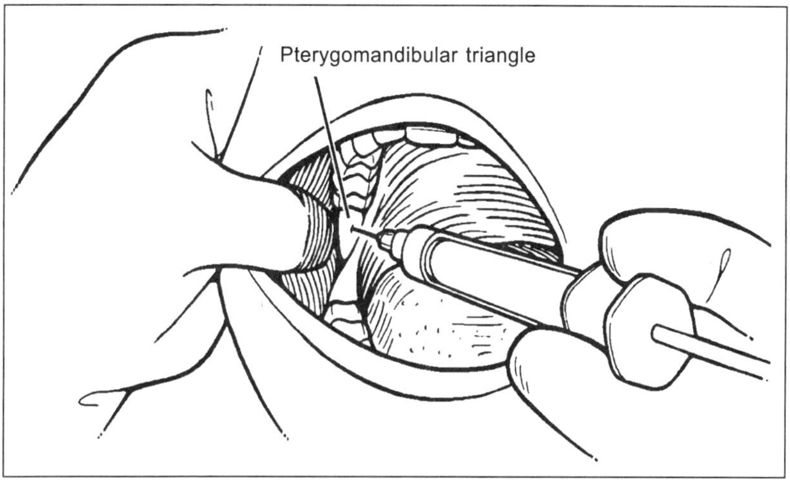

Figure A-1a: Inferior Alveolar Nerve Block.

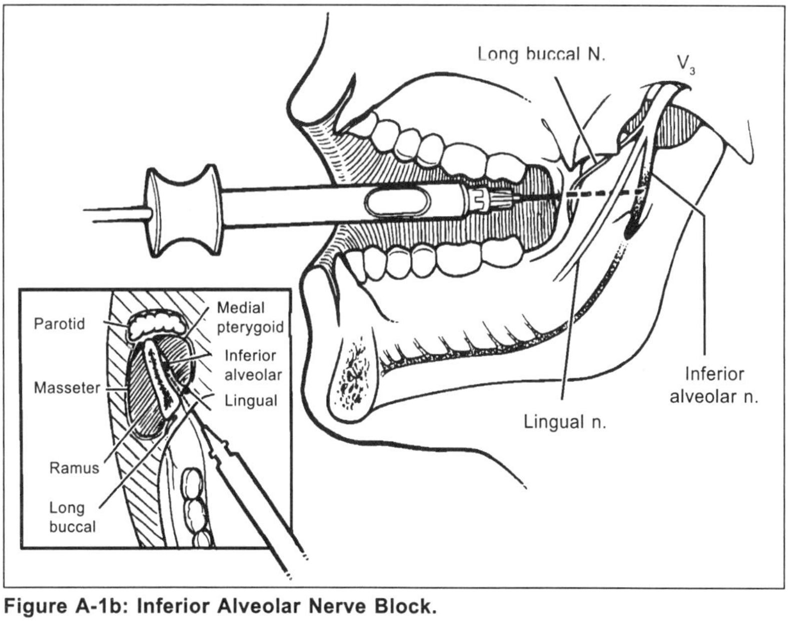

Figure A-1b: Inferior Alveolar Nerve Block.

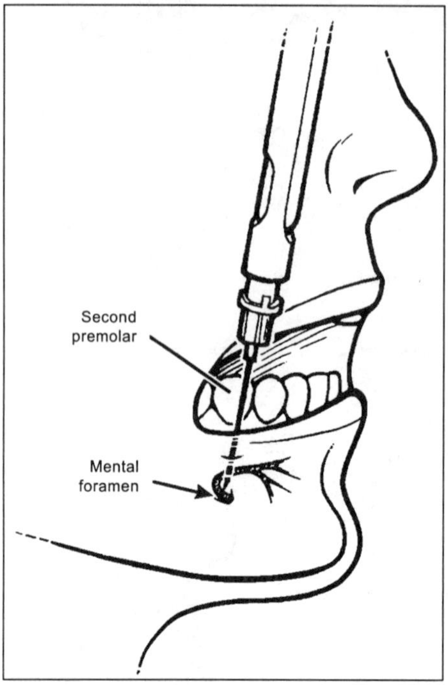

Figure A-2: Mental Nerve Block.

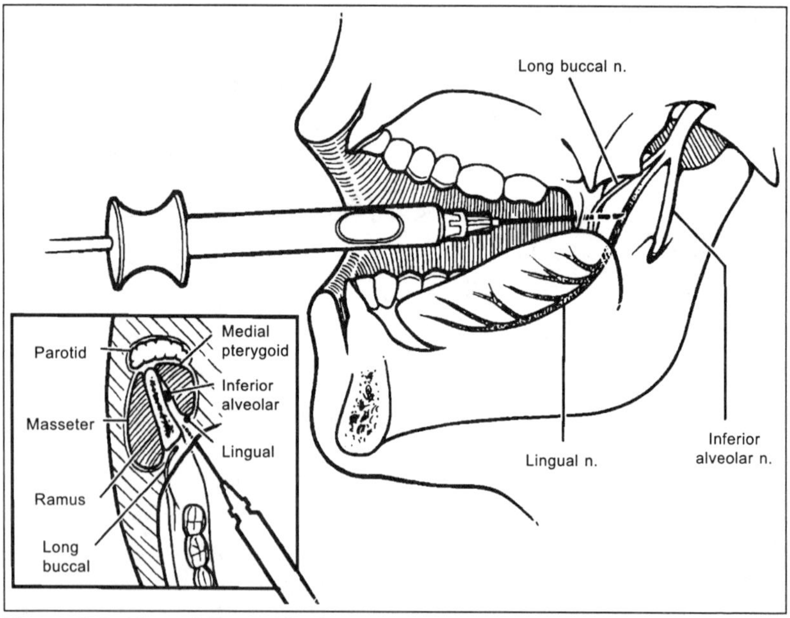

Figure A-3: Lingual Nerve Block.

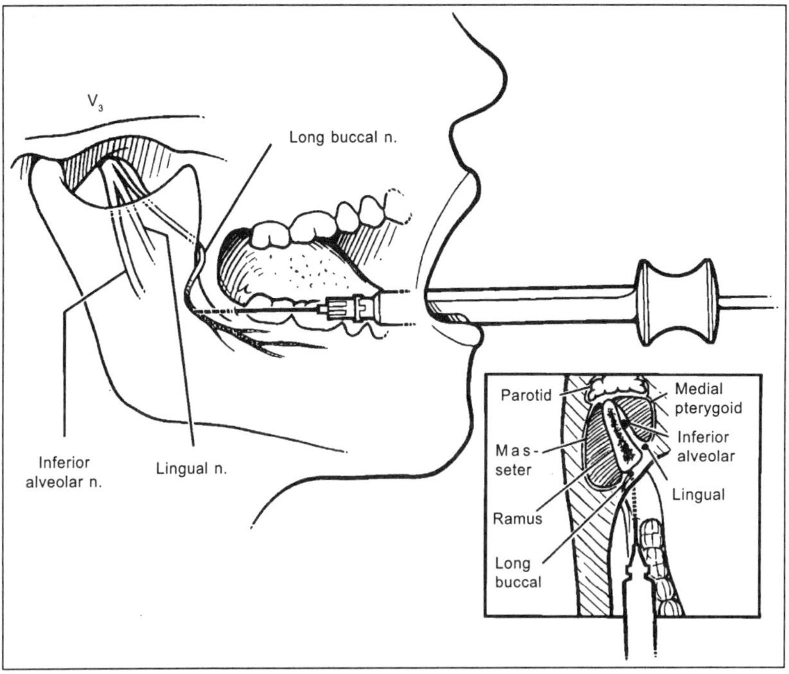

Figure A-4: Long Buccal Nerve Block.

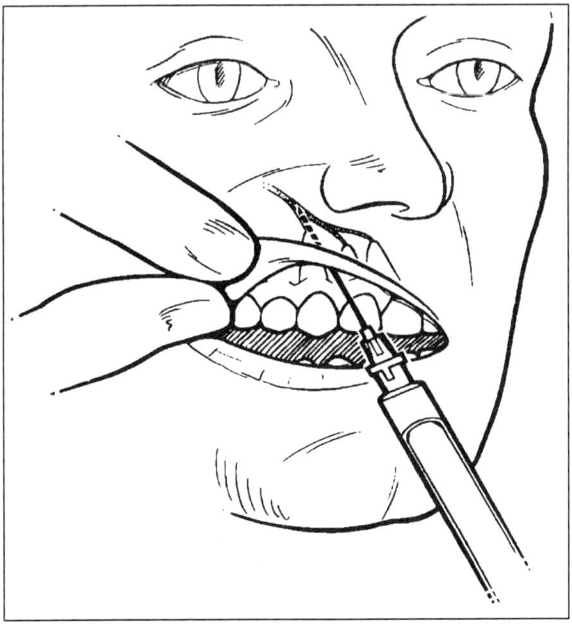

Figure A-5a: Anterior Superior Alveolar Nerve Infiltration.

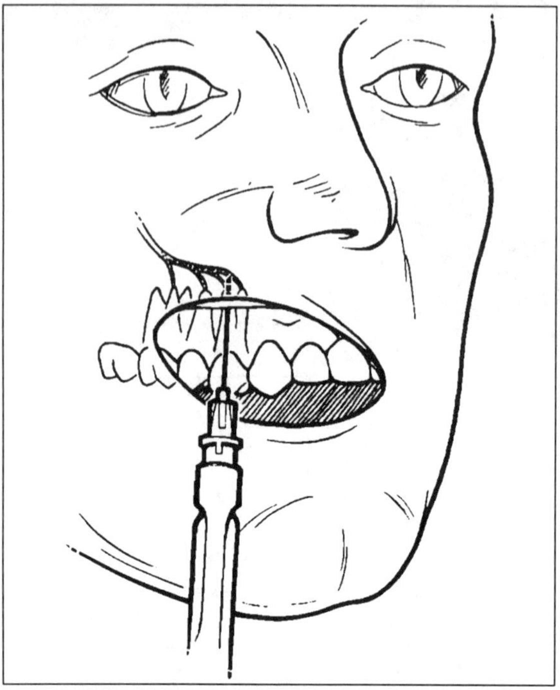

Figure A-5b: Middle Superior Alveolar Nerve Infiltration.

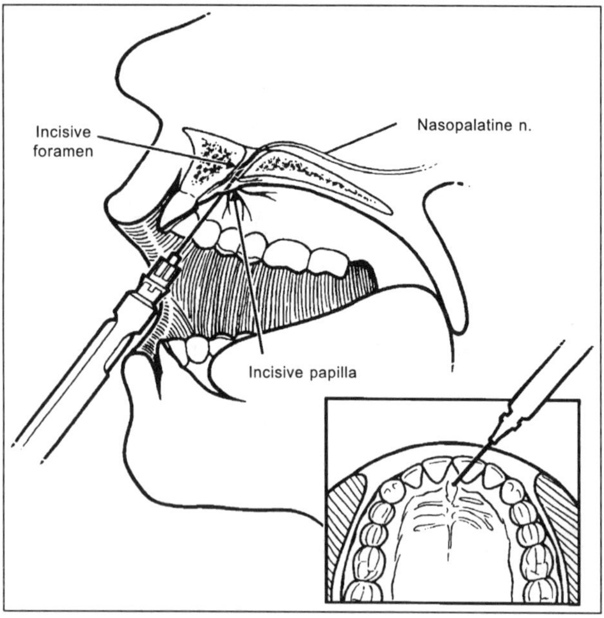

Figure A-6: Nasopalatine Injection.

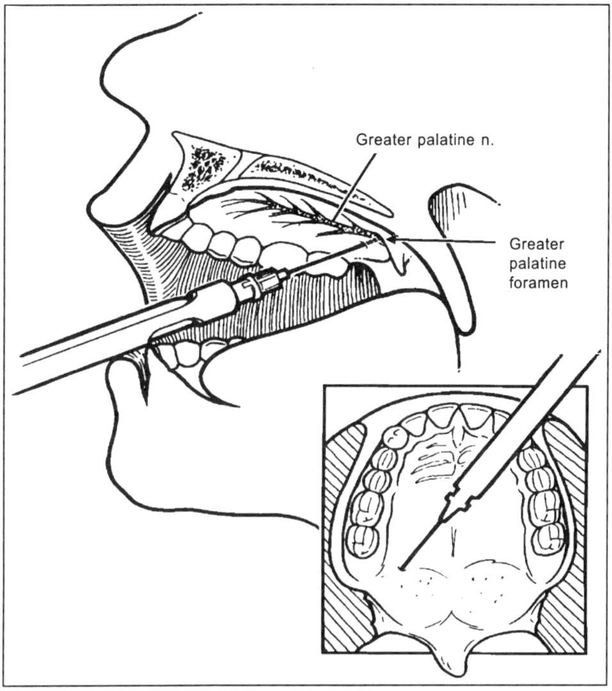

Figure A-7: Greater Palatine Injection.

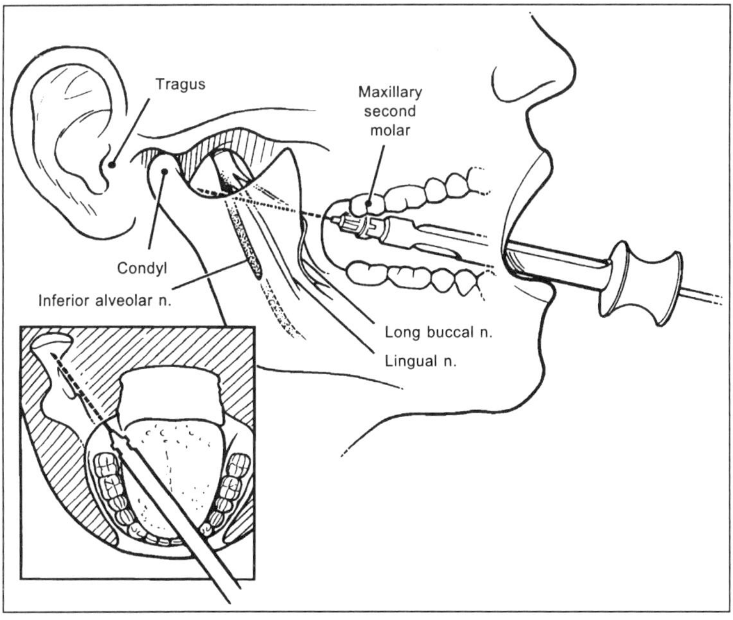

Figure A-8: Gow-Gates Technique for an Inferior Alveolar Injection.

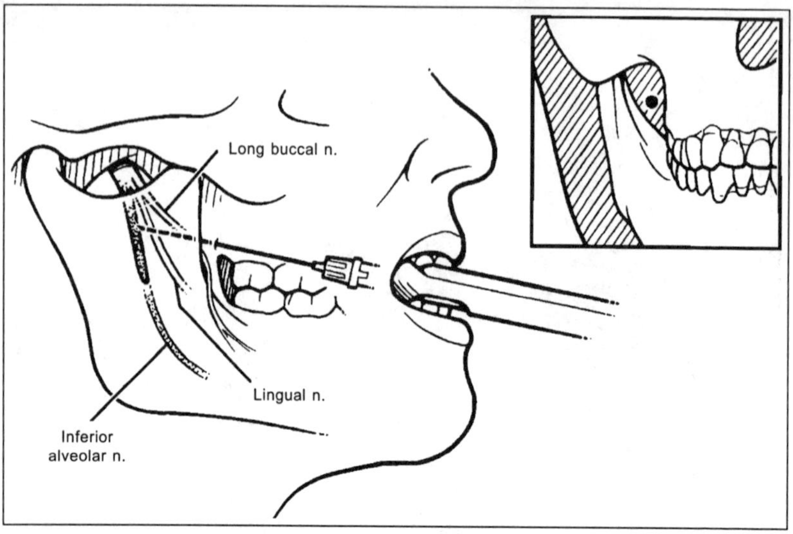

Figure A-9: Akinosi Technique for Closed-Mouth Inferior Alveolar Infections.

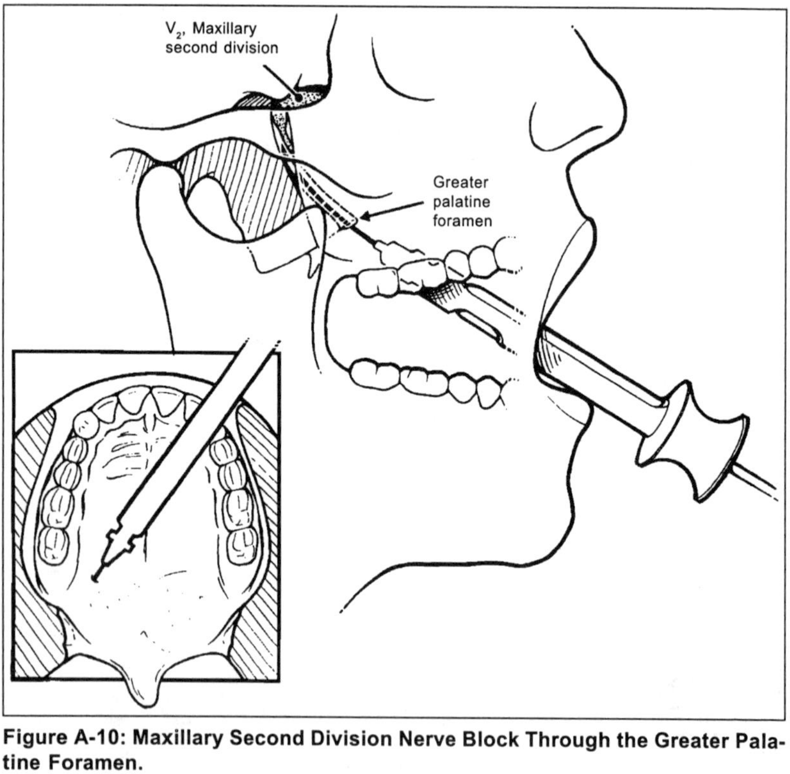

Figure A-10: Maxillary Second Division Nerve Block Through the Greater Palatine Foramen.

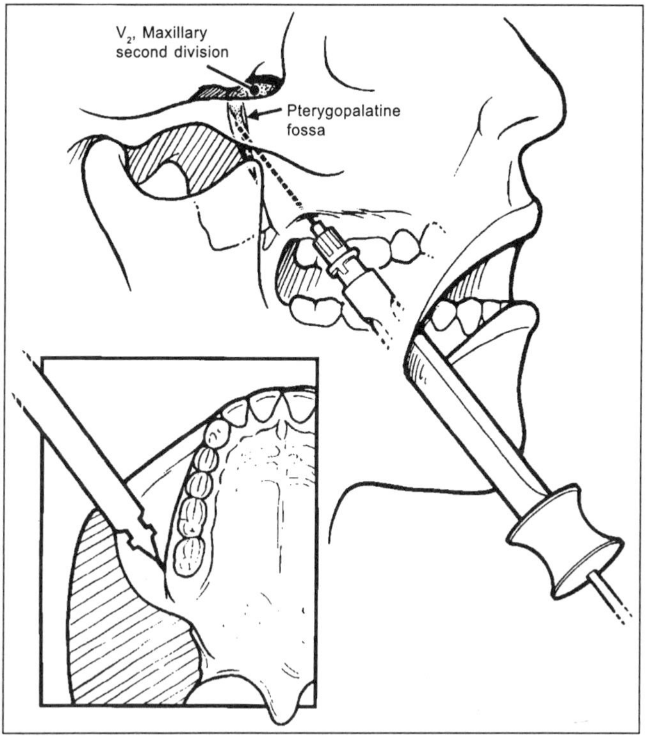

Figure A-11: Maxillary Second Division Nerve Block Through the Lateral Aspect of the Pterygopalatine Fossa.

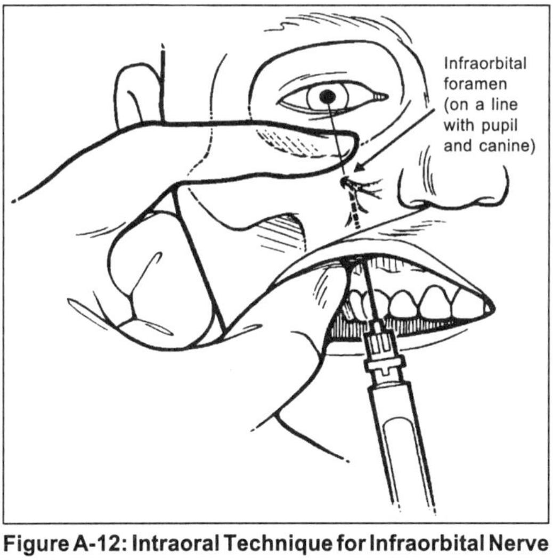

Figure A-12: Intraoral Technique for Infraorbital Nerve Block.

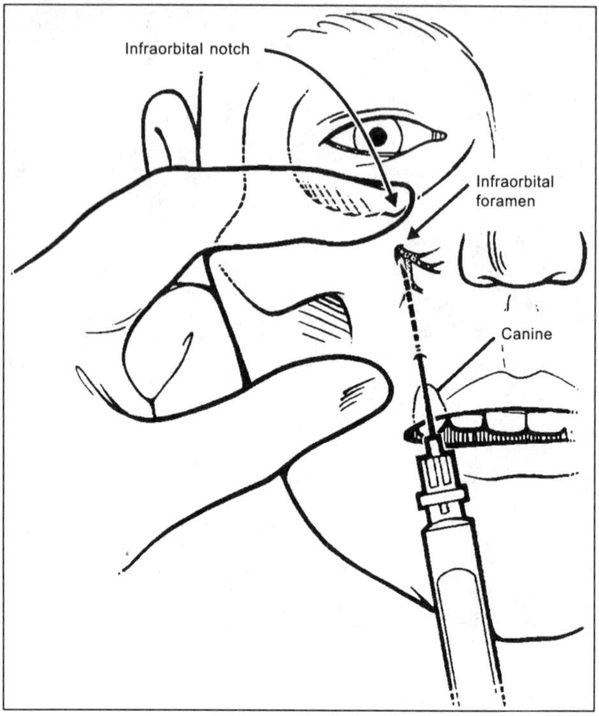

Figure A-13: Extraoral Technique for Infraorbital Nerve Block.

Appendix B

Appendix B: A Summary of Intraoral and Extraoral Dental Injections

Area to be Anesthetized	Inferior Alveolar Block (standard block, Gow-Gates & Akinosi)	Mental Nerve Block	Long Buccal Nerve Block	Lingual Nerve Block	Maxillary Superior Alveolar Nerve Block†	Nasopalatine Nerve Block	Greater Palatine Nerve Block	Maxillary 2nd Division Nerve Block	Infraorbital Nerve Block
Mandibular Molars	X								
Mandibular Premolars	X	X							
Mandibular Anteriors	X	X							
Mandibular Buccal Soft Tissue (Posterior)			X						
Manibular Buccal Soft Tissue (Anterior)	X	X							
Mandibular Lingual Soft Tissue:				X					
Mandibular Lip	X	X							
Chin	X	X							
Body of mandible	X								
Tongue (Anterior 2/3)				X					
Maxillary Molars					X			X	
Maxillary Premolars					X			X	
Maxillary Anteriors					X			X	X
Maxillary Buccal Soft Tissue					X			X	X*

Appendix B: A Summary of Intraoral and Extraoral Dental Injections

Area to be Anesthetized	Inferior Alveolar Block (standard block, Gow-Gates & Akinosi)	Mental Nerve Block	Long Buccal Nerve Block	Lingual Nerve Block	Maxillary Superior Alveolar Nerve Block†	Nasopalatine Nerve Block	Greater Palatine Nerve Block	Maxillary 2nd Division Nerve Block	Infraorbital Nerve Block
Palate (Anterior 1/3)						X		X	
Palate (Posterior 2/3)							X	X	
Maxillary Lip					X¥			X	X
Side of the Nose								X	X
Cheek								X	X
Lower eyelid								X	X

†The posterior superior alveolar nerve innervates the maxillary molars and adjacent buccal soft tissue, the middle superior alveolar nerve innervates the premolars and a part of the 1st molar and the adjacent buccal soft tissue, the anterior superior nerve innervates the anterior teeth and the adjacent buccal soft tissue.

*Maxillary anterior soft tissue only

¥With the anterior superior alveolar injection only

Appendix C

Pharmacological Sedation for Pediatric Patients

Drug	Route	Recommended Dosage		
Meperidine (Demerol)	PO	0.5 - 1.0 mg/lb		
	IM	0.5 - 1.0 mg/lb		
Diazepam (Valium)	PO	0.2 - 0.5 mg/kg*⁺		
	IM	Not recommended**		
Midazolam (Versed)	PO	Not available		
	IM	0.15 mg/kg*		
Chloral Hydrate (Noctec)	PO	50 mg/kg		
	IM	Not available		
Meperidine plus Chloral hydrate***	PO	Age	Hydroxyzine	Chloral hydrate
		<3 yrs	25-50 mg	500-1000 mg
		3-6 yrs	25-50 mg	1000 mg
		>6 yrs	50 mg	1500 mg

Patients should not be sedated until it is certain no intracranial injury is present.

Nitrous oxide inhalation sedation may be used in combination with the above agents.

---

*Malamed, 1989

**Due to pain and erratic absorption (Clinical Anesthesia Procedures of the Massachusetts General Hospital). Best given IV at a dose of 0.25 mg/kg (Braham, 1985)

***Mathewson, 1987. Hydroxyzine HCl (Atarax) available PO only. Hydroxyzine pamoate (Vistaril) available as PO & IM.

⁺For patients between 4-6 years old. Over 6 years old use 5-10 mg total dosage.

1. Oral Meperidine + Promethazine (Phenergan)

Weight	Meperidine	Phenergan
10 kg	25 mg	12.5 mg
15 kg	25 mg	25 mg
22 kg	50 mg	25 mg

Appendix D†

Tetanus Immunization Schedule & Prophylaxis Recommendations

Vaccine	Administration
DPT	< 7 years of age 1 dose q 4 - 8 weeks x 3. One additional at 1 yr
DT	> 7 years of age 2 doses 4 weeks apart followed by 1 dose at 6 months
Td	every 10 years Following DPT & DT

History of Immunization (doses)	Clean minor wounds		All Other Wounds	
	Td	TIG	Td	TIG
Uncertain	Yes	No	Yes	Yes
0 - 1	Yes	No	Yes	Yes
2	Yes	No	Yes	No*
3 or more	No**	No	No***	No

DPT (diptheria, tetanus, pertussis), DT (diptheria, tetanus - pediatric use), Td (tetanus, diptheria · adult type; use in adults to minimize adverse reactions), TIG (tetanus immune globulin, given concurrently with toxoid at separate sites, 250 units IM)

*Unless the wound is more than 24 hours old.

**Unless it is more than 10 years since the last toxoid dose.

***Unless it is more than 5 years since the last toxoid dose.

†From MMWR 1984 Vol 33:1S and 1989 Vol 38/No.13

Index

T

U

V

W

X

Z